FUNCTIONAL ELECTRONIC HISTOLOGY

FUNCTIONAL ELECTRONIC HISTOLOGY

A CORRELATION OF ULTRASTRUCTURE AND FUNCTION
IN ALL MAMMALIAN TISSUES

BY

PARIS CONSTANTINIDES, M.D., Ph.D.

Professor of Pathology, University of B.C.

University of British Columbia Medical School
Vancouver, B.C. (Canada)

ELSEVIER SCIENTIFIC PUBLISHING COMPANY

Amsterdam – Oxford – New York

1974

ELSEVIER SCIENTIFIC PUBLISHING COMPANY
335 JAN VAN GALENSTRAAT
P.O. BOX 211, AMSTERDAM, THE NETHERLANDS

AMERICAN ELSEVIER PUBLISHING COMPANY, INC.
52 VANDERBILT AVENUE
NEW YORK, NEW YORK 10017

Sole distributor in Japan:

IGAKU SHOIN LTD.,
TOKYO INTERNATIONAL P.O. BOX 5063
TOKYO, JAPAN

with 70 full-page plates

Library of Congress Card Number: 72-83202

ISBN: 0-444-40998-X

Printed in The Netherlands

FOR MY FAMILY

Contents

CHAPTER 5. MUSCLE

CHAPTER 6. NERVOUS TISSUE

CHAPTER 7. CIRCULATORY SYSTEM

CHAPTER 8. RESPIRATORY SYSTEM

Introduction

I have tried to summarise in this book most of our present knowledge about the basic ultrastructure of the cells of the mammalian and especially the human body. In doing this, I also attempted to show how intimately linked cell ultrastructure and cell function are and how the former changes with the responses of the cell to a changing environment at any given moment. For at the molecular level, biological structure and function are two aspects of the same thing; structure is really frozen function and function is nothing but structure in motion, and you cannot change the one without at the same time changing the other.

During the last half century, the science of biological structure (Anatomy) had come to be considered by most life scientists as a largely "spent" discipline in a cul-de-sac when compared to the thrilling potentials of biological chemistry. This was largely due to two things: First, the analysis of the structure of living matter had lagged far behind the analysis of its chemical composition and function; biological chemists had already descended to the level of tiny invisible building blocks of cells, *i.e.* molecules, whereas the smallest units anatomists could distinguish were packs of astronomical numbers of molecules, *i.e.* whole cells and their major parts. Secondly, the temperament and commitment of most anatomists in the past was such that they were not primarily interested in correlating structure with function; they were fascinated by the mystery of structure *per se* and were primarily preoccupied with disentangling it – a very worthy task while structure was still in a tangle. There have been, of course, sufficient exceptions to this purely structural curiosity of anatomists to show us that morphological methods need not be just descriptive, that they can give us very functional information if we use them to attack functional problems and that, as in the case of all techniques, the answers they yield depend entirely on the kind of questions we ask. Perhaps one of the most dramatic illustrations of this is the development of the extremely dynamic concept of evolution by Darwin through the proper application of the extremely descriptive methods of gross anatomy.

All that, however, has radically changed now.

The great technological revolution of electron microscopy of the last two decades has injected an unbelievably vigorous new life into the anatomical method because it uncovered an immense new cellular landscape that was completely invisible before and whose structural components are close to – and in some cases identical with – the molecular units of biological chemists. When combined with the auxiliary methods of ultrastructural autoradiography, cytochemistry and immunocytochemistry, the electron microscope makes molecular events visible within cells and enables us to trace the intracellular paths of molecules and atoms as they drive the basic function of life: assimilation, synthesis, secretion, excitation, movement and duplication. Thus, when used in properly designed studies, electron microscopy has become an invaluable tool for (a) the exploration of the normal and pathological function of cells at the molecular level, (b) the earliest possible detection of pathological tissue changes (before they become visible with the light microscope), and (c) the assessment of the effectiveness of treatments in preventing the distortion or promoting the reestablishment of normal cell ultrastructure. It has become one of the most exciting new frontiers of cell biology and medicine.

For these reasons not only the more functionally oriented present generation of anatomists but everybody else in the converging world of life scientists has now become very interested in electron microscopic histology and wants to learn it in order to use it in his own research or in order to understand the research of others: physiologists, biophysicists, biological chemists, pharmacologists, neuroscientists, pathologists, geneticists, physicians in all branches of medicine and surgeons. As a result, the study of the ultrastructure of tissues is rapidly becoming an important part of the training of biology and medical students at all levels in modern universities.

It is to facilitate the learning of this new ultrastructural world by all those who are starting out in this field at the undergraduate or graduate level that this book was written.

I chose to illustrate the entire material with drawings rather than with photographs because in my experience nothing can compete with simple diagrams for clarity, concentration on essentials and forcefulness of communication. If one studies diagrams first one will later find it very easy to recognize all salient structural details in good photographs. There is something chaotic and confusing about electron microscope photographs to the beginner that makes direct learning from them a slower and less efficient didactic procedure than the prior study of drawings followed by scrutiny of actual pictures. It should be noted that I based all diagrams on electron micrographs from the literature and that they generally represent consensus of current opinion on basic ultrastructure.

In dealing with almost every subject of special cytology, I discussed its various aspects in the following sequence: I started with a general introduction to the subject and endeavoured to provide a bridge between light and electron microscopic structure, often with the help of a simple light microscopic drawing of the tissue under consideration; this was followed by a concise description of the ultrastructural features, relating the most important ones through numerical indices to the labelled parts of corresponding drawings; finally, I discussed in that order, cytochemistry, changes of ultrastructure during function and development, and changes in response to external and internal environmental changes.

In most cases, every statement in the text represents the summary of one or more papers of the international literature of the last fifteen years, the period since the introduction of ultrathin sectioning and, therefore, high resolution electron microscopy. Most of this literature is contained in one large section at the end of the book where the references have been grouped under many short headings so that it is easy to locate within seconds all papers on a given topic. Usually, the bibliography on each cell type is classified under certain standard headings with the following sequence: (a) normal ultrastructure, (b) ultrastructural cytochemistry, (c) relationship of ultrastructure to normal function, (d) development, (e) proliferation, renewal, regeneration and ageing, and (f) effects on ultrastructure of external factors (nutritional, physical, chemical) and internal factors (metabolic, hormonal, nervous). When several references are listed under the same heading, they are arranged in chronological rather than alphabetical order so that the historical evolution of the literature on that subject can be appreciated.

In keeping with the main emphasis of this text, my selection of references favoured those that were pertinent to mammalian and especially human cells (*in situ* or in culture), but I have also included papers on lower vertebrate and invertebrate cells whenever they illustrated a particularly interesting or general biological principle.

In writing this one-volume text of electron microscopic histology, I tried to achieve a compromise between width and depth of the subject, *i.e.* between general principles and correlations on the one hand and specific details of cases on the other, because I think that both are important to the student. Despite the intense satisfaction they give to the philosophical mind, general principles seem useless without concrete applications and, conversely, attention to specific details seems sterile unless accompanied by a recognition of the basic laws at work behind them and of their relation to other things.

I learned much while I was putting this material together and I hope that by organising and illustrating it with drawings I may help others to cover the same ground faster and easier than I did so that they can devote their gain of energy and time to the advancement of ultrastructural knowledge beyond its present frontiers or to its useful application in their own fields. For this, I think, is and will remain one of the indispensable contributions of human teachers as against machines: the organisation and reduction (by selection) of the enormous, endlessly expanding volume of human experience to a rapidly transmissible concentrate that can be assimilated in a tiny fraction of the time it took to produce it.

Finally, I wish to acknowledge my debt to all those whose work was of incalculable help to me: the thousands of investigators who created this field and the writers of previous general texts on normal ultrastructure who have provided additional stimulation and enlightenment for me over the years, namely Drs. J. Rhodin, S. Kurtz, D. Fawcett, K. Porter, M. Bonneville, E. Sandborn, A. Ham, T. Leeson, J. Leeson, T. Lentz, J. Matthews and J. Martin. I also wish to thank Miss K. McDowell, Mrs. E. Botsford, Miss R. Watson and Mr. B. Winrob for their help with preparation of the manuscript and references, Mr. J. Holthejten and Mr. F. Lipfert for their help with instrumentation theory and the Medical Research Council of Canada and the B.C. Heart Foundation for research support that indirectly contributed to the creation of this book.

April 1973
Vancouver, Canada

P. Constantinides

Chapter 1

Summary of Methods

I. THE TRANSMISSION ELECTRON MICROSCOPE

The basic method used in ultrastructural research is *transmission electron microscopy*. This consists essentially of the penetration of a beam of electron rays through a small area of a very thin section of the examined tissue, its subsequent expansion through an outward bending of its rays, and its projection on a fluorescent screen or photographic film to produce a magnified image of the tissue area that was penetrated. The electronic image obtained is really a "density map" of the specimen under investigation since structural parts of low density let most of the electronic light through and appear as bright (translucent) spots, whereas parts of high density (including those rich in large or heavy molecules) keep most of it back and cast shadows, appearing as dark spots.

The instrument used in the above procedure is the *electron microscope (E/M)* which is a tubular apparatus basically similar to an ordinary (photonic) light microscope (L/M) with the following main differences:

(A) Instead of photonic light, the E/M uses a beam of electrons which are generated at one end of the tube by a heated tungsten filament and accelerated by being pulled through an anodic ring by a current of 40,000–100,000 Volts.

(B) Instead of being magnified through the refraction (bending) of light rays by a series of glass lenses, the specimen image is magnified through the bending of electron rays by a series of powerful tubular electromagnets (the "magnetic lenses") which produce considerable heat and therefore have to be constantly cooled during operation; there are usually 6 magnetic lenses in an E/M: 2 between the electron source and the specimen (condenser lens No. 1. and No. 2) and 4 between the specimen and image viewing screen (objective, diffraction, intermediate and projector lens); the 2 condenser lenses concentrate the electron beam on the specimen (and thus increase the brightness of the image), the objective lens focusses, and the diffraction-intermédiate-projector system magnifies the image that is created by the beam after it traverses the specimen; the function of all lenses can be increased or decreased by increasing or decreasing the electrical current that is fed to their coils.

(C) To avoid the scattering of electrons that would result from their collisions with air molecules, a high vacuum is produced within the E/M tube through the operation, in sequence, of a mechanical (rotary) suction pump, a mercury pump and an oil diffusion pump; the first two are preparatory while the latter produces the final high vacuum by attracting and capturing air molecules through showers of boiling hot oil.

(D) The magnified electronic image of the specimen cannot be seen by the human eye and is therefore made visible by being projected on a fluorescent viewing screen or on a photographic film.

(E) Whereas in ordinary light microscopy tissues are stiffened by freezing or by infiltration with materials such as wax and then cut into sections several μ thick that are mounted on glass slides, a different procedure is followed for the E/M: here the tissues are infiltrated by plastics such as epoxyresins that become very hard by polymerisation and make it possible to cut "ultrathin" (just a few hundred Å thick) sections which allow very much greater resolution of structural detail than the thicker sections, while still strong enough to withstand the electronic bombardment in the E/M; furhtermore, to minimize the total thickness of material traversed by the electron beam, the sections are either suspended free in the path of the beam, or they are supported by very thin films of carbon or parlodion, mounted in both cases on metallic grids.

(F) The resolving power of a good modern E/M can be as much as 1000 times greater than that of the ordinary L/M since the former can distinguish as separate entities structural points only 2 Å apart, whereas the latter cannot distinguish points less than 2000 Å (0.2 μ) apart.

Thus, the E/M has made visible a whole *new universe* (including large organic molecules) that was invisible before, and it compares to the L/M as the L/M compared to naked eye observation in the past. This does not in any way mean that the E/M has made the L/M obsolete; no level of organisation of living matter is insignificant, and correspondingly, no level of study is dispensable; the E/M study of how subcellular structures are assembled into cells, the L/M study of how cells are assembled into tissues and organs, and the naked eye study of how tissues and organs are assembled into whole animals are all indispensable stepping stones to the structural (and therefore functional) comprehension of living organisms; we cannot understand the whole if we omit the study of any one of its levels of organisation.

II. TISSUE PROCESSING FOR ELECTRON MICROSCOPY

To prepare tissues for routine examination with the E/M one usually has to fix them, *i.e.* preserve them as they are for long periods of time with the least possible change of their natural structure. This is commonly accomplished today by immersing small tissue specimens into fluids that "immobilize" them structurally such as glutaraldehyde and osmic acid solutions; both fixatives preserve cell structure but the former, when used alone, also preserves the activity of many cell enzymes, while the latter attaches to and preserves most cell lipids (including those in membranes) and thus enhances the contrast of many subcellular structures. Following fixation, tissues are (a) dehydrated by immersion in successively higher concentrations of alcohol in order to make it possible to infiltrate them by water-insoluble plastics in liquid (unpolymerized) form, (b) hardened through heating and (or) chemical catalysts which cause polymerization of the plastics, and (c) cut into ultrathin sections by the ultrasharp edges of glass chips or diamond knives; the sections are mounted on copper grids and stained by heavy metals (uranium acetate and lead citrate) which attach to the surfaces of the various subcellular structures and thus increase their density and therefore visibility (contrast) upon examination with the E/M; sometimes the contours of translucent cell components that have no affinity for stains can be made visible indirectly, *i.e.* by staining everything else around them ("negative staining").

Are the subcellular structures that we see in sections of fixed tissues real or are they artefacts produced by the chemical processing we just described?

There is good evidence that most of the structures we see, particularly the larger ones, are real entities that exist and function in living cells with shapes similar to those they exhibit on the fluorescent screen. Such evidence has been provided, among other things, by ultracentrifugal fractionation studies which have shown that most cell components seen in fixed and stained sections (*e.g.* mitochondria, microbodies, lysosomes, ribosomes, vesicles, etc.) have been isolated individually from fragmented unfixed cells and have been found to exhibit similar structural and chemical characteristics in sections as well as in ultracentrifugal fractions.

Nevertheless, fixation and dehydration through alcohol undoubtedly have several distorting effects on the molecular organisation of cell components, most evident in the case of the smallest organelles such as filaments; this is one of the reasons that the methods of freeze-fracturing, inert dehydration, freezing and freeze-drying are increasingly used as tools for the exploration of cell substructure under conditions approximating the status quo in the living and that experimentation is beginning with the new possibilities of radiation-fixation. *Freeze-fracturing* avoids fixation: the cells are chemically and structurally immobilized by instant (flash) freezing, they are fractured along a given plane to expose their internal structure, water is evaporated from their frozen fracture face (freeze-etching) to bring it out in sculptured relief, and a thin platinum–carbon film is precipitated on it and molded on its contours like a "death mask"; the latter represents an exact replica of the fracture face and is studied with a transmission E/M after the underlying tissue is dissolved away. In *inert dehydration* fixed tissues are cut after their water is replaced not by alcohol but by ethylene glycol. In *freezing* chemical fixation and in *freeze-drying* both chemical fixation and alcohol dehydration are avoided, while in both instances tissues are stiffened for cutting by freezing (cryomicrotomy). Finally, current experiments with *fixation through radiation* of very high energy and penetrance open the possibility of fixing tissues within a few billionths of a second and of avoiding the extraction of any chemicals from them since no liquids are employed.

Among the difficulties of present day E/M as compared to L/M work is the fact that one cannot study sections indefinitely. Ultrathin sections (a) tend to break under the bombardment of the electron beam and (b) they are gradually buried under a shower of hydrocarbon particles which are generated by the oil diffusion pumps and other sources, a process which is called "contamination" and can be slowed down considerably through "anticontamination devices" or improved vacuum systems but not altogether eliminated. Another nuisance is the fact that, unlike the L/M which operates for years or decades without breaking down, the much more complex and sensitive E/M (even the most expensive model) is periodically out of commission for a never ending variety of reasons. Last but not least, E/M work is very much more time-consuming than L/M work; it can take weeks to study with the E/M a series of tissues which would be surveyed with the L/M in only a few hours. For all these reasons, electron microscopists today have less peace of mind than their optical microscopist predecessors of a generation ago; their moments of reward are rare and separated by long periods of frustration.

III. SCANNING ELECTRON MICROSCOPE

When a tissue specimen is bombarded by a beam of electrons, some of the electrons go through the specimen (are "transmitted") while others bounce off its surface (are "backscattered") at various reflection angles. In addition, the bombarding stream of "primary" electrons excites some of the atoms of the specimen surface and induces them to emit "secondary" electrons. The transmission E/M, as we saw, uses those electrons that penetrate through the specimen to give us an electronic image of its internal structure, while the scanning E/M uses those electrons that bounce off the surface (and some secondary electrons) to give us an electronic image of the detailed shape of that surface in relief.

In essence, the scanning E/M operates as follows: a very narrow electron beam with a diameter of *ca.* 100 Å is generated, focussed on the intact (uncut) specimen and made by deflectors to travel zig-zag along its surface like a scanning spotlight several times a second; the reflected electrons, whose quantity depends, among other things, on the slope of the surfaces hit by the scanning beam, are picked up by a detector, amplified, translated into an electrical current and made to modulate another electron beam which is projected in a rapid scanning manner on the fluorescent viewing screen of a television tube; the image appearing on that screen is, therefore, a three-dimensional (relief) image of the surface of the specimen, with the "mountains" appearing bright and the "valleys" dark. To stiffen the irregularities of the specimen surface and to increase the generation of secondary and backscattering of primary electrones from it, the tissues or cells examined are usually fixed, dried and coated with a film of heavy metal such as gold or chromium in a vacuum evaporator. The resolving power of this instrument is obviously determined by the diameter of its electron beam (*i.e.* by the size of the "spotlight") and is in present day models of the order of about 100 Å.

The scanning E/M – alone or combined with other techniques – seems destined to make valuable contributions to the study of cell surfaces and their changes during physiological functions and disease. Its chief advantage at the moment is that by giving us a rapid overview of the surface landscape of cells and tissues, it gives us instant information of a kind that could only be gained extremely slowly and laboriously through serial sections with the transmission E/M. It should be realized, however, that despite its great potential and the esthetic appeal of its spectacular landscapes, the scanning E/M will remain essentially a tool for "ultrastructural surface anatomy", *i.e.* it will tell us what is outside. We will still have to find out what is inside cells by using the transmission E/M, and for this reason the scanning E/M will never replace the transmission E/M – it will only complement it.

IV. CHEMICAL INFORMATION TECHNIQUES

These techniques give us information on the chemical composition of the various cell parts and their changes during normal functioning and disease and enable us to visualise at the ultrastructural level the movements of an ever increasing number of chemicals into and out of cells. They show us whether a given chemical is entering the cell under study, how it gets in, where it goes and what its subsequent fate is. The most useful techniques in this area at the present time are ultrastructural cytochemistry, X-ray microanalysis and ultrastructural autoradiography.

(1) Ultrastructural cytochemistry

This method enables us to visualise several materials or compounds that are naturally electron dense or that can be made electron dense after a specific treatment. It also enables us to identify dense materials that disappear after exposure to specific enzymes or after extraction with specific solvents.

Among the naturally dense chemicals are (a) most free or bound heavy metals (*e.g.* iron, ferritin, hemoglobin), (b) certain inorganic salts (*e.g.* calcium phosphate), and (c) several groups of organic molecules such as nucleic acids (both DNA and RNA), amines and polypeptides (*e.g.* catecholamines, serotonin, vasopressin), and secretory proteins (*e.g.* pepsin, pancreatic enzymes, glucagon, insulin). Some of the above materials are not only dense but also have specific shapes through which they can be identified.

There are currently three principal ways of making translucent (invisible) compounds dense and of specifically identifying them within cells: (a) *By binding them with another chemical that has a specific affinity for them and forms a dense (visible) precipitate or complex with them;* thus *e.g.* invisible sodium ions can be bound with pyroantimonate ions to form a visible sodium pyroantimonate complex, and translucent glycogen can be bound with lead ions to form a dense lead-glycogen complex. (b) *By allowing them to act on suitable substrates to form dense products, if they are enzymes;* thus *e.g.* the protein peroxidase can be visualised by allowing it to oxidise a benzidine compound and turn it into a dense material in the presence of hydrogen peroxide, and phosphatase can be made visible by allowing it to act on phosphate esters and split off phosphate ions, which are turned into dense lead phosphate in the presence of lead ions. (c) *By binding them with specific antibodies directed against them, if they are antigens;* to make the resulting antigen-antibody complex visible, the antibodies are coupled with dense markers (*e.g.* ferritin) or with cytochemically demonstrable enzymes (*e.g.* peroxidase) before their interaction with the antigens; an example of this procedure is the demonstration of chorionic gonadotrophins in the syncytiotrophoblast by means of ferritin-marked antigonadotrophin antibodies.

Under certain conditions, as when each single antibody molecule is discernible because it is tagged by a single visible ferritin molecule, these immunohistochemical techniques make it possible not only to detect the presence but even to count the number of antigen molecules that exist in a given specimen area.

In addition to the identification of cellular components through their possession of density and special shape, or through their acquisition of density after specific treatments, several cell structures that are natively dense can be defined chemically if they disappear after treatment with specific solvents or specific enzymes – the treatment often being more effective if applied prior to fixation of the tissue. Thus, *e.g.*, cell densities that vanish after exposure to ribonuclease, desoxyribonuclease, pepsin, or chloroform–methanol represent RNA, DNA, protein or lipid, respectively.

(2) X-ray microanalysis (analytical electron probe)

This technique enables us to identify most elements (all those with an atomic weight greater than 10) and is used in conjunction with a scanning E/M. In essence, this procedure uses the X-rays that are generated when the thin electron beam of a scanning E/M hits a small specimen spot as information about the chemical composition of that spot; it is based on the fact that each atom species of the periodic system emits X-rays of a different (and characteristic) wavelength when bombarded by electrons – the lighter the element the longer the wave length emitted. In the microanalyser variant of the scanning E/M, the characteristic X-rays that come off the "illuminated spot" of the specimen are picked up by a special crystal and reflected into an amplifier, where they are translated into an electrical signal whose intensity varies with the intensity of the X-ray radiation that is emitted from a given specimen spot and, therefore, with the concentration of the emitting atom species in that spot; since X-rays of different wave lengths come off the specimen at different angles, a fractional change in the position of the crystal will select a different wavelength for reflection into the amplifier and thus enable us to monitor a different atom species at any given time.

This technique is beginning to yield invaluable information on the presence and concentration of most chemical elements in different parts of cells. Since the electron beam that produces the information scans in zig-zag fashion the whole surface of specimen, one can establish a "chemical composition map" of the tissues or cells examined. It should be emphasized, however, that X-ray microanalysis can only inform about localisation and quantities of *elements*, not compounds (inorganic or organic).

(3) Autoradiography (ARG)

This method enables us to locate radioactive (labelled) atoms in a tissue section by virtue of the fact that if a thin photographic film is spread over the section, the radiation emanating from the radioactive tissue areas will cause the formation of reduced silver grains in those spots of the film that directly overlie the radioactive sites. The most suitable types of labelled atoms for visualization with this technique are those whose radiation has a short track (of the order of a few μ) and therefore achieves satisfactory grain localisation in the film, *e.g.* ^{3}H and ^{125}I.

The common procedure is to inject animals or incubate tissue cultures with the labelled compounds whose cellular uptake we wish to study and then fix, dehydrate, embed and cut the desired tissues to produce ultra-thin sections in the customary manner; the sections are subsequently coated with a thin film of photographic emulsion in the darkroom and kept in the dark for as long as is necessary (usually weeks or months) to allow the radiation emanating from them to produce significant numbers of reduced silver grains in the overlying emulsion film. After this long exposure time, the emulsion-coated sections are treated with photographic developer and fixer to render the reduced silver grains visible as very dense structures superimposed on the radioactive areas of the tissue landscape.

This technique makes it possible to visualise the uptake of labelled compounds by cells, their migration to various cell components, their participation in various intracellular and extracellular metabolic activities, and their release from cells; thus, *e.g.* labelled thymidine, leucine, or glucose can be used to study the synthesis of DNA, protein, or polysaccharides, respectively, and labelled steroid hormones serve to visualise their entry into the nucleus. Another useful application of autoradiography is the chemical identification of various unlabelled cell components by their selective binding of certain administered labelled compounds; thus, cholinesterase can be identified through its binding of the labelled inhibitor difluorophosphate, and DNA through its binding of labelled actinomycine. Finally, under certain conditions, autoradiography can also be used for an approximate estimate of the number of labelled molecules present in a given tissue area.

One of the major hazards in autoradiography is the possibility that in some cases the radioactive atom may split off the molecule it was labelling as a result of metabolic processes, or that it may be exchanged with unlabelled atoms from other molecules in vivo; when this happens, the autoradiographic detection of labelled atoms within tissues cannot, of course, be taken to indicate the presence of the intact labelled compounds that were originally administered. Among the defenses against this difficulty are (a) the selection of labelled compounds in which the bond between the labelled atom and the molecule nucleus has been proven to be stable in vivo through previous chemical recovery studies and (b) the demonstration of disappearance of radioactivity from sections after exposure of the tissue to specific solvents that dissolve, or to specific enzymes that destroy the labelled compound under study.

V. FUTURE DEVELOPMENTS

The following developments are now under way, some of them seemingly destined for generalised use within the next ten years: (a) the 1,000,000 Volt and up transmission E/M, (b) the high resolution scanning E/M, (c) the identification of organic compounds through physical methods, and (d) the direct visualisation of small molecules and large atoms.

The *1,000,000 Volt and up transmission E/M* will have a much higher electron accelerating power and, therefore, an electron beam of much greater penetrance and resolving power than an ordinary E/M. It will *e.g.* permit the study of 2–3 μ thick sections with as good resolution of detail as that obtained in 1000 Å thick sections; since, however, the structures from all the different planes of the thick sections are projected on the same focal plane, stereoscopic photography is required for clear image formation. One of the greatest hopes for this instrument was that it would enable us to explore the ultrastructure of living cells enclosed with life-supporting fluids in thin transparent chambers; this hope does not, however, seem likely to be fulfilled at the moment since cells are damaged and killed by the high rate of intracellular ionisations caused by electron-accelerating voltages of that order of magnitude.

The *high resolution scanning E/M* will apparently be achieved through the utilisation of electron sources that can produce a much thinner electron beam than ordinary V-shaped filaments. One such source is the "field emission tip" which makes it possible to work with spot diameters (and resolutions) of 5 Å or less.

The *identification and quantitation of several organic compounds* in cell organelles may prove one day as rapidly feasible through physical methods as that of most chemical elements is today by means of X-ray microanalysis. Since many organic molecules emit characteristic energy spectra or particles when appropriately excited, or absorb characteristics zones of energy spectra when exposed to various radiations, it may be possible to make use of some of these phenomena for molecule identification purposes through a suitable combination of scanning E/M, non-electronic sources of radiation, transmission E/M and micro-spectrometric techniques.

Finally, the direct *visualisation of small molecules and large atoms* seems to be close at hand, since the dimensions of many of these particles are now within the resolution range of a powerful modern transmission E/M. Indeed, it has been recently possible in a few laboratories to obtain what appear to be convincing photographs of single heavy atoms (such as *e.g.* thorium or uranium) and of single aromatic molecules (such as *e.g.* phenolic rings in crystal lattices). Progress in this direction was slowed until recently because of the relatively low contrast of conventional bright field techniques and because of the high "background noise" created by the uneven density of even the most uniformly thick support films; the use of the much higher contrast of dark field techniques and of much more homogeneously dense support films such as crystalline graphite (which permit a higher signal to noise ratio) can be expected to facilitate research in this area. There remains, of course, one problem which can never be avoided: Some of the electrons that go through the specimen score direct hits on its atoms and cause changes that can lead to disintegration of its molecules; in other words, as elsewhere in physics, the very method of observation changes the object under observation. Since, however, the molecular changes caused by the electron bombardment do not happen at once, but accumulate gradually with increasing time of observation, it could be expected that photography of specimen structure during the very initial stages of this degradation process would minimise its distorting effects.

Chapter 2

The Cell

I. GENERAL ULTRASTRUCTURE (Plate 1, Fig. A)

(1) Plasma membrane (Plate 1)

The cell is enclosed in a *plasma membrane* (PM)[1] which is averagely 75 Å thick (range: 50–90 Å) and appears under high magnification to consist of three ca. 25 Å thick layers (an outer and inner dense and a middle light lamina), as seen after the common OsO_4 fixation methods currently in use (inset *a*). The principal functions of plasma membranes are: (a) to separate the living protoplasm from the world around it, (b) to transport into the cell interior certain selected materials from outside, and to transfer into the external space certain substances from within the cell, (c) to become "excited" in response to certain external stimuli, and (d) to change the composition of its immediate environment through enzymatic activity. Details in Sect. II of this chapter.

(2) Surface coats (Plate 1)

The plasma membranes of most cells are covered partly or totally by external coats of the following two main types: (a) the glycocalyx[2], a relatively thin layer of fuzzy material that is always adherent to the PM, and (b) the basement membrane[3], a relatively thicker layer that does not always adhere to the PM.

The *glycocalyx*[2] seems to "grow" out of the external lamina of the PM and exhibits a substructure of a fuzzy network (inset *b*). It consists of polysaccharide–protein compounds (glucoproteins) that contain acid sulfated polysaccharides and sialic acid as their carbohydrate component; it seems to be produced within the cell, "secreted" on to its surface and turned over quite rapidly (within a few hours), as shown by the autoradiographic tracing of the movements of its labelled components such as tritiated acetate, glucose and sulfate; it can be the site of intensive enzymatic activity and it also represents the surface antigens of the cells in which it occurs; it is charged electronegatively and it can be demonstrated particularly well by electron dense cations such as ruthenium – which bind its anionic groups. The antigenic glucoprotein "receptors" in the glycocalyx are thought to be branched molecules whose number depends on cell species and geographic location on the cell surface.

The *basement membrane* (BM)[3] seems to represent a moderately dense mixture of amorphous collagen with varying proportions of polysaccharides, as suggested by studies utilising collagenase, polysaccharide stains and labeled anti-BM antibodies. The ratio of these two components seems to vary greatly in different animal and cell species, ranging from mostly carbohydrate to mostly collagen. The amorphous rather than fibrillar-striated appearance of collagen within basement membranes has been attributed to the irregular orientation of the collagen molecules within the BM. Often there is a thin, uniformly wide, translucent band between the cell surface and the BM; this translucent band possibly represents a polysaccharide-rich material (perhaps a glycocalyx) that glues the BM to the cell.

A BM covers like a shirt at least part of the surface of all cell types, with the exception of almost all connective tissue cells and the hepatocytes of the liver. There are some indications that it is produced within the rough endoplasmic reticulum of the cells it covers and that certain types of injury stimulate cells to increase their production of BM; it is also possible that, at least in some cases, blood plasma components may contribute to its substance. Its function is still not completely established, but it seems to help attach cells to neighbouring structures (and thus promote tissue cohesion) as indicated by the fact that typical striated collagen fibrils[4] are often anchored in its substance. Basement membranes seem freely permeable to all molecules that cross plasma membranes.

(3) Cell joints (Plate 1)

All cells, except those of connective tissue are directly attached to one another by means of specialised junctional structures which serve variously (a) as mechanical joints between two cells, (b) as sites of impulse transmission from one cell to another, or (c) as both mechanical

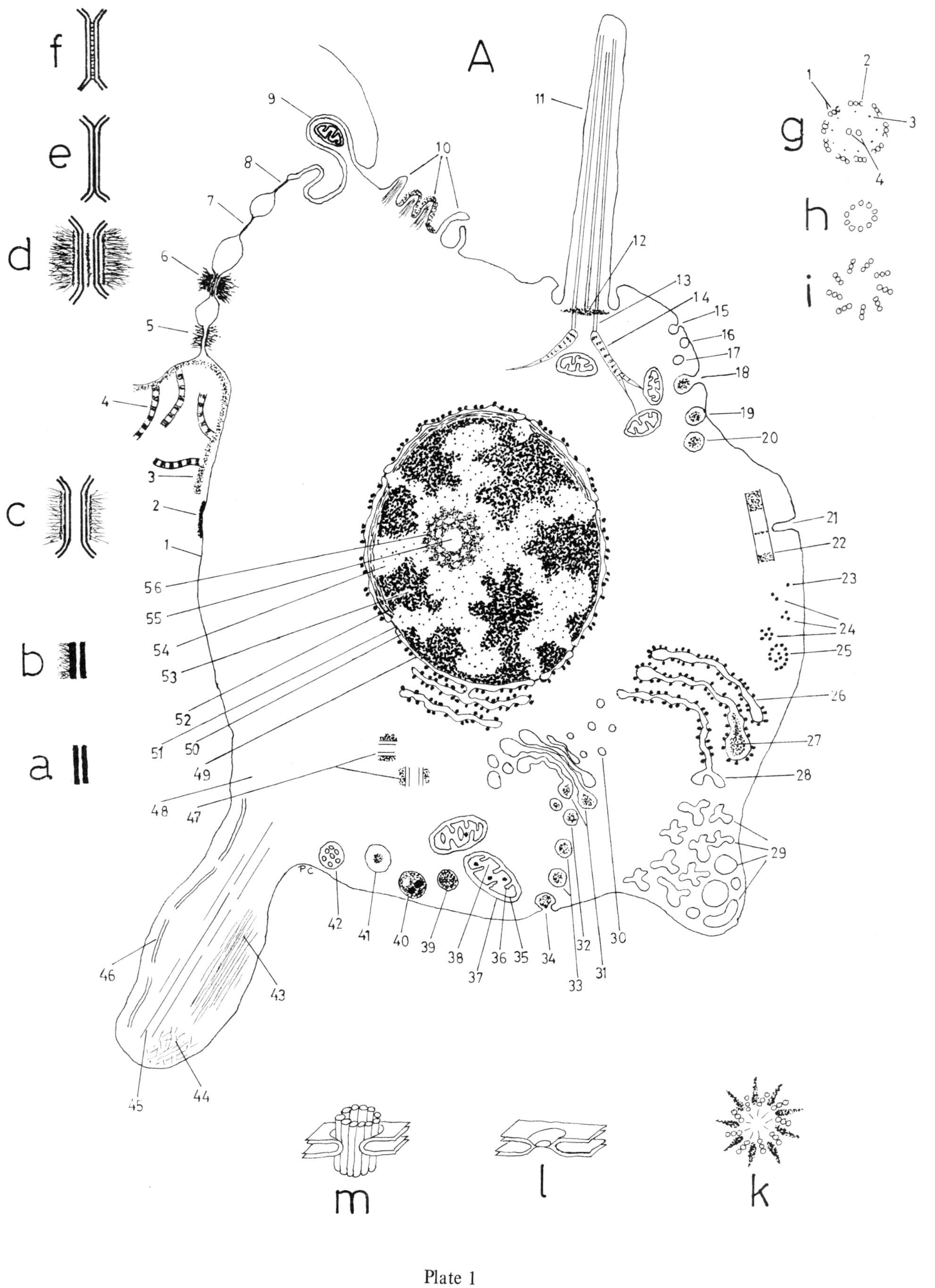
A
a
b
c
d
e
f
g
h
i
k
l
m
1
2
3
4
5
6
7
8
9
10
11
12
13
14
15
16
17
18
19
20
21
22
23
24
25
26
27
28
29
30
31
32
33
34
35
36
37
38
39
40
41
42
43
44
45
46
47
48
49
50
51
52
53
54
55
56
PC

Plate 1

joints and impulse transmission sites. Five such specialised contact structures are currently recognised: (a) the zonula adherens[5], (b) the macula adherens[6], (c) the zonula occludens[7], (d) the septate desmosome[8], and (e) the simple interlocking of adjacent cell surfaces[9].

The *zonula adherens*[5] consists of the adhesion of two cells along a long, belt-like contact area whose cross-section appears as a short approximation of the two neighbouring plasma membranes to within about 200 Å of one another (inset *c*). Delicate thin filaments of unknown function can be seen under certain circumstances to radiate into the cytoplasm from plate-like densities very close to the inner PM leaflets of the two joining cells; they usually extend into a long band of thin filaments, the "terminal web", that runs across the entire width of the cell to reach the contralateral zonula adherens (for illustration, see the drawing of an absorptive cell in Ch. 9, Alimentary System, Sect. V, Intestine, p. 111). The "glue" that fills this 200 Å cleft and holds the cells together at such a site is a translucent material of still unknown composition, possibly a glucoprotein; there are indications that calcium and perhaps magnesium are important structural components of the "glue" material within zonulae adherentes since the removal of such divalent ions by chelating agents tends to widen or open these junctions. Whatever the nature of the material within the zonula adherens cleft, it seems to be of sufficiently low molecular density so as to allow the passage of protein molecules of the size of peroxidase.

The *macula adherens*[6] (commonly also termed a "desmosome") consists of the adhesion of two cells at a circumscribed oval patch, about 4000 Å long and 2800 Å wide; the gap between the two plasma membranes at the macula is about 250 Å wide and it contains a linear density in the middle which probably represents the cross-section of a thin dense plate in mid-gap (inset *d*): Many short "tonofilaments" coarser than those of zonulae adherentes, radiate from plate-like densities close to the inner PM leaflets of both joining cells at the desmosome site. As in the case of the zonula adherens, the binding material in a macula adherens is of still unknown composition but seems to contain calcium and protein as an important building block and allows the passage of several protein molecules. Masculae adherentes seem to develop late in embryonic life. The frequent close association of mitochondria with desmosomes indicates that an energy-consuming process (probably an information transfer from one cell to another) is taking place at such sites.

It is intriguing that despite their structural similarity at the E/M level, the maculae adherentes of different tissues have apparently different chemical composition. Thus, the desmosomes of columnar epithelia can be opened by calcium-removing chelators (EDTA) but not trypsin, while the reverse is true for squamous stratified epithelia.

The *zonula occludens*[7] (also termed a "tight junction" or a "terminal bar") represents a fusion of the outer leaflets of the two adjacent plasma membranes along a long belt-like contact area (inset *e*). Such junctions are impermeable to proteins and other molecules; they exhibit low electrical resistance and hence transmit impulses from one cell to another very easily; they are reportedly absent from embryos, develop in increasing numbers with age in post-natal life and may apparently appear and disappear at various sites continuously.

The *septate desmosome*[8] consists of a very close approximation of two plasma membranes over a circumscribed area, the gap in this case being only about 25 Å and being bridged by several short septa-like bridges (inset *f*). It is currently thought that these short bridges represent the partitions of a honeycomb framework formed by shelf-like projections from the outer leaflets of both plasma membranes which meet and fuse in mid-cleft. These junctions are more frequent in invertebrates and, like the zonulae occludentes, they are absent from embryos.

The *simple interlocking of adjacent plasma membranes*[9] seems to provide some mechanical adhesion between cells, without creating a barrier to the passage of any molecule. The gap between the cells here seems to vary greatly in width; it is narrowed when the cells on both sides of it are swollen as a result of various insults (*e.g.* anoxia) and it appears to be filled by intercellular fluid; intercellular junctions of this loose type are very extensive among cells engaged in much active transport of ions and fluids (*e.g.* renal tubules, sweat glands, etc.), although their role there is still unknown.

Most epithelial cells of the body (whether they line surfaces or secrete) are joined to one another by multiple junctions of the same or different types. "Junctional complexes" consisting of sets of zonula occludens and zonula adherens – with the frequent addition of a macula adherens – occur widely in epithelia that border fluids, *e.g.* the gastro-intestinal, urogenital, thyroid, ependymal, ciliary and endolymphatic sac epithelia where they probably prevent the seepage of liquids between cells.

(4) Outward thrusting plasma membrane formations
(Plate 1)

Apart from ordinary cell processes, one must consider the following two specialized structures under this heading: (a) microvilli[10], and (b) cilia[11].

Microvilli[10] represent short projections (with or without filamentous cores) that greatly expand the cell surface and are concerned with absorption or secretion of solutions by the cell – in some as yet unexplored manner. Their surface is often covered by a glycocalyx and exhibits strong enzymatic activities. Regular arrays of numerous microvilli constitute "brush borders" and are particularly prominent in the absorptive surfaces of intestinal and renal epithelial cells.

Cilia[11] (also known as "kinocilia" or "flagella") represent long rod-like projections that perform whip-like or spiral movements and are probably the earliest specialized locomotive devices developed by cells after protoplasmic streaming. They contain several microtubules, semitubules and microfilaments which run along their entire length and are arranged in a remarkably regular pattern that is the same for all cilia throughout all unicellular and multicellular organisms. This pattern, which is best shown in a cross-section of a cilium as seen in inset *g*, consists of nine peripheral pairs of microtubules[g1] (each with an attached semitubule[g2]) nine filaments[g3] (one in front of each microtubule pair) and two centrally placed microtubules[g4]. Each microtubule has a diameter of about 250 Å, and on high magnification its wall seems to consist of 8–13 filaments about 35 Å thick each (inset *h*); it apparently contains a contractile protein "dynein" whose amino acid composition resembles that of muscle actin. At its base, each cilium is connected by means of a fuzzy "basal plate"[12] to a "basal body"[13] or "kinetosome" which is a short cylindrical structure consisting of nine microtubule triplets arranged in a turbine-like pattern (inset *i* shows cross-section of a basal body). When a cell contains many cilia, their basal bodies are interconnected by means of microfilaments that are probably concerned with coordinating ciliary activity. Sometimes striated "rootlets"[14] with a 1000 Å periodicity grow out of the base of basal bodies; mitochondria, the energy-producing organelles, are usually in close proximity to basal bodies and the branched tips of the striated rootlets. Like most cell components, cilia probably exhibit a biological cycle, some degenerating and disappearing while new ones are generated all the time.

(5) Inward thrusting plasma membrane formations (Plate 1)

Both intermittent and permanent invaginations of the plasma membrane are to be considered under the above heading.

There are two types of intermittent invaginations and they are related to the processes of pinocytosis and phagocytosis, respectively. *Pinocytic invaginations*[15] usually take in solutions from the extracellular space, are turned into 400–600 Å thick spherical *pinocytic vesicles*[16] through fusion of the invagination lips and travel into the cell interior after detaching from the plasma membrane[17]. Formation of pinocytic vesicles, and the PM consumption it entails, seems also somehow implicated in ameboid movement *Phagocytic invaginations*[18] are larger than the pinocytic ones, usually take in solid particles from the extracellular space (bacteria, debris, etc.) and are turned into *phagosomes*[19] through fusion of the invagination lips; phagosomes detach from the plasma membrane and move into the cell interior[20] where they usually fuse with enzyme sacs in an attempt to digest their contents (see Ch. 4, Connective Tissues, Sect. II, p. 35). Both pinocytosis and phagocytosis are also referred to as "endocytosis".

Typical *permanent invaginations*[21] are found in striated muscle cells, where they serve to carry the excitation (depolarisation) of the plasma membrane to the deeper lying striated myofibrils[22] and stimulate them to contract (Ch. 5, Muscle, p. 65).

(6) Cytoplasmic contents (Plate 1)

The following are the main organelles found in the cytoplasm of cells: free ribosomes[23–25], rough endoplasmic reticulum (RER)[25–28], smooth endoplasmic reticulum (SER)[29], Golgi apparatus[30–32], secretory vesicles or granules[33–34], mitochondria[35–38], lysosomes[39–40], microbodies[41], multivesicular bodies[42], microfilaments[43–45], microtubules[46], and centrioles[47]. All these structures are embedded in a cytoplasmic matrix[48].

The *ribosomes*[23–25] are tiny protein producing factories that come as single spheroid units about 150 Å in diameter[23], or as clusters, the so called "polyribosomes" or "polysomes"[24]; a special variety of spirally arranged polysomes are called "cochleosomes"[25]. The polyribosome population of a cell is roughly proportional to the amount of protein the latter produces and is particularly abundant in embryonic or growing cells. Ribosomes seem to make the protein for the construction of several other organelles such as the RER, SER and the various types of contractile and non-contractile microfilaments. The main components of ribosomes are manufactured in the nucleus, from which they are extruded into the cytoplasm. After enucleation of amebae, their ribosome population declines steadily. More details in Sect. III, Ribosomes (p. 18).

The *rough endoplasmic reticulum*[26] (RER) consists of flattened sacs or "cisternae" whose external surfaces are studded by ribosomes and whose interior is often filled with translucent or moderatly dense materials[27]. This system of organelles is particularly well developed in cells which produce proteins, glucoproteins or lipoproteins destined for release from the cell into the extracellular space (*i.e.* for "export"). Contrary to earlier speculations, it has *not* been possible to prove that the RER arises from invaginations of the plasma membrane; cell-embryological studies rather indicate that the RER cisternae are produced by the ribosomes that are attached to them. The membranes of the cisternal sacs seem to consist of enzyme proteins which contribute to the synthesis of the cisternal products (both those released into the cisternal lumen and those released into the extracisternal cytoplasmic matrix).

The *smooth endoplasmic reticulum* (SER)[29] consists of vesicles and isolated or interconnected tubes of various shapes and sizes, *i.e.* it represents a system of saccules without attached ribosomes. One way in which SER saccules are generated appears to be the development of outgrowths of RER cisternae[28] that leave their ribosomes behind and constrict off the RER system. This is supported by the frequent finding of connections between RER and SER in certain cells and by the movement of labeled membrane building blocks from the former to the latter. The SER saccules can, therefore, be viewed as enzyme-charged surfaces, produced by ribosomes, like the RER cisternae. The membranous walls of the SER are enzyme proteins involved (a) in the inactivation of foreign chemicals that hit cells, (b) in the synthesis of lipids, and (c) in the driving of various intermediate metabolic processes, including those that generate light. Thus, the SER system develops extensively, and leads to a very "spongy" cytoplasm, (a) in cells when they metabolize drugs and exogenous poisons, (b) in cells that produce lipoproteins or steroid hormones, and (c) in cells of light-generating (luminescent) organs.

The *Golgi apparatus*[31] represents a usually saucer-shaped cluster of (a) flattened saccules with dilated ends and (b) vesicles that originate from the detachment of these bulbous ends[32]. Autoradiographic studies have shown that materials which are first produced in the RER cisternae somehow travel to the Golgi saccules (by diffusion or by transport within tiny vesicles[30] detached from the RER) where they are apparently condensed, modified or coupled with other chemicals; the changed materials then leave the Golgi system within "*secretory vesicles*"[32–33] which detach from the Golgi saccules and travel to the cell surface where they fuse with the PM, open and discharge their contents into the extracellular space[34] (a secretory process which is the reverse of pinocytosis and is called "emiocytosis" or "exocytosis"). The small transport vesicles from the RER tend to arrive at the convex aspect whereas the larger secretory vesicles tend to take off from the concave aspect of the Golgi apparatus. The materials within the Golgi and the secretory vesicles, like those within the RER cisternae, can be either translucent or variably dense; when the secretory vesicles contain dense sécretion they are usually called "secretory granules"[32–33]. An example of the autoradiographic studies that have established the above described sequential events is the experimental administration of labelled aminoacids, *e.g.* [^{3}H]leucine, to enzyme-secreting cells such as those of the pancreas: the labelled aminoacid appears within 5 minutes in the RER cisternae, within 20 minutes in the Golgi complex, within one hour in the secretory vacuoles and within two hours in the extracellular space (the lumen of the pancreatic gland). Similar results have been observed with labelled glucose and sulfate in mucous or cartilage-producing cells, indicating that the production and secretion of sulfated polysaccharides involves the same RER – Golgi – secretory granules – emiocytosis sequence as that of secreted enzyme proteins. The Golgi apparatus seems to arise from and be maintained through nuclear activity via the RER; it disappears after enucleation and reappears after re-implantation of a nucleus in amebae.

The *mitochondria*[35–38] are the main organelles concerned with the production of energy from the oxidation of organic substrates, as well as a site of lipid synthesis and other functions. Each mitochondrion consists essentially of an inner sac[35] with several surface-increasing infoldings[36], which is placed within another (outer) sac[37]. The inner sac contains an amorphous "matrix"[38] which may be translucent or dense and may or may not contain dense granules of lipids or inorganic (often metallic) compounds; the wall of the outer sac is called the "outer membrane"[37] while that of the inner sac is called the "inner membrane"[35] and its infoldings "cristae"[36]; cristae may be shaped like shelves (as in the mitochondrion now described), like tubules or like concentric cylindrical projections into the matrix; the connections of the cristae with the inner membrane may be missed in the plane of the section under study so that they may appear like tiny sacs embedded within the mitochondrial matrix. More details in Sect. IV, Mitochondria, p. 19.

The membranous walls of the various saccular cytoplasmic organelles described (RER, SER, Golgi and mitochondria) have a thickness and trilaminar structure that closely resembles that of the plasma membrane (PM) which surrounds the entire cytoplasm. It is because of this structural similarity that both the membrane of the saccular organelles and the PM are collectively referred to as *"Unit Membrane"*.

The *lysosomes*[39–40] are spheroid membrane-bound bodies of homogeneous dense texture[39] which may contain vacuoles, very dense inclusions or both[40]. They represent stores of several hydrolytic enzymes which have their optimal activity at an acid pH and serve to digest phagosomes, degraded organelles or perhaps – after their extrusion – extracellular materials. More details in Sect. V, Lysosomes and Microbodies, p. 22, and Ch. 4, Connective Tissues, Sect. II, p. 35.

Microbodies[41] are vesicles with a dense central inclusion, the "nucleoid", which has a crystalline substructure. They contain oxidative enzymes and can thus be considered as a special type of lysosomes.

Multivesicular bodies[42] are spherical sacs containing several small vesicles. There are indications that one type of these organelles transport absorbed protein or other materials within the cytoplasm of neurons, kidney and other cells, where they probably arise from a conglomeration and sequestration of groups of pinocytic vesicles. There is also evidence that a different type of multivesicular bodies develops from evaginations of the outer layer of the nuclear envelope in cells such as those of the gas glands of certain fishes.

Microfilaments[43–45] are fine threads of widely varying thickness and function. They can be tightly packed[43] as in smooth muscle cells, loosely and randomly arranged[44] as in keratinised cells of the epidermis or discrete[45] as in neurons; they may vary in diameter from *ca.* 30 Å to *ca.* 80 Å, depending on the type of cells they inhabit and they may be contractile (as in muscle), structural (as in keratin) or of unknown function (as in neurons). Recently, contractile filaments of about 40–70 Å diameter have also been implicated (a) in the mediation of ATP-induced protoplasmic streaming in amebae, and (b) in the formation of the cytoplasmic cleavage furrow of dividing cells. It appears that cytoplasmic cleavage is produced by the contraction of a ring of filaments that encircle the equator of the cell, running just underneath its surface, and that this process can be selectively inhibited by Cytochalasin B, leading to suppression of cytoplasmic (but *not* nuclear) division and formation of multinucleated cells.

Other currently explored manifestations of the contractile function of some microfilaments include (a) the contraction of microfilament-endowed endothelial cells, (b) the simultaneous development of 40 Å microfilaments and invasive mobility in certain cells that become cancerous as a result of chemical carcinogen treatment, and (c) the microcontraction of parts of the cell surface that is associated with the development of pinocytic and phagocytic vesicles, the latter process being reportedly inhibited by the anti-filament chemical cytochalasin. Finally, one of the most fascinating new functions attributed now to microfilaments is their inhibitory effect on cell secretion, as seen *e.g.* in the pancreatic β-cells where cytochalasin greatly increases the emiocytosis of insulin. Perhaps in this case dense webs of sub-surface microfilaments retard the discharge of secretion-containing vesicles because they represent a physical barrier which is interposed between the latter and the cell surface.

Microtubules[46] throughout the cytoplasm of various cells have a diameter of 200–280 Å and their wall seems to consist of microfilaments arranged in a circle like the staves of a barrel, as already described in the case of the ciliary microtubulus (see inset *h*). They are found in many types of cells, ranging from blood cells to neurons; their various functions are still not settled but it seems that one of their roles is to provide a structural framework for certain cells and their processes, *i.e.* a shape-maintaining "cytoskeleton". Other probable functions are (a) contractility (as in cilia and flagella), (b) translocation of organelles to which they attach (*e.g.* chromosomes), and (c) directed transport of materials from one site of the cytoplasm to another. Microtubules seem to be constrantly renewed at one end and "worn out" at the other, and they appparently disappear and reform all the time. Among the environmental conditions that greatly influence these organelles are temperature changes: cooling to 2°C completely degrades mitotic spindle and platelet microtubules while rewarming leads to their reappearance.

Centrioles[47] are pairs of short cylindrical structures disposed at right angles to one another. Each of these cylindrical structures is very similar to the basal body of a cilium, *i.e.* it consists of nine triplets of microtubules arranged in a circle like the blades of a turbine (see inset *k* for a cross-section). Dense amorphous material is attached to the external surface of the centrioles and forms fine regular patterns within their lumen. These organelles, like mitochondria, are semi-autonomous structures *i.e.* they possess DNA of their own and can duplicate themselves, presumably by virtue of the above fact. Their two known functions seem to be (a) their duplication during mitosis and the formation of a microtubular support-movement framework for the dividing chromosomes, the "mitotic spindle", and (b) the formation of ciliary basal bodies by a duplication (copying) process. More details in Sect. VI, Centrioles, mitotic spindle and microtubules, p. 23.

The *cytoplasmic matrix*[48] is the material filling the space between the organelles. It is usually translucent and amorphous but it may be dense and have a fine fibrillogranular texture, depending on the methods of tissue processing and the types of cells involved. When its matrix has a high density and its ribosome population is large, the cytoplasm of a cell appears very dark. Neither the composition nor the function of the cytoplasmic matrix is settled at the present.

Scattered in the matrix of certain cells are various *inclusions* of diverse functions which are illustrated in the subsequent chapters, namely glycogen, lipids, pigments (*e.g.* hemoglobin, melanin, lipofuscin) and crystalloids (*e.g.* yolk, Reinke crystalloids, Charcot–Böttcher crystalloids). In normal cells (a) glycogen and lipids represent stores of metabolic fuels, (b) *yolk* provides building blocks for cell membrane sysnthesis, (c) *lipofuscin* apparently consists of bags of accumulated metabolic or structural wastes in cardiac muscle and neurons which resembles in several ways lysosomal "residual bodies (see Sect. V, Lysosomes and Microbodies, p. 22 and Ch. 4, Connective Tissues, Sect. II, p. 35), (d) *hemoglobin* and *melanin* play active roles in controlling metabolic processes and radiation effects, respectively, and (e) the function of most crystalloid inclusions is obscure at the moment.

The two commonest inclusions are glycogen granules and lipids. *Glycogen* consists of spheroid granules

150–450 Å thick that occur as single units ("β-particles"), tight clusters of varying degrees of aggregation (rosettes, or "α-particles"), or massive pools, depending on animal and cell species and physiological conditions. Although of low native electron density, glycogen granules can become very dense after staining with lead ions and they appear to represent conglomerates of 30 Å filaments. Since some of the enzymes concerned with the handling of glycogen are located on SER membranes, pools of glycogen particles are intimately mingled with lattices of interconnected SER cisterns (as *e.g.* in hepatocytes) or with concentric whorls of SER cisterns (as *e.g.* in the case of the "glycogen bodies" of ciliated cells). *Lipids* consist of usually spherical but sometimes star-shaped droplets which acquire various degrees of density after osmium fixation, depending on their nature or state of metabolic degradation; there are indications that lipids with unsaturated fatty acids appear much more dense than lipids with saturated fatty acids after osmium, and that as lipids are broken down metabolically they may lose electron density. Osmium not only fixes lipids (like formaldehyde and glutaraldehyde) but is also stains them, *i.e.* it gives them electron density, and it makes them less soluble in lipid solvents; when osmium does not reach the center of lipid droplets the latter is extracted by the lipid solvents used during the tissue dehydration and embedding procedures and the droplets appear as dense rings surrounding empty centers. Usually, most lipids – particularly those synthesized within the cell – are not bound by membranes while those that are absorbed or phagocytized from outside are membrane-enclosed, but there are exceptions; thus, lipoprotein globules apparently synthesized in liver cells are membrane-bound, and in the late stages of fat absorption by intestinal cells some lipid may appear free in the cytoplasmic matrix.

(7) Nucleus (Plate 1)

The nucleus consists of a nuclear envelope[49–50] which encloses the chromatin[53–54] and the nucleolus[55–56].

The *nuclear envelope*[49–50] is a double-walled sac that is continuous with and represents an extension of the rough endoplasmic reticulum (RER). Of its two membranes, the *outer membrane*[49] is always studded with ribosomes, while the *inner membrane*[50] is sometimes (notably in invertebrates) underlaid by an *inner fibrous lamina*[52]. The envelope appears to be perforated at several sites by small *nuclear pores*[51], which however, upon higher magnification and with special techniques are shown in most cases to be sealed by thin diaphragms (see inset *l*) or more rarely, to be plugged by short cylinders with a palisade-like substructure (see inset *m*). There are indications that an exchange of materials between the nucleus and the cytoplasm occurs through the nuclear pores even when they are sealed by thin diaphragms.

The chromatin[53–54] contains the genetic (DNA) material of a cell, *i.e.* the set of operational instructions and reflexes it inherits from its ancestors. It comes in two forms: (a) the *heterochromatin*[53], a genetically dormant, dense material, and (b) the *euchromatin*[54], a genetically active, translucent material. The nucleic acids of chromatin are bound to certain proteins, notably histones.

The *nucleolus*[55–56] represents a local accumulation of mainly ribosomal RNA on its way to the cytoplasm, *i.e.* of chemical building blocks that are used in the construction of ribosomes. It usually consists of (a) a light amorphous component, the "pars amorpha"[55], and (b) a dense knot-like component, the "pars granulosa" or "nucleolonema"[56].

More details about the nucleus are contained in Section VII of this Chapter.

II. PLASMA MEMBRANES

(1) Composition

Plasma membranes (PMs) are primarily lipoproteins but also seem to include relatively smaller quantities of other chemicals such as adenine nucleotides (AMP, ADP, ATP). As regards the lipid component of PMs, 80% of it is phospholipid (in order of decreasing percentage: phosphatidylcholine, phosphatidylethanolamine, phosphatidylserine, sphingomyeline), the remaining 20% being cholesterol. As regards the protein component of PMs, much of it seems to consist of enzymes (*e.g.* ATP-ase, alkaline photophatase, peptidases, nucleotidases, invertase). The PM phospholipid seems to be essential to the enzymic activity of PMs (*e.g.* the ATP-ase activity of red cell membranes) since the latter disappears when the phospholipid is removed or degraded. The union between phospholipid and enzymic proteins seems to be a freely reversible process in the case of the lipoprotein forms of several enzymes, such as cytochrome oxidase.

(2) Structure (Plate 2)

Several hypothetical models of the molecular structure of the PM have been proposed but none of them has yet been proven. If in the adjacent diagrams *protein* molecules (amino-acid chains) are shown as long accordioned carbon chains and their hydrophilic (polar) segments as white spheres (Fig. A), while the hydrophilic ends of *phospholipid* molecules are represented by black spheres and their hydrophobic (fatty acid) parts as double tails

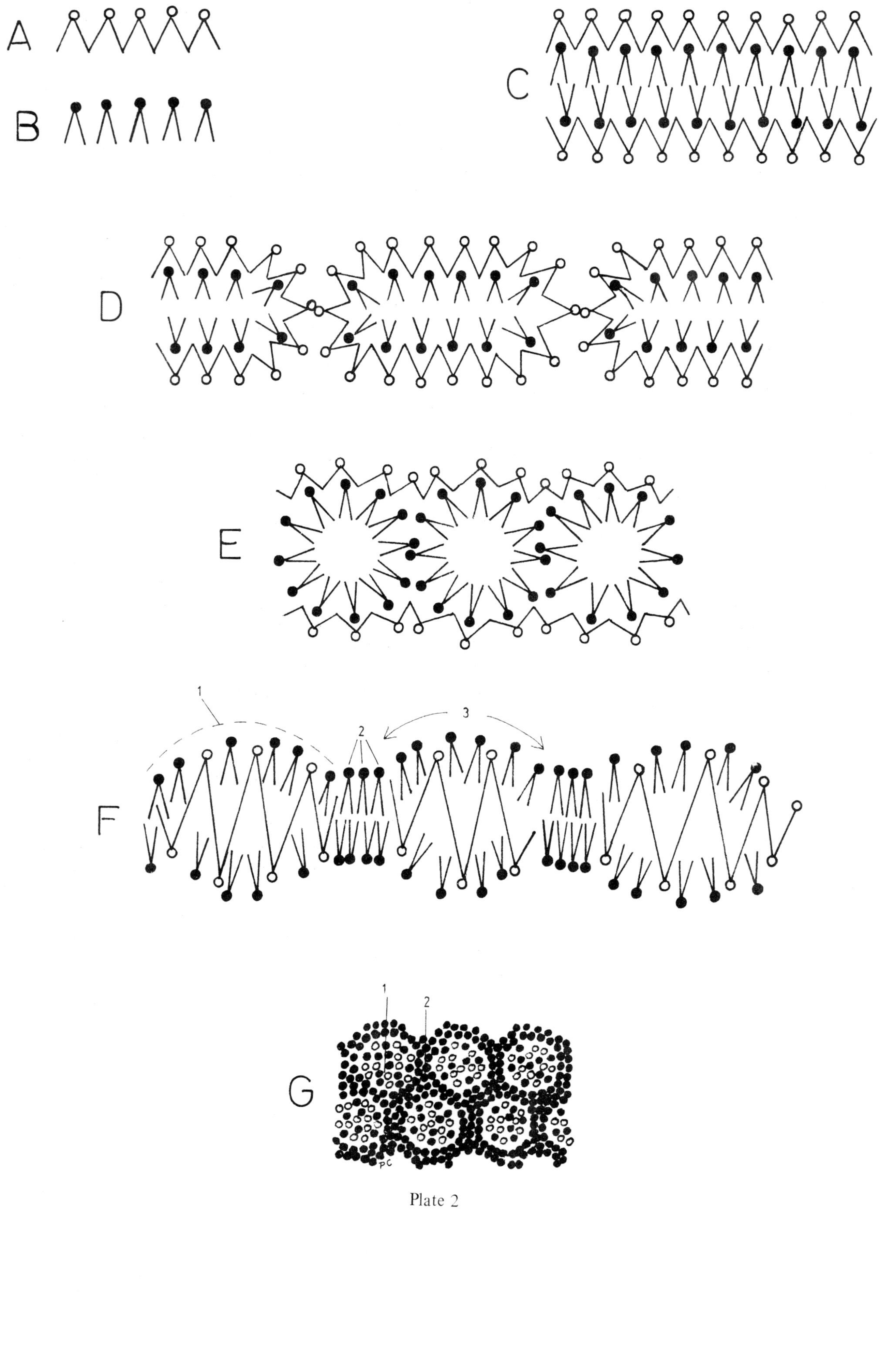

Plate 2

(Fig. B), then the currently four main models of PM structure postulate the following configurations:

(A) *The Davson–Danielli model* (Fig. C)

The oldest of the four models proposes that the PM consists of two monolayers of lipids with facing hydrophobic parts, flanked on the outside and inside by two protein monolayers. It is based on early chemical findings that the PM of red cell ghosts (red blood cells without cytoplasm) contains sufficient lipid for only two monolayers along their entire surface, and on the reasoning that the very low surface tension (0.1 dyne/cm^2) exhibited by these cells can be explained best if protein rather than lipid forms their outermost boundary. One of the difficulties of this model is that if it were correct one would expect a light-dense-light E/M image in PM cross-sections after OsO_4 fixation (since the dense element osmium is known to attach to lipids) and yet the reverse is true: one obtains a dense-light-dense E/M image. The above difficulty has been countered by experiments involving the osmium staining of artificial bimolecular leaflets of heavy metal-fatty acid soaps which indicate that osmium has perhaps a greater affinity for the hydrophilic (polar) groups of proteins and lipids than for the hydrophobic (non-polar) lipid parts.

(B) *The Stein–Danielli modification of the Davson–Danielli model* (Fig. D)

This modification postulates the existence of multiple "protein-lined", 8–15 Å wide hydrophilic pores in a PM otherwise structured as proposed in the Davson-Danielli model just described. The pores are postulated in order to explain the observed rapid passage of water and water-soluble molecules (*e.g.* glucose) through a PM possessing a lipid barrier in its mid-zone, and it is thought that they need occupy only 0.01–0.1% of the total cell surface in order to accomplish this function.

(C) *The globular micelle model of Lucy–Glauert* (Fig. E)

This model proposes that the PM consists of a layer of lipid globules oriented with their hydrophobic parts in the centers and their hydrophilic parts at the periphery of the globules and flanked by two layers of protein; the globular lipid micelles would be held together by hydrogen bonds forming between adjacent polar groups. The whole concept is based on (a) the observation that suspensions of lecithin and cholesterol in water (which imitate the chemical composition of PMs) form globular molecular patterns, visible at about 300,000 × magnification, and (b) suggestions of a discontinuous, globular substructure seen in certain PMs under conditions of freezing-drying at 200,000–600,000 × magnification.

(D) *The mosaic model of Sjöstrand* (Figs. F, G)

This latest of all models views the PM as a mosaic of lipoprotein globules[1] separated by lipid "septa"[2]; both protein and lipid molecules are oriented in such a manner that their hydrophilic (polar) parts are at the surfaces and their interacting hydrophobic (non-polar) parts in the mid-zone of the PM; the lipoprotein globules would represent many different enzyme-protein units and they could interact through thermal rotational oscillations in various directions[3] (see Fig. F for profile and Fig. G for "en face" view of this model). This concept has the considerable functional attraction that it presents the biochemist with locations for the numerous proteins and enzymes that he can isolate from the PM, and, like the preceding one, it fits E/M suggestions of globular PM substructure, obtained under technical conditions that are thought to minimize denaturation of proteins.

The strongest support for a globular substructure of at least certain areas of the PM has recently come from freeze-etch studies, which have demonstrated the existence of distinct globular units of *ca.* 75 Å (or more) diameter within the PM, the "intramenbranous particles". These particles are best visible in fresh unfixed cells, can also be seen in aldehyde-fixed cells, but are not visible after OsO_4 fixation. They vary in numbers and distribution pattern depending on cell species, geographic part of the cell surface, phase of cell development, and environmental conditions; thus, *e.g.* the intramembranous particle concentration of the lymphocyte PM is different from that of the erythrocyte, it is much greater in parts of the PM which are involved in cell junctions than elsewhere and in adult rather than embryonic cells, and it can be changed by certain enzymatic treatments. The intramembranous particles probably represent enzyme units within the PM; they may also represent sites of ion transfer across the PM and they may help the transfer of information from one cell to another at junctions. There is recent evidence that each glucoprotein surface receptor in the glycocalyx of a cell is continuous with a corresponding intramembranous particle in the underlying PM: if one labels the glycoprotein receptors with *e.g.* ferritin–phytohemagglutinin, their distribution pattern on the PM surface corresponds exactly to that of the intramembranous particles in the underlying PM (as seen in freeze-etch studies) and furthermore, if one changes the latter through some means one changes the former in identical fashion.

It is considered more and more likely that the PM structure does not follow one rigid pattern for all cells and all times but rather that different cells have different PM structures to serve different functions. In fact, there are several indications that even the same cells may change their PM structure (or parts of it) at various times to accommodate changing functional requirements. Thus *e.g.* it is known that the PM of granular leucocytes binds pyroantimonate while that of non-granular leucocytes does not; furthermore, the PM of muscle and nerve cells changes during excitation and recovery and it is possible that the process of memory may be associated, among other things, with structural and functional PM changes at neuronal synapses ("membrane memory").

Everything that has just been said about the structure of plasma membranes also applies to the structure of the "unit membrane" which is found in all intracytoplasmic membranous structures.

(3) Functions

The following main functions are associated with PMs:

(a) Separation and protection of the living protoplasm from its non-living environment. Life seems to be incompatible with a permanent break in the continuity of the PM.

(b) Transport of materials from outside into the cell and *vice versa*. Four basic transport mechanisms are recognized at present: (a) "Simple diffusion" of mostly very small molecules along concentration gradients (from high to low concentration sites) through thermal agitation; it is thought that polar compounds would enter the PM slower than non-polar compounds because they would have to rupture their hydrogen bonds with the water outside cells and because of their lack of affinity for the lipid layer within the PM, whereas non-polar compounds would be slower than polar ones in leaving the PM for the opposite reasons. (b) "Facilitated diffusion" of certain polar molecules along concentration gradients at a much faster rate than would be expected in view of their hydrogen bonding activity and the lipid "barrier" within the PM. Thus, glucose seems to cross the red blood cell PM about 10,000 times and glycerol about 100 times faster than would be expected on the basis of the above. It appears that facilitated diffusion promotes easy entry of energy sources into the cell and easy removal of metabolic wastes from it. The presence of protein-lined (and water-filled) pores in the PM has been proposed as one way of explaining facilitated diffusion. (c) "Active transport" of certain molecules against concentration gradients (from low to high concentration sites) requiring the expenditure of energy, as evidenced by its inhibition by metabolic inhibitors. Such transport (*e.g.* the transport of Na out of the cell through a "sodium pump" after the end of excitation) is supplied with energy from the splitting of ATP through an ATP-ase in the PM and is inhibited by inhibitors of ATP-ase (*e.g.* ouabain); it is thought to involve the action of enzymes at both surfaces of the PM (for the capture and release of the transported molecule) as well as shuttling "carriers" (for crossing the width of the PM). (d) "Vesicular transport", *i.e.* transport by infolding of the PM to capture extraneous materials into small or large pockets which become small or large vesicles (pinocytosis and phagocytosis, respectively). This mechanism of "endocytosis" seems to be reserved for the entry of larger molecules and particles into a cell; its reverse ("exocytosis" or "emiocytosis") seems to serve the elimination or secretion from the cell of larger molecules and particles. One type of pinocytotic vesicles (the "coated" or "alveolate" vesicles) seems to be covered externally by a coat of bristles which has been found to represent an intricate basketwork that somehow plays a role in driving the PM invagination process.

(c) Excitation. The excitation of excitable cells is associated with a series of reversible structural and functional changes of their PMs (see Chapters on Muscle and Nerve Tissue).

(d) Enzymatic action on the external environment. By virtue of the enzymes built into them, some PMs can act chemically on their immediate environment.

(e) Division and fusion. Cell membranes can divide to form new cells or new vesicles, and they can fuse to unite two cells or a vesicle with a PM. The two processes seem to be intimately associated for one never sees the one without the other. They can be physiological (as in mitotic cell division, the sperm-ovum fusion and the pinocytosis and secretion phenomena) or pathological (as in virus-induced cell fusion).

All above functions are shared to variable degrees by both the external cell membrane (the PM) and the internal membrane of the various saccular organelles, *i.e.* they are basic properties of the unit membrane.

III. RIBOSOMES (Plate 3, Figs. A–D)

Ribosomes are miniature protein-synthesizing factories consisting of ribosomal protein and ribosomal RNA. It is currently thought that within each ribosome amino acids are assembled into proteins through the action of messenger RNA and transfer RNA as follows: As a long messenger RNA ribbon passes through the ribosome, transfer (soluble) RNA triplets carrying amino acids enter the ribosome, attaching to the messenger RNA ribbon along a sequence determined by their affinity for different segments of that ribbon; the amino acids carried by the transfer RNA triplets are then assembled into a protein chain following a sequence dictated by the sequence of the transfer RNA triplets (which in turn is dictated by the base sequence of the messenger RNA). As each amino acid is welded into the growing protein chain, it is "unhooked" from its carrier transfer RNA, which is released from the ribosome, and when the protein synthesis is completed both the newly produced amino acid chain and the messenger RNA ribbon are likewise extruded from the ribosome.

Polyribosome clusters (Fig. A) can be unravelled by certain techniques (spray shadowing) and shown to consist of rows of ribosomes attached to and strung along a messenger RNA thread (Fig. B). Ultracentrifugal fractionation, X-ray analysis and other methods suggest that each ribosome consists of a smaller "light" fraction (Fig. C^1) and a larger "heavy" fraction (Fig. C^2), and that each of these two fractions is made up of 32–40 Å thick globular subunits of ribosomal protein embraced by a loop of ribosomal RNA (Fig. D); the light fraction consists of about 20 and the heavy of about 60 such globular protein subunits which probably represent enzymes concerned with guiding the protein synthesis process that goes on within the ribosomes – the ribosomal RNA loop around each globular subunit probably having synthesized it. Running through the ribosomes between their two fractions is the messenger RNA ribbon that determines the sequence of the amino acid chains manufactured in them.

Ribosomes are usually found very close to the cell organelles whose protein they manufacture; they are thus abundant in the immediate vicinity of RER sacs, developing myofilaments and other cytoplasmic structures during their biogenesis.

IV. MITOCHONDRIA

(1) Functions

Mitochondria produce the energy needed to drive numerous cell functions such as contraction, ciliary and sperm movement, impulse transmission, synthesis of protein and lipids and "uphill" ion transport (against concentration gradients). They produce this energy through oxidation, *i.e.* by removing hydrogen and electrons from fatty acids and other organic substrates and by transferring them through a series of hydrogen and electron acceptors (*e.g.* NAD, FAD, the cytochromes) to oxygen. More specifically, they dehydrogenate fatty acids, etc., through Krebs' cycle and transfer their electrons through cytochromes b, c_1, c, a and a_3 (in that sequence) to oxygen, by the action of the "respiratory chain" enzymes. The energy derived from the above oxidative process can (a) be used directly to drive various cell functions, or (b) it can be used to synthesize ATP by the phosphorylation of ADP (through the mediation of coenzyme "Q" or ubiquinone) and ATP can later be split, releasing the energy stored in it for the driving of energy-requiring cell activities. The combined process resulting from the coupling of oxidation (electron transport along the respiratory chain) to the phosphorylation of ADP (ATP synthesis) is referred to as "oxidative phosphorylation", whereby the precise nature of the coupling mechanism is still under debate; one of the results of "uncoupling" of oxidation from phosphorylation can be the induction of maximal respiration and heat production (thermogenesis), as accomplished in the mitochondria of brown adipose tissue. In addition to energy production and ATP synthesis, the mitochondria of some cells also seem to manufacture lipids (*i.e.* yolk production in ova by mitochondrial masses). Finally, these organelles behave like miniature nuclei: they synthesize and replicate DNA (as indicated by their uptake of labeled thymidine) and they can synthesize RNA (as indicated by their uptake of labeled uridine). These latter functions make mitochondria autonomous not only in the production of their own enzyme-proteins but also in self-replication and regeneration, in many cases.

(2) Chemical composition

The following chemicals have been isolated from the main parts of a mitochondrion: (1) Matrix: NAD (pyridine nucleotide) and coenzyme A; NAD-linked dehydrogenases; fatty acid–coenzyme A synthetases and dehydrogenases; Krebs cycle enzymes; DNA and RNA (apparently used for self-replication and local enzyme synthesis, as discussed below). (2) Inner membrane: cytochromes b, c_1, c, a and a_3; coenzyme A; enzyme systems of the respiratory chain (electron transport) system; enzyme systems concerned with ATP synthesis; ion translocating enzyme systems; fatty acid dehydrogenases, transferases and elongating enzymes. (3) Outer membrane: cytochrome b_5 and NADH-cytochrome b_5 reductase; monoamine oxidase; fatty acid–coenzyme A synthetase and fatty acid elongating enzyme systems; phospholipid-handling enzymes; nucleoside diphosphokinase.

The inner membrane appears to have a low permeability for small molecules when the mitochondrion is "at rest" whereas the outer membrane seems freely permeable to them.

(3) Ion translocations and conformational changes during function (Plate 3)

In vitro studies of recent years have shown that when mitochondria respire they undergo the following changes: (a) calcium and other divalent cations, phosphate and other anions and water from outside move across their membranes into their matrix, (b) potassium cations simultaneously move out of them, (c) they swell slightly, (d) their surface potential drops from about 180 mV to about 40 mV, and (e) their membranes develop changes of fluorescence (in the presence of fluorochromes) indicative of structural changes. These phenomena express oxidations occurring without (uncoupled from) ATP synthesis.

The above changes are reversed when the mitochondria return to a "resting" state, apparently with the help of a "calcium pump" that pumps calcium out of and potassium into the mitochondria again; they can be prevented or inhibited (a) by metabolic inhibitors, (b) by agents such as oligoamines which bind to the phospho-

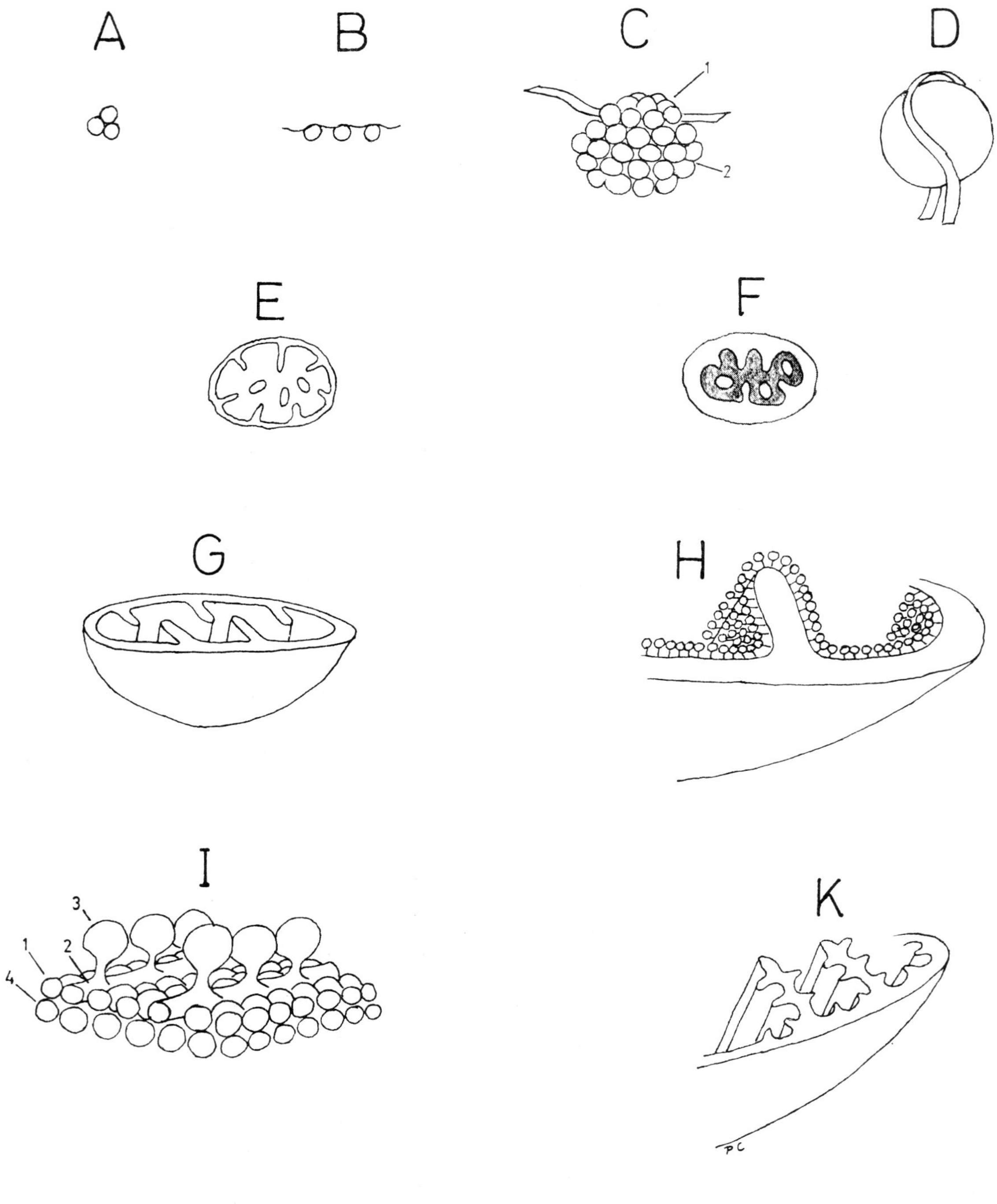

Plate 3

lipids of mitochondrial membranes thus "blocking" the transport of calcium across them, and (c) by absence of calcium from the medium. Since calcium stops ATP synthesis, the "resting state" favours it.

The movement of calcium across the mitochondrial membrane is thought to involve (a) the attachment of this cation to phospholipids at the external surface of the membrane, (b) its transport across the membrane thickness through some "shuttle carrier", and (c) its unloading at the inner membrane surface and capture by anions in the matrix. Calcium stops ATP synthesis by binding phosphate and stopping ADP phosphorylation.

Prolonged and excessive calcium action or prolonged and marked hypoxia lead to severe ATP depletion within the mitochondria and their membranes. This paralyzes the mitochondrial cation pumps (which require ATP for their function) and thus causes extreme swelling and destruction of these organelles.

Apart from the very rapid physiological changes of volume and membrane fluorescence which accompany their respiratory activity, mitochondria undergo relatively slower and more dramatic structural changes following the addition of ADP *in vitro*: they change from an "orthodox" configuration (Fig. E) to a "condensed" one (Fig. F) in which the inner membrane contracts and the matrix becomes much denser. The "condensed" state expresses marked ATP synthesis from ADP through coupling of energy to ADP phosphorylation.

(4) Structure (Plate 3, Figs. G–I)

The outer and inner membranes of the mitochondrial envelope have, in recent years, revealed a number of functional differences which hint at significant differences in their substructure. Thus, the *outer membrane* has proven (a) more resistant to proteolytic digestion, (b) much more permeable to small molecules, (c) much less resistant to membrane insults, and (d) more endowed with phospholipids than the inner membrane; when mitochondria are exposed to very hypotonic solutions or to certain membrane-injuring agents (phospholipase, fatty acids, peroxides) the outer membrane soon ruptures while the inner membrane bulges through the breaks and expands until the inner compartment swells to 10 or 11 times its original size. Furthermore, the finding that autoantibodies directed against the inner – but not the outer – membrane circulate in the blood of persons suffering from biliary cirrhosis has been interpreted as evidence of an antigenic difference between the two membranes.

The cristae represent a considerable increment of the inner mitochondrial membrane, the main site of oxidative phosphorylation (Fig. G). Under high magnification and with negative staining the inner surface of the entire inner membrane proves studded with small *stalked particles* (Fig. H) which can be torn off by sonication.

Recent studies suggest that the *inner membrane* consists of two layers of globular lipoprotein units (Fig. I): (a) an inner layer[1] of smaller globules with fibers[2] that carry the stalked particles[3], and (b) the outer layer of slightly larger globules[4]. These globular units represent the various enzyme units and coenzymes of the inner membrane: the inner layer includes cytochrome b and c_1 units, the knobs of the stalked particles contain the coupling factor F_1 (the terminal enzyme in ATP synthesis), and the outer layer includes cytochromes c, a and a_3. Electron transport from one unit to another is thought to be facilitated through oscillatory movements of the globular units in lateral and transverse directions. Thus, the "elementary particles" that exhibited both respiratory and phosphorylating activity and that were isolated from comminuted mitochondria in earlier biochemical studies consisted most probably of fragments of inner membrane.

The general shape and the shape and number of the cristae of mitochondria vary considerably depending on the metabolic activity of the cells that host them. Thus, the mitochondria of heart muscle cells (which have a very high level of respiratory activity) exhibit many more cristae than those of cartilage cells (which have a low level of respiration). Furthermore, in cells of hypermetabolic patients and in muscle cells with extremely high contraction frequency, as found *e.g.* in the heart of canaries and the cricothyroid of bats (which literally vibrates to produce ultrasound), the mitochondrial cristae develop multiple triangular folds which even further increase the surface area and therefore the metabolic capacity of the inner membrane (Fig. K).

The overall *size* of mitochondria also depends greatly on their physical and metabolic environment. Thus, *e.g.* they grow to literally gigantic dimensions under the influence of electro-magnetic fields, various nutritional deficiencies (*e.g.* protein, cystine) and toxic factors (*e.g.* alcohol excess).

Among the least studied structural components of the mitochondrial *matrix* are its various inclusions which greatly influence its density. These can be globular, fine granular, microtubular, filamentous or crystalloid and of variable density and number; they may be completely absent or they may fill up the entire mitochondrial matrix space. Some of them consist of lipids, others of inorganic salts (*e.g.* iron, $Ca_3(PO_4)_2$), and many are of unknown composition. Massive $Ca_3(PO_4)_2$ deposits, ATP depletion and mitochondrial destruction can be induced by high calcium levels (*e.g.* in hypervitaminosis D) and by magnesium deficiency (which has the same effects as high calcium levels).

(5) Destruction, autophagy and replication

There are indications that some mitochondria are dying and new ones are born all the time, *i.e.* that there is a "turnover" of these (and other) organelles. This turnover may be more rapid in some tissues than in others and it may be accelerated by toxic destruction of mitochondria as *e.g.* by calciferol overdose, severe magnesium deficiency, intravenous detergents such as triton etc.

When mitochondria are dying they are wrapped up (segregated) in a sac (which is perhaps derived from the SER) to form *"autophagosomes"* or *"segresomes"* that fuse with lysosomes to form *(auto-)phagolysosomes*; within the latter, the dead organelles are degraded in stages to amorphous, lamellar or filamentous residues or vacuoles, as if they were digested foreign bodies.

Considerable study has been devoted to the regeneration mechanism of mitochondria in recent years. It now seems certain that in some cases (*e.g.* in annelids) new mitochondria can be created "de novo" in mature cells through nucleus-guided biogenic activity involving the extrusion of a probably RNA-containing dense granular material from the nucleus into the cytoplasm (the "mitochondrial cement") within which cristae and envelopes materialize piecemeal before being assembled into whole mitochondria. It now also seems certain that in other cases (*e.g.* in several plant cells and vertebrates), mitochondria are capable of self-replication through growth and elongation and subsequent division into two daughter organelles or through budding, with or without the help of a nucleus-derived catalytic "cement" material. It is thought that the autochthonous DNA and RNA of mitochondria guides their replication through the fission or budding mechanism.

V. LYSOSOMES AND MICROBODIES

Lysosomes contain the following hydrolytic enzymes, all effective optimally at an acid pH: (a) enzymes acting on nucleic acids and other phosphorylated compounds, *i.e.* desoxyribonuclease, ribonuclease and acid phosphatase, (b) enzymes acting on proteins, *i.e.* cathepsin and collagenase, (c) enzymes acting on carbohydrates, *i.e.* α-glycosidase, glucosaminidase, glucuronidase, galactosidase and mannosidase, and (d) enzymes acting on sulfated compounds, *i.e.* arylsulfatase. They don't seem to contain any lipases.

These organelles are present to a varying degree in many cells, most notably in macrophages and polymorph leucocytes. Their origin has been disputed but they now seem to arise primarily in the Golgi complex, thus representing secretory vesicles.

Microbodies probably represent a special type of lysosomes and, like the latter, are found in many cell types. They contain oxidative enzymes, *i.e.* catalase, amino acid oxidase and urate oxidase. Their crystalloid "nucleoids" consist of uricase; microbodies without nucleoids lack this enzyme.

Enzymes are released from *lysosomes* by procedures and agents that break up the lysosomal membrane such as acid pH, sonication, osmolysis, lecithinase, lipid solvents, detergents, ultraviolet irradiated uroporphyrin K, and etiocholanolone. This release seems to be inhibited by certain agents that "stabilise" the lysosomal membrane such as cortisone, acetyl salicylic acid (aspirin), chloroquin and cholesterol.

A main proven function of these organelles is their role in the digestion of (a) foreign particles and materials (*e.g.* bacteria, debris) taken up by the cell through phagocytosis and enclosed in "phagosomes" or (b) endogenous structures and materials (*e.g.* dead organelles, metabolic wastes) segregated within the cell and sealed in membranous sacs, the "cytosegresomes" or "autophagosomes". Lysosomes have been documented to fuse with phagosomes and digest them gradually – if they contain organic material that can be attacked by their enzymes; any undigested contents of the resulting "phago-lysosomes" (*e.g.* lipids, iron) are either discharged from the cell through emiocytosis or retained in it as "residual bodies" (*e.g.* lipofuscin). Phagosomes can probably stimulate the generation of lysosomes in the cell (see also Ch. 4, Connective Tissues, Sect. II, p. 35).

The ability to promote autophagocytosis seems to account for the particularly abundant development of these organelles in rapidly regressing tissues (*e.g.* post-partum uterus, post-lactation mammary gland) and rapidly differentiating or regenerating tissues (*e.g.* embryonic limb buds). In the former case lysosomes promote the shrinkage and degradation of cells that are no longer needed, while in the latter they are thought to remove old ribosomes (templates) and organelles in order to make room for new ones.

Lysosomes have also been held responsible for the autolysis (decomposition) of cells that occurs following complete loss of their oxygen supply (*e.g.* after death of the animal of which the cells are part). It has been speculated that anoxia causes a drop of cytoplasmic pH which activates the proteolytic enzymes within the lysosomes so that they digest the lysosomal membrane and break out, like "tigers out of a cage", to digest the whole cytoplasm as well. It has not been possible, however, to prove this attractive hypothesis so far. In special experiments that studied the autolytic process in stages, the plasma membrane was found to break long before the lysosomal membranes, and the two lysosomal enzymes that were scanned histochemically (acid phosphatase and aryl sulfatase) did not move out of the lysosomes throughout the autolytic process.

Lysosomes have been shown to be released from polymorph leucocytes when the latter are exposed to certain bacterial toxins such as streptolysin ("degranulation" of polymorphs).

In recent years, lysosomes have been increasingly implicated in a number of human diseases, such as the following: (a) rheumatoid arthritis, a disease attributed in part to the increased release of lysosomal enzymes within joint cavities as a result of the action of streptolysin on polymorph leucocytes, (b) Chediak–Higashi disease, a condition associated, among other things with defective lysosomes in polymorphs and increased infection tendency, (c) glycogenosis of children, an accumulation of glycogen in tissues resulting from the absence of α-clucosidase from lysosomes, and (d) metachromatic leukodystrophy, a disorder leading to accumulation of sulfated polysaccharides in the brain and associated with the absence of aryl sulfatase from lysosomes.

VI. CENTRIOLES, MITOTIC SPINDLE AND MICROTUBULES (Plate 4)

Upon higher magnification, the cross-section of a centriole reveals an intricate substructure (Fig. A): Its 9 triplets of microtubules are interconnected by means of dense bands[1] and the *intracentriolar material* forms a wheel with spokes that bear terminal nodular densities and connect with one another as well as with the microtubules. The *pericentriolar material* forms a crown of "satellite" masses that vary in shape, size and number in different centrioles: they may represent solid[2] or segmented[3] arms radiating from the centriole, or irregular densities[4] with no visible connection to the centriole. The microtubules of the 9 triplet systems have a diameter of about 200 Å and their wall is about 40 Å thick; each microtubule consists of about 10–13 hollow microfilaments arranged in a circle, as in cilia and their basal bodies. In a longitudinal plane, centrioles are about 3000–5000 Å long and *ca.* 1500 Å wide; one of their ends is open and the other often seems closed by an amorphous material.

Both DNA and RNA are present in centrioles, thus conferring upon these organelles an unusual autonomy for self-replication and protein synthesis, as in the case of mitochondria. It is possible that the nucleic acids are located in the pericentriolar and intracentriolar structures.

Centrioles appear to have two main functions: (a) they form basal bodies of cilia in differentiating ciliated epithelium, and (b) they form the mitotic spindle in dividing cells.

When they form the hundreds of *basal bodies* of a ciliated cell, centrioles replicate themselves repeatedly; the resulting basal bodies then "induce" the generation of ciliary microtubules above them. Like centrioles, these organelles can also duplicate themselves, the new basal body developing first at a right angle to the old basal body and then gradually turning by 90° to become perpendicular to the cell surface and shoot off a new cilium.

When a cell enters mitosis, its pair of centrioles is doubled by self-replication and the resulting two centriole pairs (the two "poles") move away from one another while generating the spindle apparatus that supports the chromosomes in its center (Fig. B). Centriole replication may occur repeatedly when there is repeated replication of genetic nuclear material without corresponding cytoplasmic divisions; thus more than two centriole pairs (sometimes several dozen) may be found in polyploid cells (*e.g.* in some liver cells, in megacaryocytes, etc.).

The *mitotic spindle* (Fig. C) consists of several hundred microtubules[1] which are structurally identical with those found in cilia; they originate in the pericentriolar satellites[2] rather than the centrioles themselves[3] and they move towards the chromosomes[4]; it is uncertain at present whether they attach to the chromosomes or go right through them and it is likely that some microtubules go from one pole of the spindle to the other. Spindle microtubules seem capable of aminoacid incorporation and they exhibit strong ATP-ase activity, a feature that relates them to myofilaments. Their function in mitosis is still unknown; they seem to elongate during the unfolding of metaphase (probably through protein incorporation at the centriolar end) and they shorten and disappear during anaphase, with the exception of continuously dividing cells, where they persist throughout the interphase.

All *microtubules* in cells (*e.g.* the microtubules of basal bodies, cilia, centrioles, mitotic spindles, and neurotubules) appear to have identical structure even though their functions are quite diverse. They have been variously implicated in (a) cell shape maintenance (cytoskeletal role), (b) intracytoplasmic transport of materials from one cell area to another and cytoplasmic streaming (*e.g.* in amebae or in axons), (c) movement of their own (*e.g.* in cilia), and (d) causation of movement in other organelles (*e.g.* the saltatory movements of certain organelles in cultured cells).

The ubiquitous microtubules consist of proteins of *ca.* 120,000 molecular weight called "tubulins" which together with actin, myosin and collagen make up about half of the total body protein and seem to vary with the tubule species; mitotic spindle tubulins *e.g.* are immunochemically different from those of neurotubules. As in the case of mitotic spindle tubules, the microtubules of cilia arise from dense amorphous masses that are satellites of basal bodies and seem to "seed" the polymerisation of these tubular organelles. The motility of microtubules appears to be associated with their ATP-ase ac-

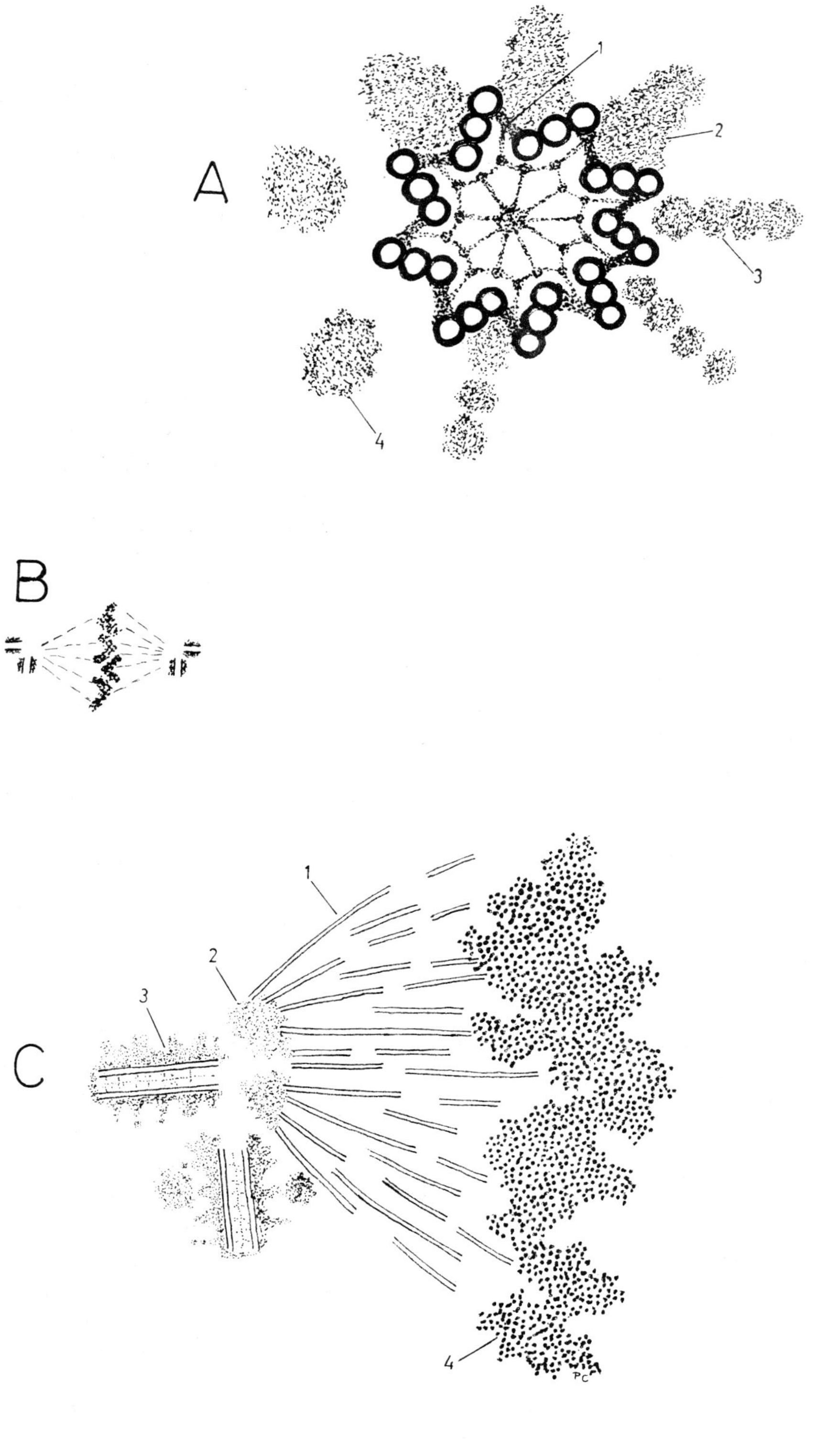

Plate 4

tivity – the addition of ATP makes cilia beat. On the other hand, the coordinated movement of a group of microtubules (as *e.g.* in a cilium) seems to depend on the integrity of fine filamentous bridges that have been found to join individual tubule pairs to one another; the enzymatic destruction of these bridges leads to loss of coordination – the dissociated tubule doublets slide past one another. Finally, microtubules have been recently implicated in the promotion of secretion in certain endocrine cells; it is thought that these tubular organelles somehow induce movement of the secretion-containing vesicles towards the cell surface.

Many agents can depolymerise microtubules (by combining with tubulin or otherwise) and cause their disappearance: colchicine, vinblastine, podophylline, griseofulvin, low temperature, hydrostatic pressure and chloral hydrate. These agents bring about not only the structural disappearance of microtubules and the cell processes whose shape they support (*e.g.* cilia, axopods) but they also cause the loss of all cell functions associated with them, such as protoplasmic streaming, mitosis, saltatory movements of organelles and secretion. It is fascinating that all above changes are completely reversible, *i.e.* that the microtubules are re-assembled and cilia, streaming, mitosis, movements and secretion reappear, following elimination of the tubulo-lytic agents.

Contrary to previous beliefs, microtubules and microfilaments seem to consist of different proteins and are not thought to be interconvertible.

VII. NUCLEUS

(1) Basic functions (Plate 5)

There are two main functions of the nucleus and both are the functions of the DNA (chromatin) it contains.

Firstly (Fig. A), DNA[1] manufactures in its own image and sends into the cytoplasm a constant stream of messenger RNA[2] ("m-RNA") through which it directs the synthesis of cytoplasmic proteins in the ribosomes: Short three-base segments of transfer RNA[3] (soluble or "s-RNA"), each carrying a different aminoacid[4], attach to the m-RNA in a sequence dictated by the base sequence of the latter, thus building an amino acid chain whose composition ultimately depends on the composition of the particular DNA segment (gene) that manufactured the m-RNA; DNA similarly manufactures s-RNA and ribosomal RNA. Evidence that most RNA is synthesized in the nucleus (except for a small amount synthesized by the sparse cytoplasmic DNA) can be found, among other things, (a) in the fact that little or no RNA synthesis occurs in cells that have been enucleated experimentally or that have lost their nucleus physiologically (*e.g.* the blood reticulocytes), and (b) in elegant autoradiographic studies following the administration of labelled RNA building blocks which have shown that newly synthesized labelled RNA first appears in the nuclei and later moves into the cytoplasm.

The *second* function of DNA is to duplicate itself in cells that are about to divide (just before mitosis), in order to transmit to each daughter cell an exact copy of itself and thus of the genetic know-how of the mother cell. DNA duplication is realised by the splitting of the molecule into two halves and the reconstitution of each half to a whole through the addition of the proper building blocks in the proper sequence (Fig. B).

(2) Genes, DNA and chromosomes (Plate 5)

Genes are short segments of the long double-stranded DNA molecules while chromatin and chromosomes represent masses of one or more whole lengths of DNA molecules, coiled and "knotted" to find space in the crowded nucleus. It appears (Fig. C) that the most coiled and knotted parts of a DNA strand[1] are the inactive, dormant parts, while its most stretched-out parts[2] (the "puffs") are its active, RNA producing parts, at any given moment. The non-homogeneous, "geographic" pattern of chromatin in formaldehyde or glutaraldehyde fixed nuclei is evidently due to the alternation of tightly knotted and, therefore, dense DNA areas, with stretched-out and therefore, more lucent areas.

When an increased need for protein arises, the newly born RNA does not wait until it crosses over into the cytoplasm but starts turning out protein right in the nucleus (Fig. C). Thus, considerable amounts of "cytoplasmic" proteins[3] can accumulate within nuclei, in close association with nuclear RNA[4] and DNA[2], *e.g.* hemoglobin in the nuclei of bird erythrocytes. In certain instances, the demand for protein is of such staggering dimensions that it can be met only by an enormous multiplication of the DNA factories within a cell's nucleus. Such is the case, *e.g.* with the larvae of diptera at the time they secrete their cocoon (puparium), when a few hundred salivary gland cells must manufacture huge amounts of cocoon protein – several thousand times their own volume – within a relatively short time (a few hours). To accomplish the above task, the DNA content of each salivary gland cell nucleus is increased 1024 times over its normal amount through 10 successive DNA duplications, without accompanying mitosis or cytoplasmic divisions; the resulting chromosomes are gigantic and are called "polytene" because of the multiple DNA strands they contain.

(3) Control of genetic activity

There is considerable recent evidence, particularly from experiments with unicellular organisms, that genes are

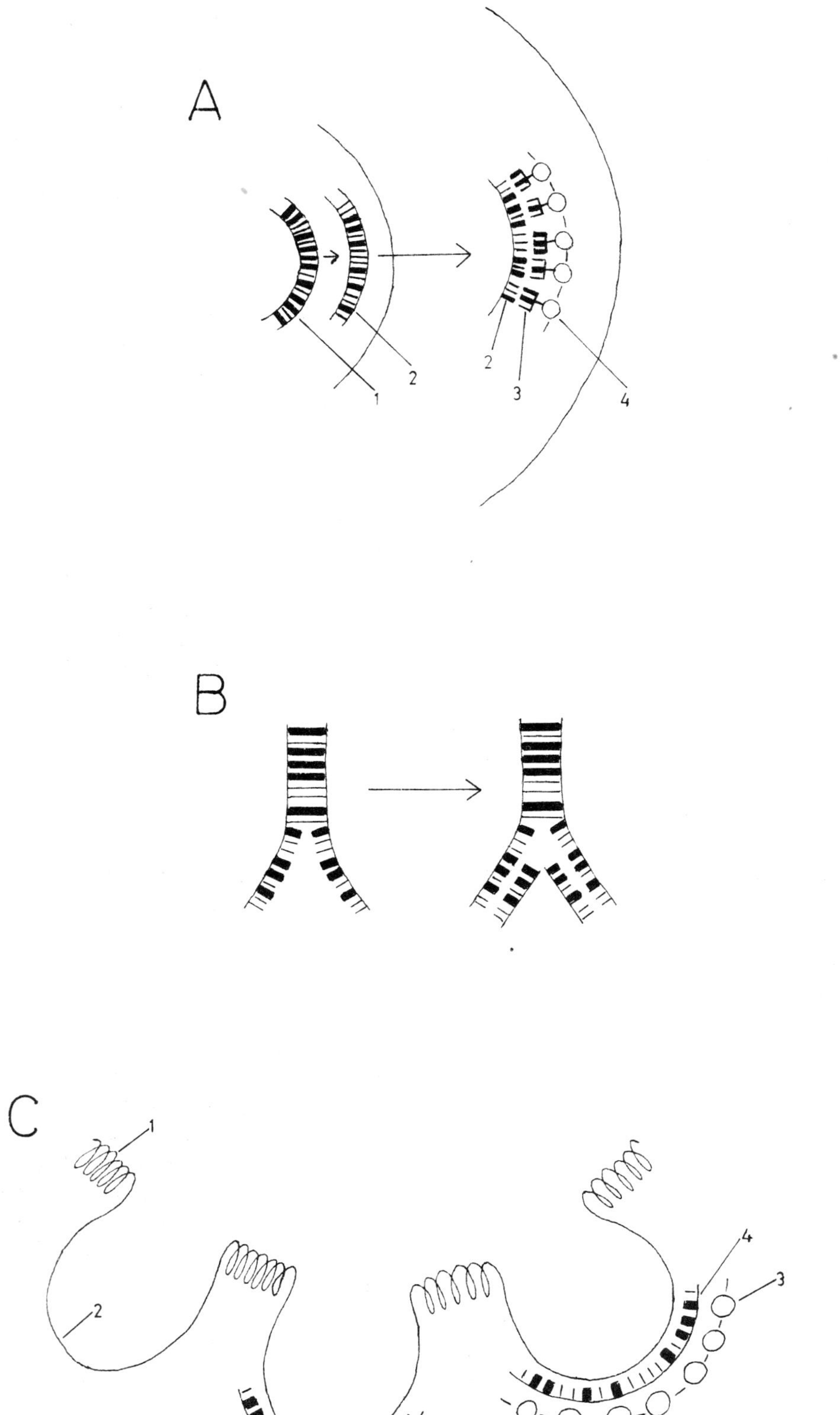

Plate 5

not all active at all times, but that at any given moment only some of them are "turned on", depending on the needs and the environment of that movement. It has been found *e.g.* that DNA activity responds and adjusts to changes of available metabolic substrates (feedback effects) and to hormonal stimulation.

Thus, as an example of positive feedback by substrate, lactose will turn on the gene that makes the m-RNA that produces the enzyme (lactase) that can break it down – and when lactose is replaced by a different substrate, the lactase-making gene is turned off and another gene is turned on. An example of negative substrate feedback can be found in substrates produced by cells such as tryptophane: tryptophane is produced by the enzyme tryptophane synthetase, which in turn is produced by an appropriate gene through the appropriate m-RNA; large amounts of this substrate will turn off the gene that makes the enzyme that synthesizes it and thus eliminate its unnecessary continued production.

Examples of hormonal control of genetic activity are found in both invertebrates and vertebrates. Thus, the premature injection of the puparium-forming hormone "ecdysone" into insect larvae will lead to penetration of this substance into the nuclei of its target gland cells, where it will activate within a few minutes the genes that produce cocoon proteins (as evidenced by the development of the characteristic chromosomal puffs) and will precipitate the rapid production of a cocoon out of season; there is some evidence that this invertebrate hormone activates genes by changing the Na/K ratio within the nuclear sap. Similarly, steroid and protein hormones enter the nuclei of vertebrate secretory cells where they apparently stimulate the production of specific proteins by activating the appropriate nucleic acid polymerases.

(4) Nuclear pores, nucleocytoplasmic traffic and inner fibrous lamina

Nuclear *pores* are round holes in the nuclear envelope, usually underlaid by euchromatin. Their inner diameter is about 200–700 Å and their frequency ranges between approximately 35 and 135 per square micron nuclear surface, although it is probable that both their size and their number change continuously in adaptation to different cellular functions. Under high magnification, the pores in the nuclei of most plant and animal cells are found to be sealed by thin diaphragms ("septal pores"), while in a few cell types (*e.g.* amphibian ova) they seem to contain hollow cylinders with an inner diameter of about 150 Å. A remarkably standard substructure has been discovered in the majority of septal pores that have been studied so far: It appears that in most cases (a) the rim of each pore is occupied on its external surface by 8 granules disposed at equidistant intervals to form a ring or "annulus" around the circular diaphragm, (b) 1–3 granules are occupying the center of the diaphragm, and (c) filaments run in a chain from one annulus granule to the next and radially from the central granules to each of the annulus granulus. Often the granules seem to be replaced by filament knots or by rodlets and all these accessory structures (granules, knots and rodlets) contain RNA, possibly in transit out of the nucleus at points of increased permeability. It is interesting that the number of nuclear pores per μ^2 nuclear surface increases greatly during mitosis.

Studies with microelectrodes implanted in cells have shown that the nuclear envelopes with septal pores exhibit a very high electrical resistance (indicating that they represent a continuous barrier between nucleus and cytoplasm) while those without diaphragms in their pores display a very low electrical resistance, indicating the absence of a nucleocytoplasmic barrier. There is evidence, however, that even in the presence of diaphragms, extensive molecular traffic is taking place between the nucleus and the cytoplasm, in both directions.

As far as *traffic from the nucleus to the cytoplasm* is concerned, autoradiographic studies have shown that RNA is first made in the nucleus and moves from there to the cytoplasm, and that when labeled nuclei are transplanted into enucleated cells, labeled compounds pass from the former to the host cytoplasm. The precise mechanism through which these nuclear materials move, however, through the nuclear envelope into the cytoplasm is still not established for most cell species. In the case of some invertebrate and lower vertebrate cells (*e.g.* in silkworm glands and lung fish oocytes) the nucleoli approach the inner nuclear membrane, focal gaps are seen to develop in the nuclear envelope at the points of contact and nucleolar material "pours out" through these breaks into the perinuclear cytoplasm. In the case of several mammalian cells, on the other hand, RNA granules are seen to approach septal pores and elongate into filaments or rodlets that seem to "squeeze through" small holes in the center of pore diaphragms. In still other cases, clouds of dense nuclear material are clearly "oozing out" of nuclear pores. It appears that pore diaphragms have a loose molecular texture that makes them readily permeable to RNA and other molecules.

As far as *traffic from the cytoplasm to the nucleus* is concerned, (a) it has been shown autoradiographically that labeled amino acids, purines, pyridines, steroids and other molecules enter nuclei from outside, (b) it has been reported that inorganic ions diffuse freely into nuclei and (c) colloidal gold particles of 25–55 Å diameter that were injected into the cytoplasm were found to enter nuclei with variable speed, depending on cell species – they penetrated into nuclei of amebae faster than into nuclei of amphibian oocytes. It has also been found that during mitotic division (when nuclear envelopes dis-

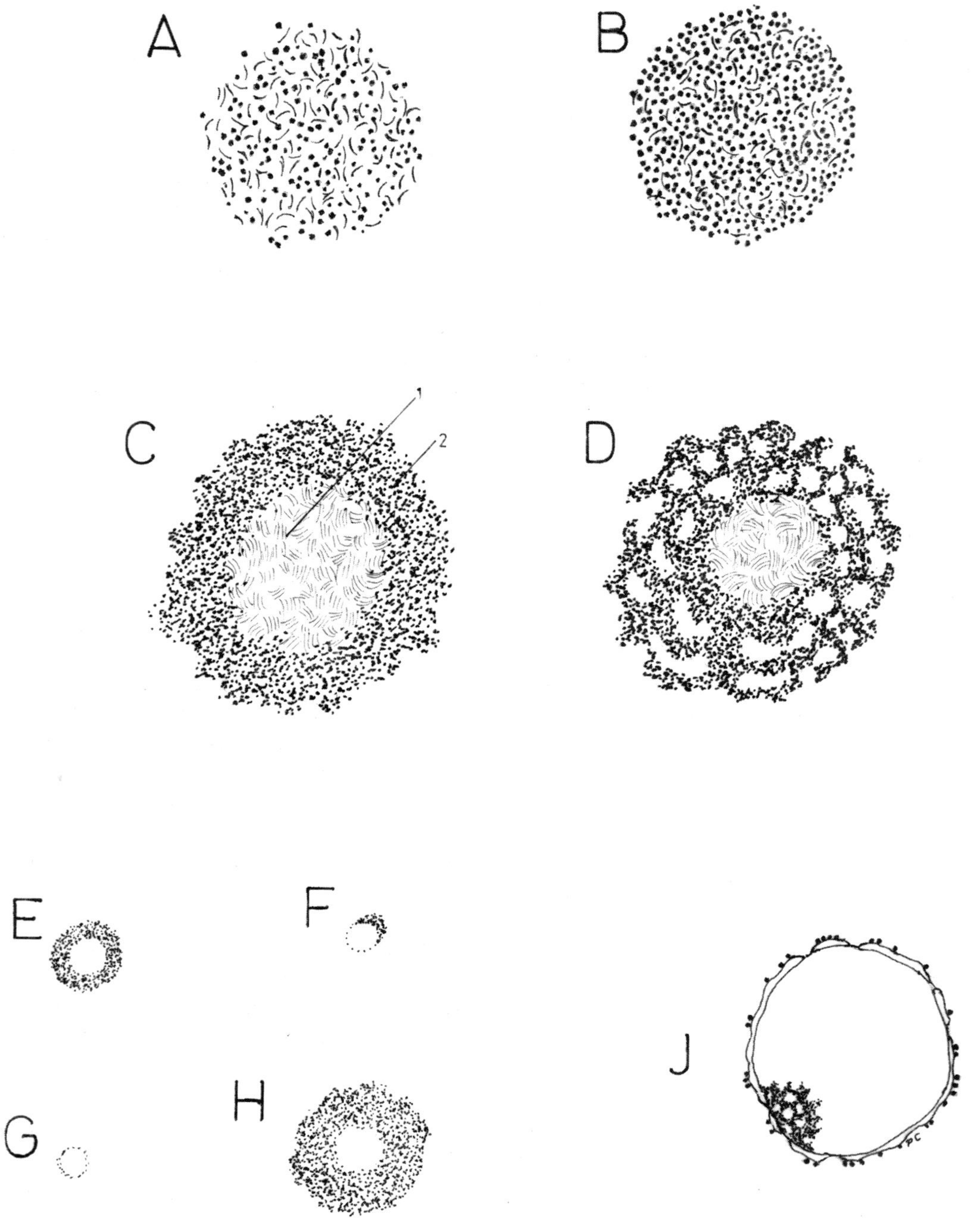

Plate 6

appear temporarily) nuclei can incorporate much greater cytoplasmic particles and much more easily than during interphase – a fact that makes them particularly vulnerable to virus penetration during mitosis.

Finally, the *inner fibrous lamina* represents a fibrillar layer that (a) is closely apposed to the inner nuclear membrane, (b) is about 400–600 Å wide in vertebrates (and thicker in invertebrates) and (c) disappears under every nuclear pore. Its function is unknown at the present; it has been suggested that it may be involved in the maintenance of the nuclear envelope.

(5) Chromatin (Plate 6)

The apparent structure of chromatin depends largely on the fixation method used. It is always a mixture of fibrils and granules, but it is more fibrillar after primary glutaraldehyde (with or without osmium post-fixation) and more granular after osmium fixation. Furthermore, the two chromatin types (eu- and heterochromatin) are much more evident after primary glutaraldehyde than primary osmium fixation.

After glutaraldehyde followed by osmium, *euchromatin* (Fig. A) appears as a loose, cotton-like tangle of short, *ca.* 200 Å thick filaments interspersed with granules of variable density and size (100–350 Å), single or in clusters (inappropriately termed the "interchromatinic granules"), whereas *heterochromatin* (Fig. B) contains many more granules and is much more tightly packed, resembling the structure of a chromosome; in both chromatins, the translucent material that occupies the space between the filaments and granules is called the "interchromatinic matrix".

Both the thick filaments and the granules of chromatin contain DNA. The reasons the long, slender (*ca.* 20 Å wide), thread-like DNA molecule is not visible in chromatin even at E/M resolutions of 10 Å or less seem to be (a) that the DNA molecules are hidden by their association with RNA and protein (the whole assembly being particularly susceptible to distortion and fragmentation after fixatives such as OsO_4), and (b) that much of the DNA (the temporarily inactive part) is coiled into tight knots. Long, thin filaments of DNA with a diameter approaching that postulated by current chemical concepts of its structure can be seen (a) in nuclei containing little or no RNA and protein (*e.g.* those of spermatozoa), (b) in deproteinised nuclei, (c) when chemically extracted and purified DNA is spread on thin films, "shadowed" and photographed at very high magnification (100,000 × or more), and (d) when similarly treated labelled DNA (after [^{3}H] thymidine uptake) is spread and radio-autographed.

Under conditions that lead to greatly increased RNA (and therefore protein) synthesis, as *e.g.* during active cell response to injury and during repair processes, most or all of the dense heterochromatin often turns into light euchromatin, as a visible expression of DNA "activation" (uncoiling).

In addition to chromatin, certain large, about 200–400 Å thick RNA-containing corpuscles, the so-called *perichromatin granules,* are scattered diffusely throughout the nucleus, usually situated at the periphery of heterochromatin islands. These structures are believed to carry m-RNA; their numbers increase close to activated DNA areas ("puffs").

Finally, 3 main types of true *nuclear inclusions* are occasionally seen embedded within the chromatin: (a) cytoplasmic organelles (RER cisternae, Golgi, mitochondria), (b) saccules and (c) spheroid bodies ("spheridia"). The cytoplasmic organelles probably become trapped in the nucleus during mitosis; the saccules seem to arise from invaginations of the inner nuclear membrane that lose their connections with the nuclear envelope; the spheridia are 0.3–1.5 μ thick corpuscles of fibrillar, globular, membranous or mixed substructure and unknown origin and function.

(6) Nucleolus (Plate 6)

A nucleolus is basically a production site and accumulation of mainly ribosomal RNA in the nucleus, synthesized under the guidance of DNA and destined to cross into the cytoplasm to build ribosomes. It is thus understandable that nucleoli are most prominent in cells at times of maximal ribosomal protein-synthetic activity, *i.e.* in the growing and differentiating cells of embryonic tissues and in regenerating or injured cells that respond to various insults with increased enzyme-producing and other synthetic activities. Under the above circumstances, nucleoli not only increase greatly in size but also attach to the nuclear envelope, apparently in order to transfer their materials faster into the cytoplasm (Fig. J). Depending on the species and other factors, cells may possess one or more nucleoli; thus the yolk-poor mammalian ova possess only one nucleolus whereas the yolk-rich amphibian ova possess several hundred.

Chemically, nucleoli contain more RNA than DNA and the fact that they incorporate uridine indicates that they can also produce RNA. Some nucleoli also contain protein, lipids and carbohydrates, as *e.g.* the nucleoli of ova during yolk formation; the finding that certain nucleoli incorporate [^{3}H] leucine, indicates that they can manufacture some of the protein they contain. A typical rat hepatocyte nucleolus has been found to consist of about 11% or DNA, 20% RNA and 69% protein, in contrast to the overall composition of the hepatocyte nucleus, which is approximately 29% DNA, 5% RNA and 66% protein.

Structurally (Fig. C), a nucleolus consists of two parts: (a) the *pars fibrillaris*[1], a tangle of *ca.* 50 Å thick filaments, which is relatively light and corresponds to the "pars amorpha" of low magnifications, and (b) the *pars granulosa*[2], a mass of *ca.* 150–200 Å dense granules, which probably represent filaments wound into knots, and which seem to be connected to one another and to the surrounding euchromatin through fine fibrils. Both parts normally contain RNA but there are some indications that the pars fibrillaris also contains DNA whereas the pars granulosa contains only RNA. When [^{3}H] uridine is made available to nucleoli, its incorporation (and, therefore, the RNA synthesis) begins in the pars fibrillaris and extends from there to the pars granulosa; this would fit the hypothesis that the pars fibrillaris contains the DNA template for the production of RNA, while the pars granulosa represents merely a temporary storage site to which the recently produced RNA moves before its shipment into the cytoplasm; it might also explain the hitherto rather mysterious "segregation" of pars fibrillaris from pars granulosa which has been observed to occur after treatments which inhibit RNA production by DNA (*e.g.* actinomycin). In addition to the above two main parts of the nucleolus, a minor third component of *argentaffine material* can be shown to be scattered diffusely in both the pars fibrillaris and the pars granulosa; this material may represent lipoprotein and, therefore, nucleolar enzymes.

The pattern formed by the two nucleolar components varies with species, functional state, time and other factors. Nucleoli can be (a) compact, with both components mixed or, more commonly, the pars fibrillaris surrounded by the pars granulosa (as in Fig. C), or (b) spongy, with the spongy framework or "*nucleolonema*" formed by both components or, more commonly the pars granulosa (as in Fig. D). Normally, there is no sharp demarcation between the two nucleolar parts, or between the nucleolus and the immediately surrounding euchromatin, which represents a nucleolus-supervising portion of nuclear DNA (the so called "nucleolus-associated chromosome" or the "pars chromosoma" of a larger nucleolus-DNA complex). Occasionally, nucleoli contain certain accessory structures of obscure function such as the system of membrane-walled channels that develops within the nucleoli of endometrial epithelial cells during the secretory (luteal) phase of the menstrual cycle. These channels probably represent invaginations of the inner layer of the nuclear envelope into the nucleolar mass in order to increase the contact between nucleolus and nuclear envelope.

There are many indications that the structure and the position of the nucleolus changes continuously in relation to different functional states of cells. After the ovum development is completed, its nucleoli become inactive and lose their pars granulosa, which indicates that a prominent pars granulosa is the expression of intense nucleolar activity.

The relationship of ribosomal RNA to the nucleolus is demonstrated in several ways: A mutational deletion of ribosomal cistrons (genes) in the nucleolus-associated chromosome of *Xenopus* causes loss of all or most of the pars granulosa of the nucleolus and simultaneously an absence of ribosomes and death of the embryo mutants; a similar "degranulation" of the nucleolus by ultraviolet irradiation likewise inhibits cytoplasmic RNA formation; finally, there is a linear relationship between nucleolar volume and cytoplasmic RNA in neurons. It is possible that nucleoli are production sites of relatively small fragments of ribosomal RNA (*e.g.* 18 S or 28 S RNA) which cross the nuclear membrane and are assembled in the cytoplasm into the larger molecules of definitive ribosomal RNA. By contrast, messenger RNA and soluble (transfer) RNA are currently thought to be produced throughout the whole nuclear chromatin rather than by the nucleolus-associated chromatin.

Several agents have dramatic effects on nucleolar structure. Thus, compared to the normal (Fig. E), actinomycin reduces the pars granulosa to a tiny "cap" on the pars fibrillaris (Fig. F) and simultaneously causes disappearance of ribosomes, evidently because it inhibits RNA synthesis by DNA and, therefore nucleolus and ribosome formation; heat of 42°C applied for a few minutes to cells in culture causes complete nucleolar 'degranulation" through an unknown mechanism (Fig. G); streptomycin and thioacetamide (which inhibit protein synthesis by RNA) induce marked growth of the pars granulosa and therefore "giant" nucleoli (Fig. H), probably because they eliminate the negative feedback effect of protein on RNA (and therefore nucleolar) formation; finally, acute starvation greatly reduces nucleolar size and ribosome number (perhaps because it removes the building blocks that make the enzymes which are necessary for RNA synthesis) while refeeding reestablishes both.

(7) Nuclear and cytoplasmic duplication

When a cell is about to divide, its nuclear DNA is first duplicated and then coiled tightly and packed into two sets of chromosomes which are shipped to the two daughter cells during a process we call mitosis, with the help of the centriole-induced microtubule (spindle) apparatus. During mitosis, notably its metaphase, (a) the nuclear envelope disappears, *i.e.* breaks up into sacs (cisternae) that merge with the RER in the cytoplasm, (b) the entire chromatin converts to the dense heterochromatin type and is concentrated in a few chromosomes (*i.e.* the entire DNA with its companion material is tightly wound into knots) and (c) the nucleolus disappears. During meiotic prophase, the homologous chromosomes are joined into "bivalent" pairs by specialised structures, the "synaptinemal complexes" which appear to be harnessing devices vaguely resembling desmosomes and consist of (a) two parallel "lateral plates", each attached to one of the two facing chromosomes, (b) a "central plate" situated in the middle of the gap between the two lateral plates and parallel to them, and (c) many short transverse connections between the central and the two flanking lateral plates. During metaphase, some spindle tubules seem to be attached to specialized regions of the chromosomes, the "Kinetochores". At the end of mitosis or telophase, (a) a nuclear envelope reforms around the chromatin material of each daughter cell through the coalescence of RER cisternae, (b) large parts of the DNA in the daughter nuclei "unwind" and start producing RNA, and (c) the nucleoli reappear.

In addition to the main mitotic type of cell division, a much more rare amitotic type of cell division has been documented to occur in some cases. In this latter process, the nucleus retains its envelope and "resting" internal structure and is cleaved into two daughter nuclei by the contraction of an encircling ring of filaments and microtubules, similar to that which causes cytoplasmic cleavage. This constricting peri-nuclear ring seems to arise from the centriole.

At the end of mitosis, each daughter cell contains about half as many organelles as its mother cell did. Its organelle population subsequently grows to the size that prevailed in the mother cell through apparently two processes: (a) some new organelles are produced "de novo" through the organising activity of ribosomes (*e.g.* the myofilaments) or other organelles such as the basal bodies (*e.g.* the ciliary microtubules), and (b) other organelles seem to replicate themselves through fission, budding and appositional growth, *e.g.* the mitochondria, the chloroplasts and the centrioles. Self-replication in organelles of the latter autonomous type appears to be guided by the DNA which they have been shown to possess through a variety of techniques including local $[^3H]$thymidine uptake and binding of ^{14}C-labeled actinomycin.

(8) Cell fusion

It has been an intriguing discovery of recent years that when cells, even those of different species, are treated with an ultraviolet-inactivated virus of the Sendai type, they can be induced to fuse. Fusion takes place most easily between cells that have many microvilli – and, therefore, increased contact surfaces – and it is initiated by the formation of many small cytoplasmic bridges between the fusing cells (see section on formation of giant cells through macrophage fusion in the connective tissue chapter).

When cells of different species are fused, the resulting binucleated "heterocaryons" show antigens of both parent cells on their surface, in random distribution. Furthermore, when a highly undifferentiated cell that keeps producing DNA and RNA (*e.g.* a HeLa cell) is fused with a highly differentiated cell that has ceased producing both nucleic acids (*e.g.* a nucleated hen erythrocyte), the former induces resumption of DNA and RNA synthesis and a corresponding volume increase in the nucleus of the latter. In other words, the grafting of an undifferentiated cell on to a differentiated one causes the latter to dedifferentiate, perhaps because it acts as an injury.

Chapter 3

Epithelial Tissues

I. GENERAL

The term epithelial tissue is purely descriptive and it comprises compact cell formations which (a) form *membranes* that cover the external body surface or line the inner and outer surface of its hollow viscera, and (b) form *glands* that develop from inpocketings of the epithelial membranes; the great cohesion of both epithelial membranes and glands is due to the abundance of intercellular junctions (particularly zonulae occludentes and adherentes and maculae adherentes) among them. Epithelial structures arise from various embryonic primordia and have an enormous variety of functions, mostly secretory. They will be discussed in detail with the regions in which they occur, in subsequent chapters; only their basic architecture at the L/M level will be summarised now.

II. EPITHELIAL MEMBRANES (EPITHELIA) (Plate 7, Figs. A–F)

These consist of either a single cell layer (simple epithelia) or multiple cell layers (stratified epithelia).

Simple epithelia are squamous (Fig. A), cuboidal (Fig. B) or columnar (Fig. C), depending on their thickness. They are found only in the interior of the body, where cuboidal or columnar epithelia line the inner surfaces of most hollow viscera, while squamous epithelium lines their outer surfaces ("mesothelium") and the inside of all vessels ("endothelium"); functionally, they are concerned primarily with the absorption, secretion or filtration of materials.

Stratified epithelia are squamous stratified (Fig. D), cuboidal stratified ("transitional") (Fig. E) or columnar stratified (Fig. F), depending on the shape of the cells in their most superficial layer. They are found mainly on the external body surface or close to it (*i.e.* lining the initial or terminal segments of canals communicating with the latter); functionally, they are primarily concerned with physical cover and protection, particularly the squamous stratified epithelium whose superficial layers harden through keratinisation and other changes in order to increase their protective properties in the skin.

All epithelia (*e.g.* Fig. C) are underlaid by a layer of connective tissue (the *lamina propria*[1]) from which they are demarcated by a basement membrane[2] that is attached to their basal surface; together with its lamina propria, any epithelium that lines a wet surface is referred to as a *"mucous membrane"* (mucosa) since it is usually covered by a film of mucus.

III. GLANDS (Plate 7, Figs. G–P)

Glands develop from single or repeated infoldings of secreting segments of epithelial membranes into the protected underlying connective tissue, and thus represent great increments of total secreting epithelial surface (Figs. G–J). Even the simplest, unbranched glands (Fig. K) differentiate into a *secretory portion*[1] that specialises in secretion and a *duct*[2] that conveys the secretion to the epithelial surface.

Exocrine glands (Fig. K) release their secretion on an epithelial surface; *endocrine glands* (Fig. L) develop from exocrine ones through obliteration of their duct[1] and they release their secretion into the surrounding capillaries[2], *i.e.* in the blood.

Exocrine glands are classified into simple (Fig. K) and compound types (Fig. M) depending on the number of their secretory portions, and into tubular (Fig. N), alveolar (Fig. O) or acinar (Fig. P) types, depending on the shape of their secretory portions. The connective tissue bed (Fig. M) (stroma)[1] in which compound glands are embedded wraps up groups of secretory portions into *lobules* and groups of lobules into *lobes* and forms partitions between the latter (the interlobular[2] and interlobar septa[3], respectively).

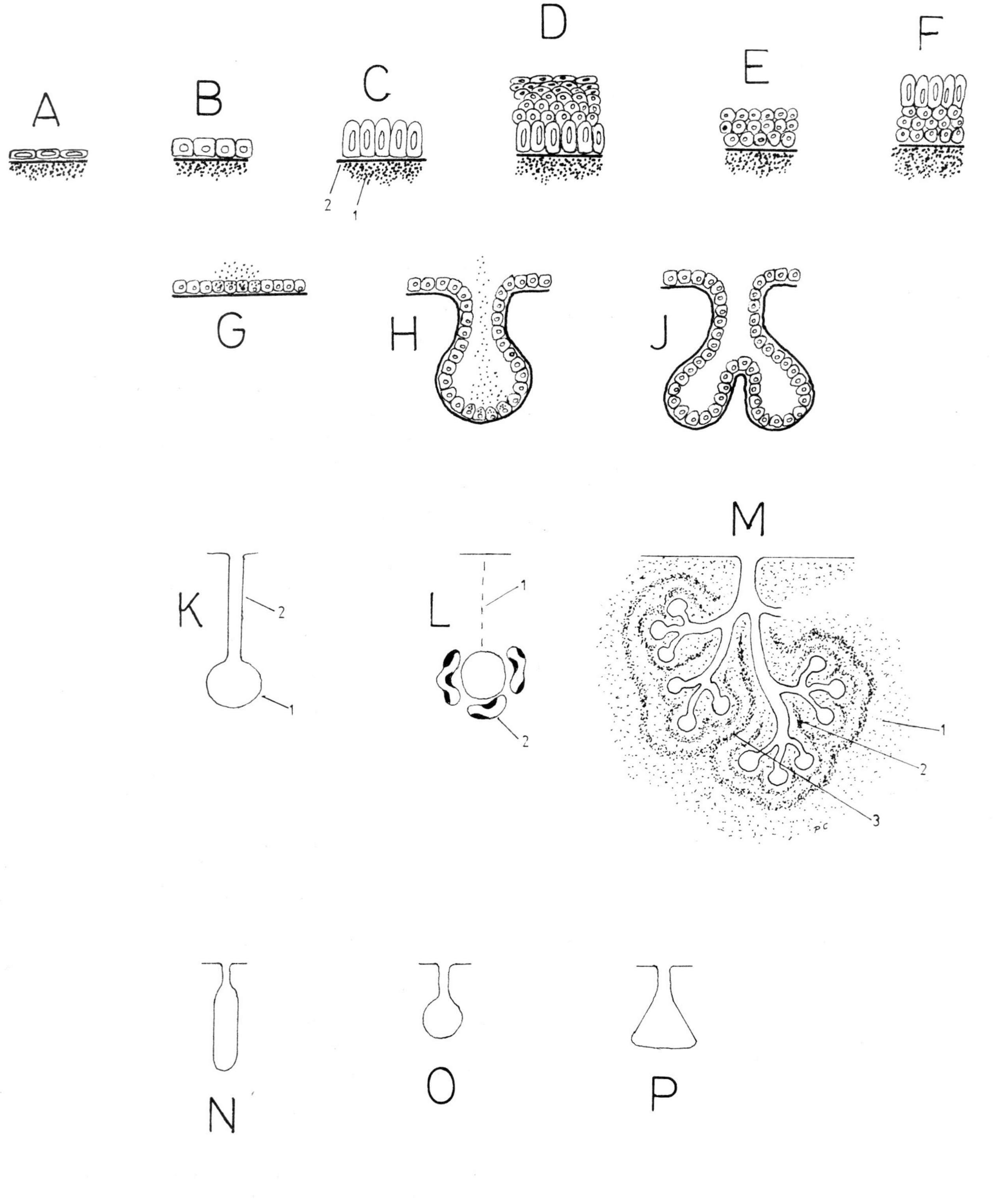

Plate 7

Chapter 4

Connective Tissues

I. GENERAL

This heading comprises a wide variety of tissues which have a common embryological origin (the mesenchyme) and generally hold the body together or service its various parts by transporting vital materials to them and defending them against invaders. Histologists traditionally recognise the following connective tissues: (a) *areolar tissue* that fills the space between various structures and contributes to their defense, (b) *dense fibrous tissue* that wraps up (encapsulates) and connects various structures, (c) *adipose tissue* that stores surplus energy and makes it available in times of need, (d) *the skeleton tissues* (cartilage and bone that make and maintain the body's shape), and (e) *the hemopoietic tissues* (blood and blood-forming tissues) that transport vital materials to and drain wastes from the body's organs in addition to defending them against invasions. The consistency of the connective tissues varies enormously in relation to their extracellular materials, which range from fluids and jellies to fibers and hard mineral masses.

II. AREOLAR AND DENSE FIBROUS TISSUE

(1) General

Areolar tissue fills up the space between the various specialized cell groups and vascular channels of the body. It, therefore, separates all body structures from one another and, at the same time, holds them together. If one compares the various specialized structures with raisins embedded in a pudding of areolar connective tissue, one realizes that all vital chemicals reach the specialized cells (and all metabolic wastes leave them) by crossing this connective tissue pudding; and that any serious change in the quality, density or quantity of the connective tissue caused by ageing or disease will affect the survival of the cells embedded in it. The cells found in this tissue are mostly fibroblasts, with a variable admixture of macrophages and mast cells, while the extracellular materials of areolar tissue consist of the unyielding collagen fibers and a variable amount of elastic fibers, all embedded in a jelly, the "amorphous ground substance". Certainly all collagen and elastin and, apparently, most of the jelly components are manufactured by the fibroblasts, as can be shown in developing or regenerating connective tissue and in fribroblast cultures. In addition to the above two main types of fibers, "microfibrils" of less than 100 Å diameter, which seem to be neither collagen nor elastin, have been described occasionally in embryonic connective tissue and around the edges of mature elastic fibers; this third fibrillar component may represent a filamentous form of glucoprotein and is still under exploration.

Dense fibrous tissue contains the same elements as areolar tissue but collagen usually prevails in it and it is very densely packed; it makes up tendons, ligaments and the tight fibrous capsules of most organs.

(2) Collagen (Plate 8)

This is a fibrous protein in which the aminoacids glycine, proline, hydroxyproline and hydroxylysine are prominent building blocks – the latter two being specific for this material. Seen with the E/M, a mature collagen "fiber" of the L/M consists of numerous banded "fibrils" (Fig. A), each *ca.* 400–700 Å wide and with a periodicity of 600–690 Å, *i.e.* about 640 Å (one period being one dense plus one light segment). Every collagen fibril in turn, consists of an assembly of long, thin molecules called "tropocollagen" units, which are *ca.* 2800 Å long and 15 Å wide (Fig. B); collagen fibrils can be broken up into tropocollagen units and reassembled from them, under certain laboratory conditions. Finally, each tropocollagen molecule consists of three long polypeptide chains wound into a triple helix (Fig. C), which can be unravelled by heat or fragmented transversely by collagenase. The cause of the striking 640 Å cross-banding of collagen fibrils is not yet established; it was thought to be due to a staggered arrangement of their tropocollagen units, separated by gaps as wide as half a period (Fig. B), or to a regular succession of polar and non-polar side chains along the tropocollagen molecules,

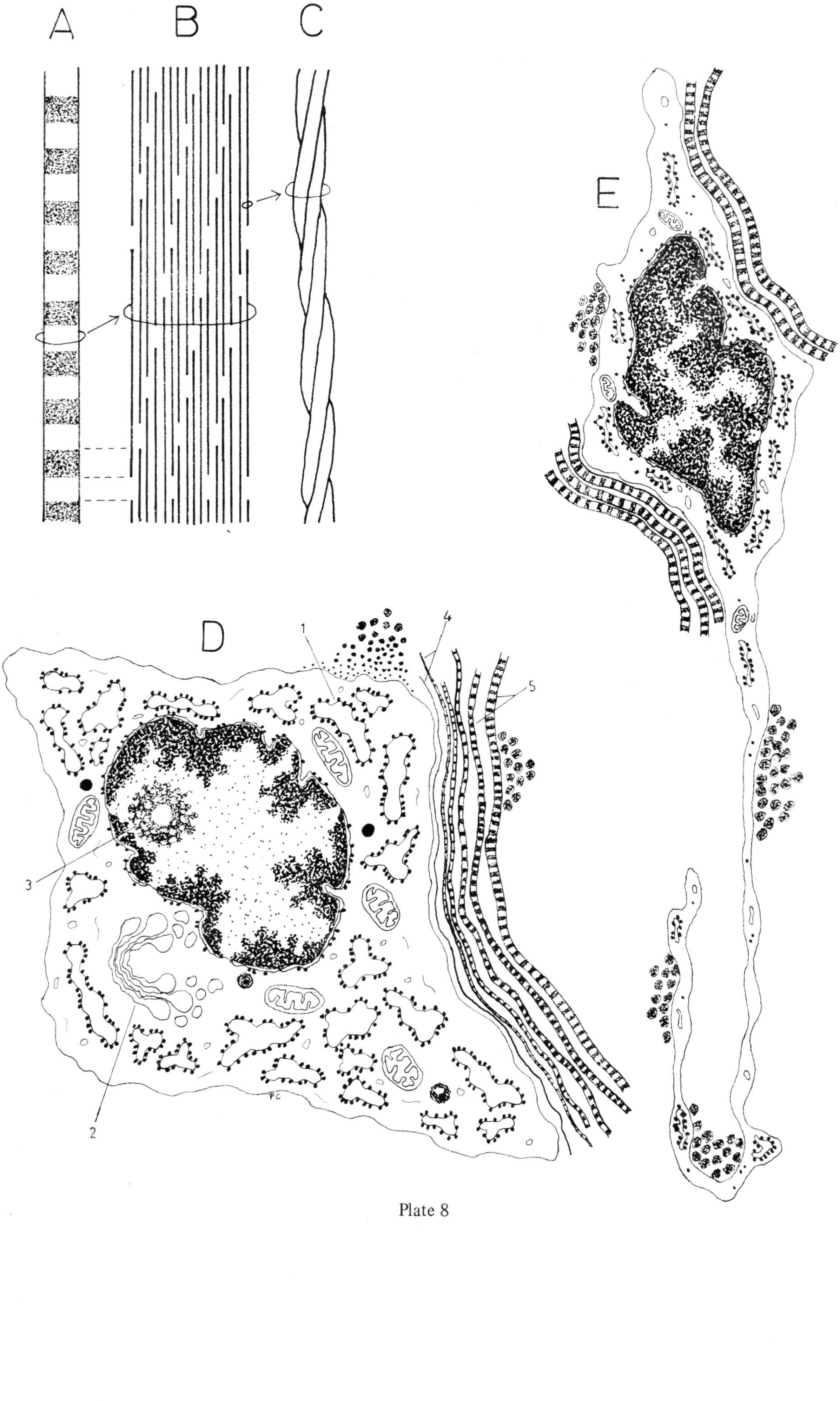

Plate 8

in register. Recent studies with developing (embryonic) collagen of skin, however, also suggest that it may be caused by bead-like links joining *ca.* 40 Å thick tropocollagen aggregates every 640 Å, in register – the linking structures apparently containing carbodydrate and lipid in addition to protein.

When new collagen is formed, it is preceded by the formation of amorphous ground substance which perhaps contributes structural components (carbohydrate glue?) to its make up. Young collagen consists of thin (100–250 Å), often unbanded fibrils, is easily extractable with saline and has a very rapid turnover: labelled hydroxyproline given to growing animals appears first in the peridental fibroblasts, a few hours later in the peridental collagen fibrils and disappears within a few weeks. By contrast old collagen is very difficult to extract or unextractable with saline and it exhibits a very slow turnover. Ageing causes (a) the formation of increasing numbers of stable and irreversible cross-linkages between the polypeptide chains of the triple helices (apparently between the oxidised lysine units of the adjacent amino-acid chains), (b) a marked drop in the hydration state of the collagen molecules, and (c) a trend towards their increasing polymerisation.

(3) Elastic fibers

These have almost remained unstudied in the loose areolar tissue and have been investigated so far mainly in the elastin-rich ligamentum nuchae and in the walls of arteries. They seem to consist of thin, tubular fibrils of a 100–130 Å diameter, embedded in masses of an amorphous low-density matrix, so that they appear as amorphous clumps rather than fibers; they are rich in dicarboxylic acids.

Mature elastin apparently consists of branching and cross-linked amino-acid chains that include the amino-acids lysine, desmosine, isodesmosine, glycine, alanine and valine. Desmosine and its isomer isodesmosine most likely constitute the bridges (cross-links) between these chains; desmosine represents a tetra-amino and tetra-carboxylic cross-shaped molecule with 4 side-chains coming off a central benzene nucleus, each side-chain carrying at its end one amino and one carboxyl group; it probably arises from the modification and condensation of 4 lysine molecules. The precursor of elastin is a more soluble material called "proelastin" which represents straight amino-acid chains and contains much more lysine than mature elastin.

When new elastic fibers or lamellae are formed, elastin seems to combine with polysaccharides to form elastic granules of *ca.* 70 Å diameter; the latter line up in chains and fuse to form elastic fibrils, which fuse with one another and become embedded in an amorphous polysaccharide matrix to produce elastic clumps; finally several elastic clumps fuse to form the plump, low-density elastic "fibers" or lamellae of the L/M.

Like collagen, maturing elastin is strengthened by the development of cross-links between oxidised lysines in its amino-acid chains. Since lysyl oxidase, a copper-requiring enzyme is essential for this process in both elastin and collagen, copper deficiency prevents the maturation of (and weakens) these materials.

(4) The amorphous ground substance (AGS)

This substance consists largely of polymerised sugars (polysaccharides) which seem to combine with protein to form glycoprotein complexes. The chief sugar is an unsulfated polysaccharide (polymerised hyaluronic acid) with a smaller admixture of sulfated sugar polymers. In addition to these glycoproteins, the AGS is also permeated by variable amounts of plasma which filters out of the capillaries and makes up the "tissue fluid".

Under the E/M, the AGS is invisible as it forms a highly hydrated, very loose molecular sponge, the meshes of which allow a free and easy traffic of metabolites between capillaries and specialized cell groups (epithelia, glands, muscle, neurons).

(5) Fibroblasts (Plate 8)

When they are in an *active state of collagen production*, as *e.g.* during wound healing or in embryonic tissues (Fig. D), fibroblasts exhibit (a) an activated RER, *i.e.* numerous and dilated RER cisternae[1], (b) a prominent Golgi[2], (c) several mitochondria, (d) a few peripheral microfilaments, lipid inclusions and lysosomes, (e) a conspicuous large nucleolus[3], and (f) more euchromatin then heterochromatin in the nucleus, as an expression of vigorous DNA activity. They apparently manufacture tropocollagen molecules within the RER cisternae which are then somehow secreted onto the cell surface where they are gradually polymerised into visible collagen fibrils[4] that become increasingly thicker with increasing distance from the cell[5], reflecting continuing polymerisation towards mature diameter outside the fibroblast; vitamin C seems to be necessary at some stage of this process. The finding that injected labelled collagen building blocks (*e.g.* glycine) appear within 30 minutes in RER cisternae of collagen producing cells and within four hours among the extracellular developing collagen microfibrils supports the above production sequence. In the dense fibrous tissue that attaches teeth to their bony sockets (the "peridental membrane"), collagen turnover is so rapid that acute protein or vitamin C deficiency for only a few days causes loosening of the teeth, in guinea pigs. Furthermore, in animals that cannot synthesize ascorbic acid (guinea pig, man) vitamin C deficiency leads to the formation of immature, *i.e.* very thin (60–70 Å)

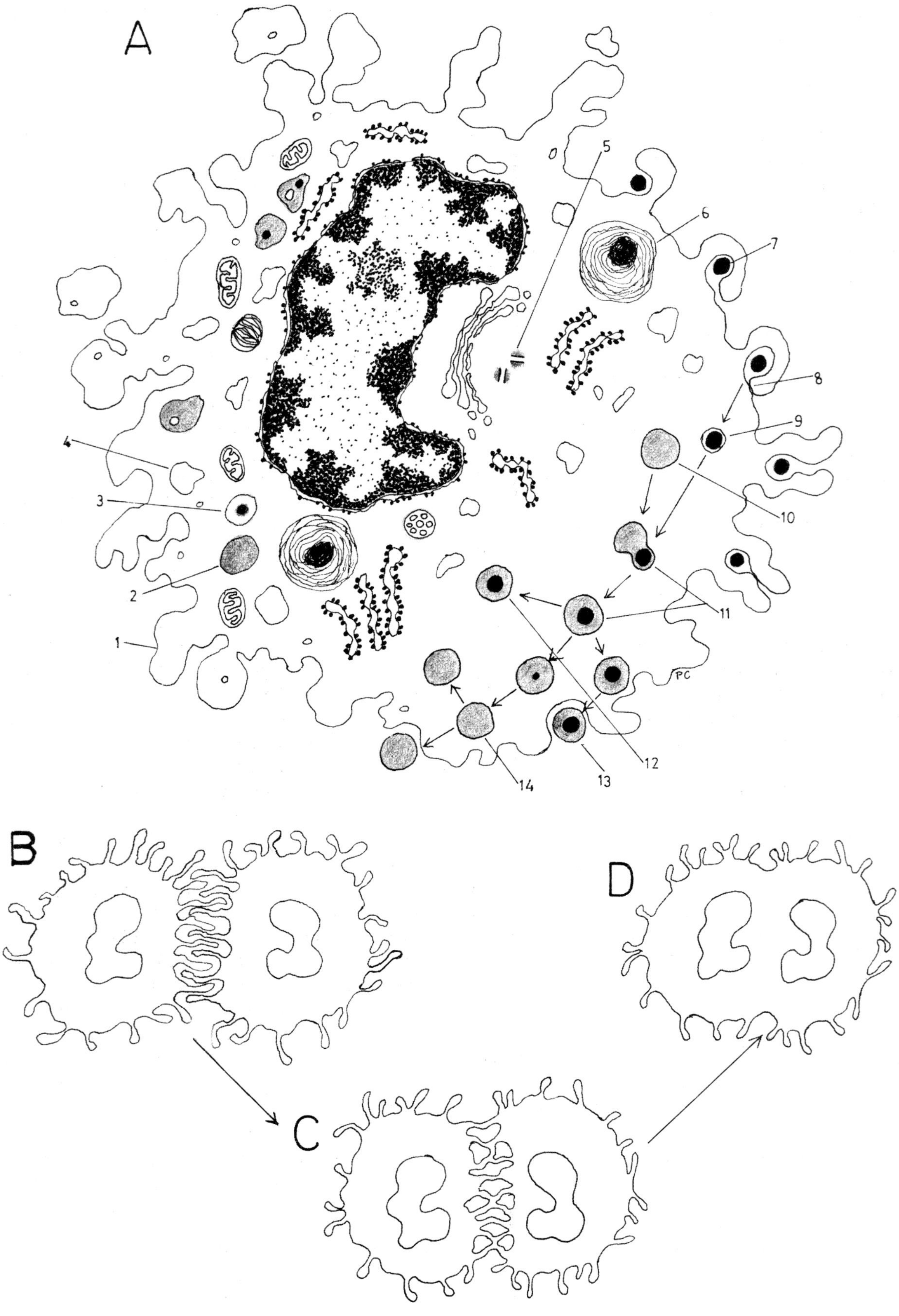

Plate 9

and unbanded collagen fibrils – a defect that can be rapidly corrected by the administration of vitamin C.

Fibroblasts *resting after collagen production* (Fig. E) (also called "fibrocytes") display a very sparse cytoplasm and an atrophy of the RER, Golgi, mitochondrial and nucleolar systems. These cells are capable of enormous proliferation under the influence of many stimuli; when mitosis is inhibited through colchicin however, their centrioles may differentiate into basal bodies and form cilia.

There is some evidence for the possibility that new fibroblasts can arise not only from local pre-existing fibroblasts by mitosis, but also from immigrant blood cells (perhaps monocytes) by transformation.

(6) Basement membrane

Much or all of the surface of epithelial, muscular, and other cells which are embedded in connective tissue is covered by a Basement Membrane (BM). The BM, which demarcates epithelia, muscle, nerves and capillaries against the surrounding connective tissue, consists of an inner sheet-like glucoprotein layer and an outer layer of matted collagen fibrils. The inner glucoprotein layer seems to be produced by the specialized cell it covers – as indicated by its immunochemical similarity to antigens within that cell – whereas the outer collagen layer is produced by the surrounding fibroblasts. The only cells without a BM are those of the various connective tissue species (areolar, dense fibrous, blood, cartilage and bone), with the exception of the adipose cells.

(7) Macrophages (histiocytes)

(A) Structure (Plate 9, Fig. A)

The most prominent features of macrophages are (a) the numerous blunt ridges and pseudopods[1] sprouting off their surface and (b) the abundant enzyme-storing dense bodies (lysosomes[2] and microbodies[3]) and vesicles[4] within their cytoplasm. In addition to the above, they exhibit (a) appreciable numbers of RER cisternae and mitochondria, (b) a distinct Golgi, (c) often conspicuous centrioles[5], (d) various often lamellated phagosomes[6], and (e) appreciable ATP-ase activity on their plasma membranes. Recently, macrophages have also been found to be coated by a prominent glycocalyx (ruthenium positive acid polysaccharides).

The *lysosomes* are sacs enclosing a dense material which is known to contain the following groups of hydrolytic enzymes, all of which act at an acid pH: (a) nucleic acid splitting (desoxyribonuclease, ribonuclease, acid phosphatase), (b) proteolytic (cathepsin, collagenase), (c) carbohydrate splitting (α-glycosidase, mannuronidase), and (d) sulfate ester splitting (aryl sulfatase). The *microbodies* are membrane-bound corpuscles with dense cores (nucleoids) which probably represent a lysosome variant and contain oxidative enzymes (catalase, aminoacid oxidase, urate oxidase). The origin of the lysosomes is not entirely clear; it seems that they can arise either within vesicles of the smooth endoplasmic reticulum system (including the Golgi) or in the cytoplasmic matrix between ribosomes; they are termed "primary lysosomes" before their involvement in phagocytosis.

The macrophages originate from two sources: (a) from pre-existing local macrophages by mitosis, and (b) from immigrant blood monocytes by "transformation".

(B) Function – (hetero) phagocytosis (Plate 9, Fig. A)

Macrophages remove foreign particles (bacteria, viruses, minerals, debris) by swallowing them up (phagocytosis) or by surrounding them in large numbers and thus isolating them from the rest of the organism.

The foreign particles to be engulfed are trapped in pockets between adjacent cytoplasmic projections or between embracing projections and the macrophage surface[7]; in either case they are sealed into sacs formed by the fusion of the lips of the pocket in which they are trapped[8]; the sacs containing the engulfed foreign particles are termed "phagosomes"[9] and they evidently consist of macrophage plasma membrane. Protein coating of particles aids their phagocytosis by macrophages.

Once phagosomes appear in the cytoplasm, they somehow attract primary lysosomes[10] which approach and fuse with them to form the complex "phagolysosomes" or "secondary lysosomes"[11]. Such fusion has been actually documented in all its stages in experiments involving the phagocytosis of bacteria or particles marked by their density (*e.g.* red cells, DNA) or by histochemical reactions (*e.g.* peroxidase) and it results in the immersion of the foreign particles into tiny pools of lysosomal enzymes. The further destiny of these complex corpuscles depends on the digestibility of the foreign material they contain. If the foreign material is of a type that cannot be broken down by the lysosomal enzyme battery (*e.g.* iron or carbon), the phagolysosomes will persist unchanged within the cytoplasm as "residual bodies"[12] or they will be ejected out of the cytoplasm by emiocytosis[13] (reverse phagocytosis). If the foreign material is of a type that *can* be lysed by the lysosomal enzymes (*e.g.* a bacterium), the phagolysosomes that contain it gradually revert to lysosome-like structures[14] and are either retained or ejected. Either way, phagocytosis evidently requires a considerable turnover of lysosomes and it is believed that the formation of the latter is somehow stimulated by phagosomes.

(C) Function–autophagocytosis

Like other cells, macrophages will under certain conditions (*e.g.* after toxic influences such as chloroquine) develop autophagosomes, *i.e.* they will envelop several of

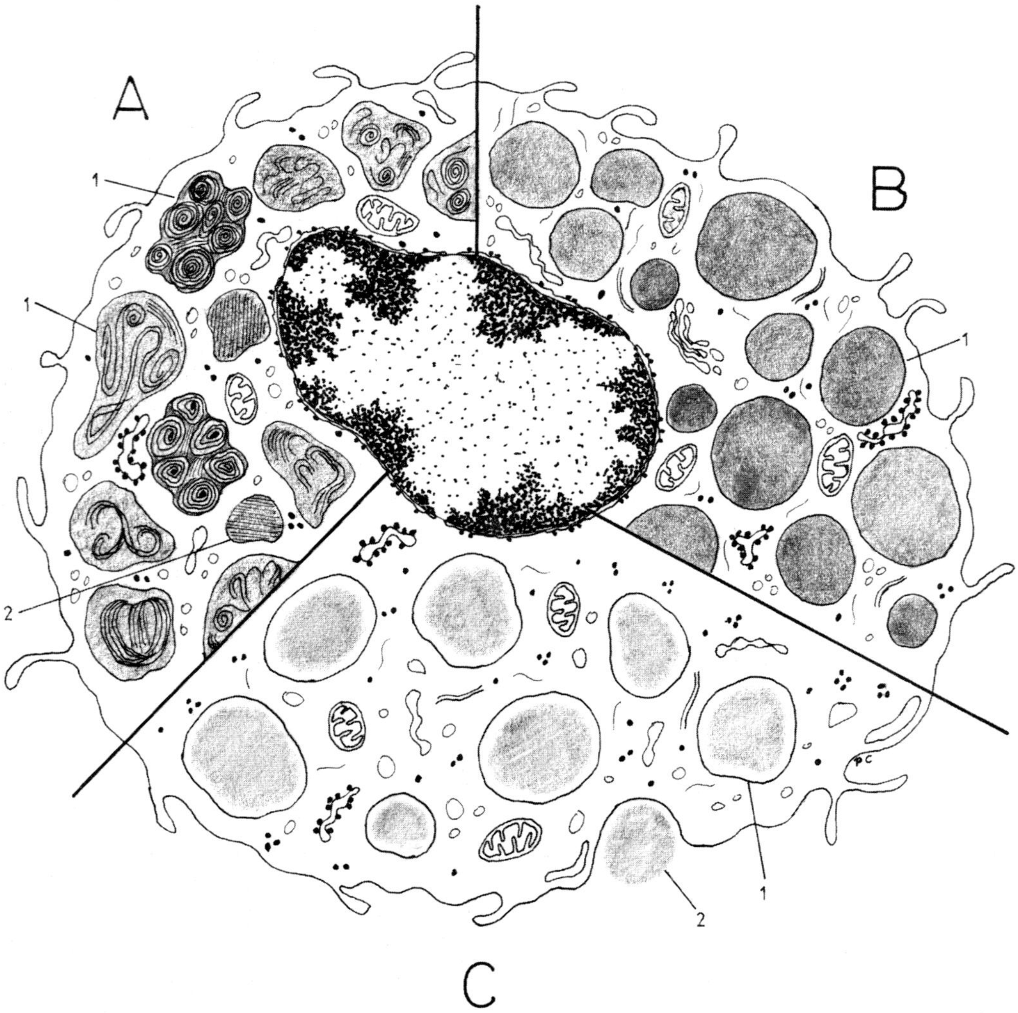

Plate 10

their own damaged organelles by membranes and digest them by fusing them with lysosomes.

(D) Function – giant cell formation (Plate 9, Figs. B–D)

Under certain conditions, *e.g.* when the foreign masses and debris are too large, or under the influence of certain chemicals and viruses, macrophages crowd together ("epithelioid cells") and fuse with one another to form giant cells (Figs. B–D) which attempt to surround the foreign material. During giant cell formation the macrophages approach each other, their processes become long and thin, they interdigitate and their plasma membranes break down leading to cytoplasmic fusion. It is believed that giant cells develop in this manner rather than by nuclear without cytoplasmic division, because they never exhibit mitosis and because macrophage fusion has been observed in tissue cultures.

(8) Mast cells

(A) Structure (Plate 10, Figs. A and B)

The mast cells have no basement membrane and their plasma membrane forms microvilli and small folds. Their most prominent feature is the large (0.5 μ) dense granules that fill the cytoplasm. In man (Fig. A), they have irregular shape and contain lamellar[1] (whorls or scrolls) or crystalloid[2] structures but in the rat (Fig. B) they are homogeneous and round[1]; in most cases they seem enclosed in membranes, apparently because they originate within the vesicles of the Golgi system. Ribosomes, RER, Golgi and mitochondria are very inconspicuous in mature cells and the nucleus is very rarely seen to synthesize new DNA; thus mature mast cells seem to have a low level of metabolic activities and they do not appear to divide as a rule.

(B) Function (Plate 10, Fig. C)

The normal function of the mast cells is still not entirely elucidated, even though we possess several clues from their contents, their location and their involvement in anaphylactic shock.

It is now certain that the human mast cell granules contain heparine and histamine, probably bound to each other by virtue of their opposite electric charges; in the rat, the granules also contain the amine serotonine. The evidence for this rests in the chemical extraction of the above substances from isolated granule populations, and in the good correlation between the mast cell concentration of a given tissue and its content of heparin and histamine. The manufacture of the sulfated polysaccharide heparin explains why mast cells quickly take up labelled sulfur (*e.g.* ^{35}S) when it is offered to them.

Certain compounds, *e.g.* stilbamidine or cpd. 48/80, will induce mast cells to release histamine from their granules into the extracellular space. As this happens, the density of the granules diminishes (Fig. C) and a space appears between the granules and their envelope, making the latter much more visible than normally[1]; if the stimulation is strong enough, whole granules are thought to be discharged, apparently by emiocytosis[2].

Mast cells also seem to be responsible for most of the body's histamine which is released during anaphylactic shock and causes its key symptoms. It is believed that antibodies produced in response to the organism's first exposure to an antigen become adsorbed to the mast cell surface, and that when the body is exposed for a second time to the same antigen the latter binds to the antibody attached to the mast cell surface, forming an antigen-antibody complex which triggers the release of histamine.

The fact that mast cells are normally attached to capillary walls or form chains between densely packed collagen bundles has long suggested that they may secrete some substance into the bloodstream or that they contribute to the formation or maintenance of some extracellular materials of connective tissue, although no clear cut evidence for either possibility has yet been produced.

Finally, mast cells have recently also been found capable of phagocytosis since they take up thorium particles and sequester them in large phagosomes.

III. ADIPOSE TISSUE

(1) General

Adipose tissue turns fatty acids, amino acids and glucose into fat and thus stores vast amounts of energy. Fat represents the most space-saving form in which energy can be stored since one gram of fat yields the highest number of calories of all usable organic compounds. In man, under normal conditions all adipose tissue is of the so-called "white" variety whereas in rodents and hibernating animals some adipose tissue belongs to the so-called "brown" variety.

(2) White adipose tissue

(A) Structure (Plate 11, Fig. A)

Under conditions of maximum lipid storage most of the cell is occupied by one huge lipid globule[1] that displaces the nucleus to one corner; this lipid mass of usually appreciable electron density is either enclosed in a fenestrated (sieve-like) sac or embedded "naked" in the cell matrix, often surrounded by a regular array of fine (80 Å thick) apparently supportive filaments[2]. Although most of the cytoplasm is reduced to a thin film around the fat mass, it contains a moderate number of free ribosomes, some short profiles of smooth endoplasmic reticulum and small SER vesicles, several long thread-

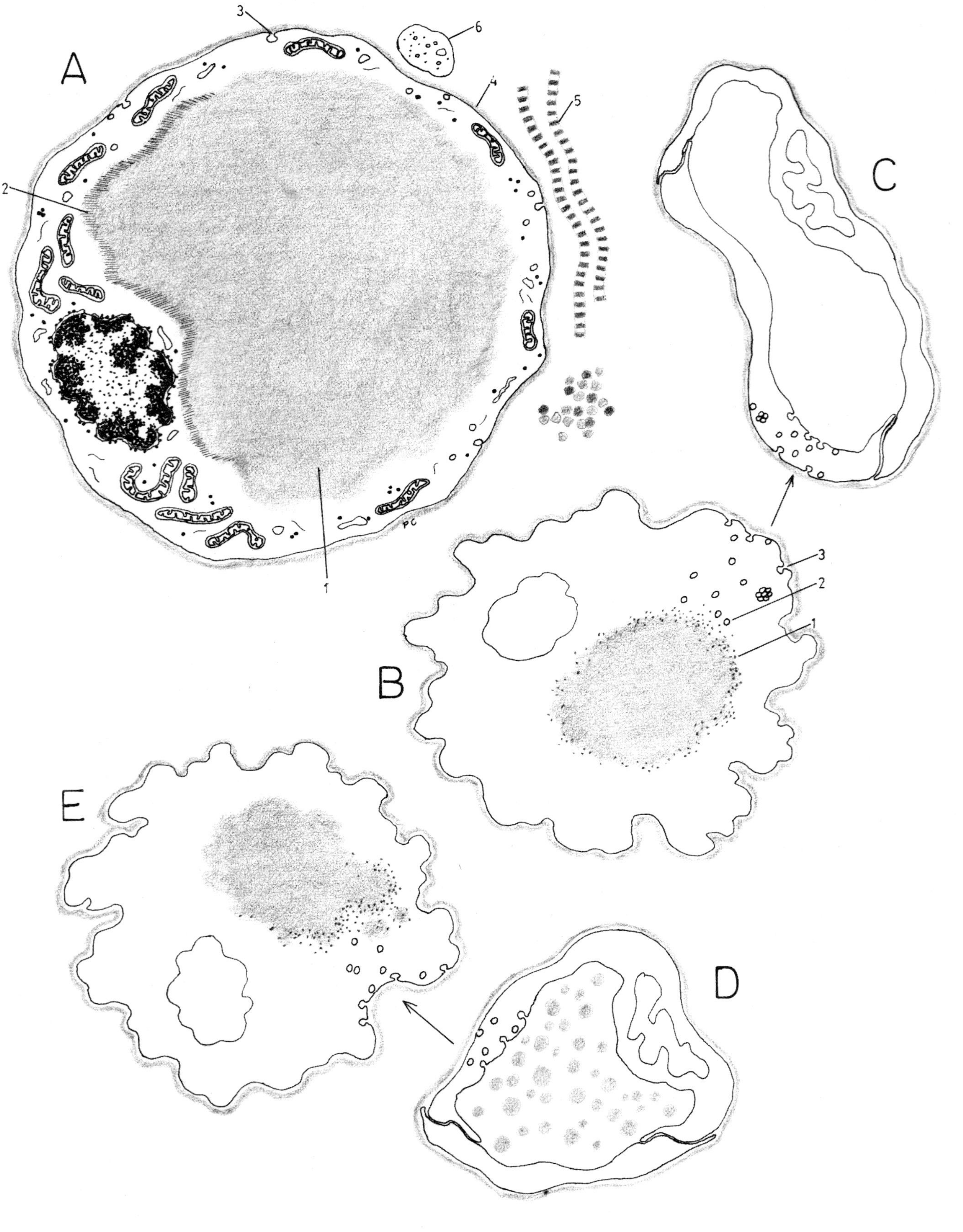

Plate 11

shaped mitochondria, and a few fine filaments; there are several pinocytosis-type invaginations[3] at the cell surface, which is covered by a basement membrane[4] (a glycoprotein layer), unlike the surface of all other connective tissue cells. The space between adipose cells contains, in addition to collagen fibrils[5] and amorphous ground substance, several unmyelinated nerves[6] (axons) which sometimes can be seen to approach the fat-storing cells very closely.

(B) Functions in lipid depletion (Plate 11, Figs. B and C)

When a need develops for the energy it stores (as *e.g.* during starvation), or when the adipose cell is stimulated by injected epinephrine or a sympathetic nerve discharge, an enzyme (presumably lipoprotein lipase) appears to be activated within its cytoplasm resulting in the splitting of tiny particles of triglycerides at the dark rim of the fat globule[1] (the "lipomicrons") into free fatty acids and glycerin; the free fatty acids thus liberated are probably carried to the cell surface as invisible cargo within small vesicles[2] and are discharged into the extracellular space by emiocytosis[3] (reverse pinocytosis) after crossing the BM of the adipose cell; from there they seem to cross the BM of the capillary (Fig. C) and the whole endothelium (by pinocytotic uptake at its basal and emiocytotic release at its luminal surface) before reaching the bloodstream which carries them, presumably complexed with albumin, to the skeletal muscle, heart and other tissues where they are burned as fuel.

(C) Function in lipid repletion (Plate 11, Figs. D and E)

When fat is absorbed from the gut, it enters the blood stream mostly in the form of chylomicrons, *i.e.* 0.5–2 μ thick dense globules which represent lipoprotein aggregates assembled in the intestinal epithelium, although some fatty acids also enter the blood unesterified, complexed to albumin. The fat in the chylomicrons appears to be split into free fatty acids and glycerin by the enzyme lipoprotein lipase, acting in the blood or at the surface of capillary endothelium; the free fatty acids released from chylomicrons as well as those that entered the blood independently seem to be ferried across the endothelium by pinocytosis-emiocytosis (Fig. D) and to be taken up by the adipose cell through pinocytosis (Fig. E); they are then esterified in the cytoplasm with glycerin to form visible tiny fat particles, the lipomicrons, which fuse with and add to the large intracellular fat mass. The proposal that chylomicrons are chemically degraded before they cross the endothelium and enter the adipose cell is supported by the fact that particulate lipid has never been seen in the capillary endothelium or in the space between adipose cells during fat absorption from the gut. The adipose cell can likewise manufacture lipid from the aminoacids and the glucose that enter its cytoplasm. All fat seems to be produced within the cytoplasmic matrix, not within vesicles or endoplasmic reticulum cisternae. Adipocytes also seem capable of taking up proteins; the process as studied in insects with peroxidase (a small protein molecule of approximately 40,000 MW) involves the uptake of protein in pinocytotic vesicles which coalesce to form large vesicles and finally multivesicular bodies; similar mechanisms of protein uptake seem to operate in several other tissues, *e.g.* mammalian neurons or renal glomeruli.

(3) Brown adipose tissue

Cells of this tissue are characterised by (a) many small lipid globules or "liposomes" which are enclosed in membranes – unlike the lipid in white fat cells, (b) many large spherical mitochondria with numerous tightly packed cristae that do not, however, appear to exhibit much oxidative phosphorylation and are charged with certain brown-orange pigments (hence the color of this tissue), (c) appreciable numbers of glycogen granules (in neonatal cells), (d) extensive micropinocytosis (as in capillary endothelium), and (e) a surrounding BM, as in the white fat cells. They seem to be innervated by axons of an adrenergic type whose terminals contain cored vesicles and often dip into invaginations of the brown adipocytes, attaining synaptoid contact with the BM of these cells.

Brown fat tissue seems to be concerned with thermoregulation. Intensive *thermogenesis* in this tissue is thought to result from the "uncoupling" of oxidative from phosphorylative processes in its mitochondria. Exposure of an organism to cold causes a discharge of lipid into the blood from its brown fat cells, which is thought to be mediated through norepinephrine (via the adenyl cyclase system) and can be inhibited with β-adrenergic blockers. The synthesis of new *liposomes* has been studied in the rat after a seven day fast that caused complete depletion of lipid from the brown adipocytes; refeeding (of glucose) in such animals caused in these cells (a) a rise in pinocytotic activity, (b) an enormous proliferation and dilatation of the SER vesicles, and (c) the development of numerous liposomes within the SER vesicles (as in hepatocytes and adrenal cortex cells).

IV. CARTILAGE

(1) General

Traditionally, three types of cartilage are recognised: hyaline cartilage, fibrocartilage and elastic cartilage. The main type of cartilage, and the one described here, is the hyaline variety. The whole embryonic skeleton in man consists of hyaline cartilage and is replaced in the adult

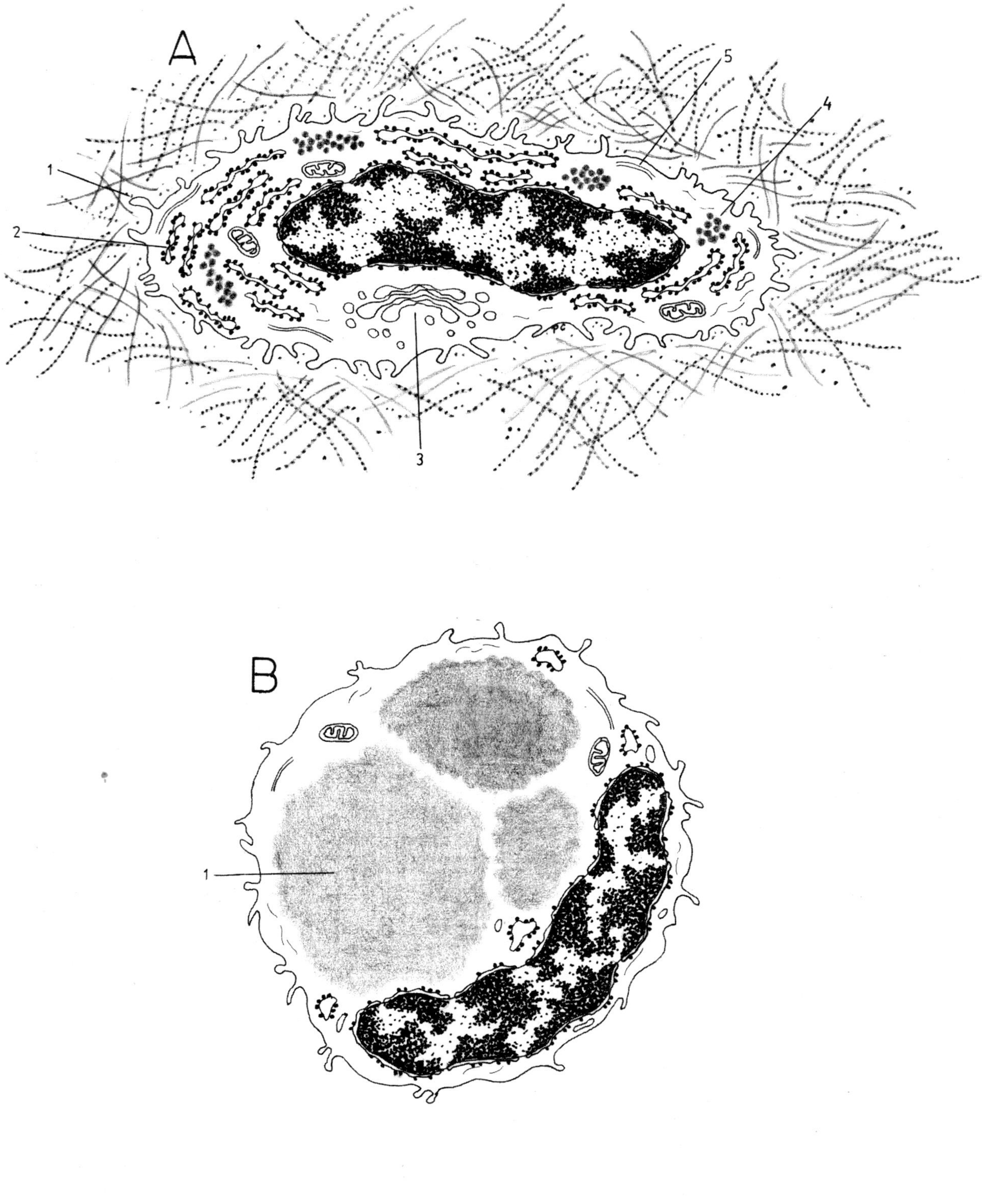

Plate 12

almost entirely by bone tissue, except at the articulating ends of the bones and around certain canals in the anterior end of the body (the nasal, tracheal and auditory canal cartilages), where it prevents collapse of orifices by virtue of its rigidity.

(2) Matrix

The extracellular material or matrix of cartilage makes up the bulk of its mass; embedded in it are the cells that produce and maintain it, the chondrocytes. The matrix of hyaline cartilage consists of a framework (lattice) of unusually thin collagen fibrils (100–200 Å diameter) with indistinct or invisible striations; this framework is in turn embedded in (and masked by) a stiff amorphous jelly of glucoprotein whose sugar component is a sulfated polysaccharide (chondroitin sulfate A and C). In the matrix of hyaline cartilage there is more glucoprotein than collagen, while the reverse is true for the matrix of "fibrocartilage", a variety found in some major tendons and ligaments joining muscle to bone or bone to bone. Finally, the matrix of the third, "elastic" cartilage variant, which is found in the epiglottis, has been traditionally believed to contain abundant elastin on the basis of certain L/M tinctorial criteria but no E/M studies of this have yet been forthcoming.

(3) Chondrocytes (Plate 12, Figs. A and B)

The main features of young, active (*i.e.* matrix synthesizing) chondrocytes or "chondroblasts" (Fig. A) are (a) numerous surface microvilli or "footlets"[1] and a glycocalyx, (b) a prominent RER[2] and Golgi[3], (c) relatively few mitochondria, (d) a few glycogen granules[4], and (e) some microtubules[5]. The changes that occur in ageing, inactive chondrocytes (Fig. B) consist of the dramatic shrinkage of the RER and Golgi and the frequent accumulation of a large mass of lipid[1], as in adipose tissue cells. Since capillaries do not run inside cartilage but in the connective tissue coat that surrounds it (the perichondrium), the chondrocytes are supplied with oxygen and nutrients by diffusion of these molecules across long distances of semi-solid matrix; this fact imposes a limit to the size cartilage can reach before its center begins to die, and it also makes the chondrocytes vulnerable to changes in matrix composition and density. When cartilage ages and is about to be replaced by bone, its matrix becomes calcified, burying the chondrocytes in hard mineral tombs and thereby killing them. Calcification of the matrix seems to be preceded by the development and coalescence of "PAS positive bodies" within which the calcium crystallites first appear; it is also thought to be associated with the manifestation of alkaline phosphatase activity by chondrocytes.

There is good evidence from autoradiographic studies that the sulfated polysaccharide component of the amorphous matrix is assembled in the Golgi system where it is also coupled with the protein component, then ferried to the cell surface in vesicles and discharged into the extracellular space, presumably by emiocytosis. Thus, labelled glucose and labelled sulfate ions offered to chondrocytes *in vitro* reach the Golgi in a few minutes and then move in vesicles towards the cell surface.

The protein component of the amorphous matrix is synthesized in the ribosomes of the RER and moves from there to the Golgi, where it is apparently coupled with the sulfated polysaccharide and then travels in vesicles with the latter (as a glycoprotein complex) to the cell surface where it is unloaded. This sequence of events is suggested by the finding that when labeled amino acids such as proline are taken up by chondrocytes they first appear in the RER within about 10 minutes, move from there to the Golgi in approximately 20 minutes, reach vesicles in the cell periphery 2–3 hours later and after a few more hours materialize in the matrix space outside the cell.

Finally, studies with labeled amino acids indicate that the collagen of the matrix is manufactured in a manner similar to that already described for fibroblasts: proline and lysine-rich polypeptide chains are synthesized in the RER, move rapidly to the Golgi, are hydroxylated into hydroxyproline and hydroxylysine chains through the action of an oxygen-activated hydroxylase and somehow leave the chondrocytes to be polymerised extracellularly.

V. BONE

(1) General

Bone develops either directly in sheets of mesenchyme (membranous osteogenesis), of indirectly in the middle of disintegrating hyaline cartilage, which it replaces (endochondral osteogenensis). In both cases, bone matrix is manufactured by osteoblasts, which soon become embedded in bone substance to be then called osteocytes, and in both cases bone can be broken down by the action of usually multinucleated giant cells, the osteoclasts.

(2) Bone matrix – composition

Bone matrix consists of (a) "osteoid", *i.e.* an organic framework of collagen fibrils of very variable diameter plus some amorphous and translucent mucopolysaccharide–protein complex, and (b) an electron dense mineral component, namely hydroxyapatite crystals (a complex

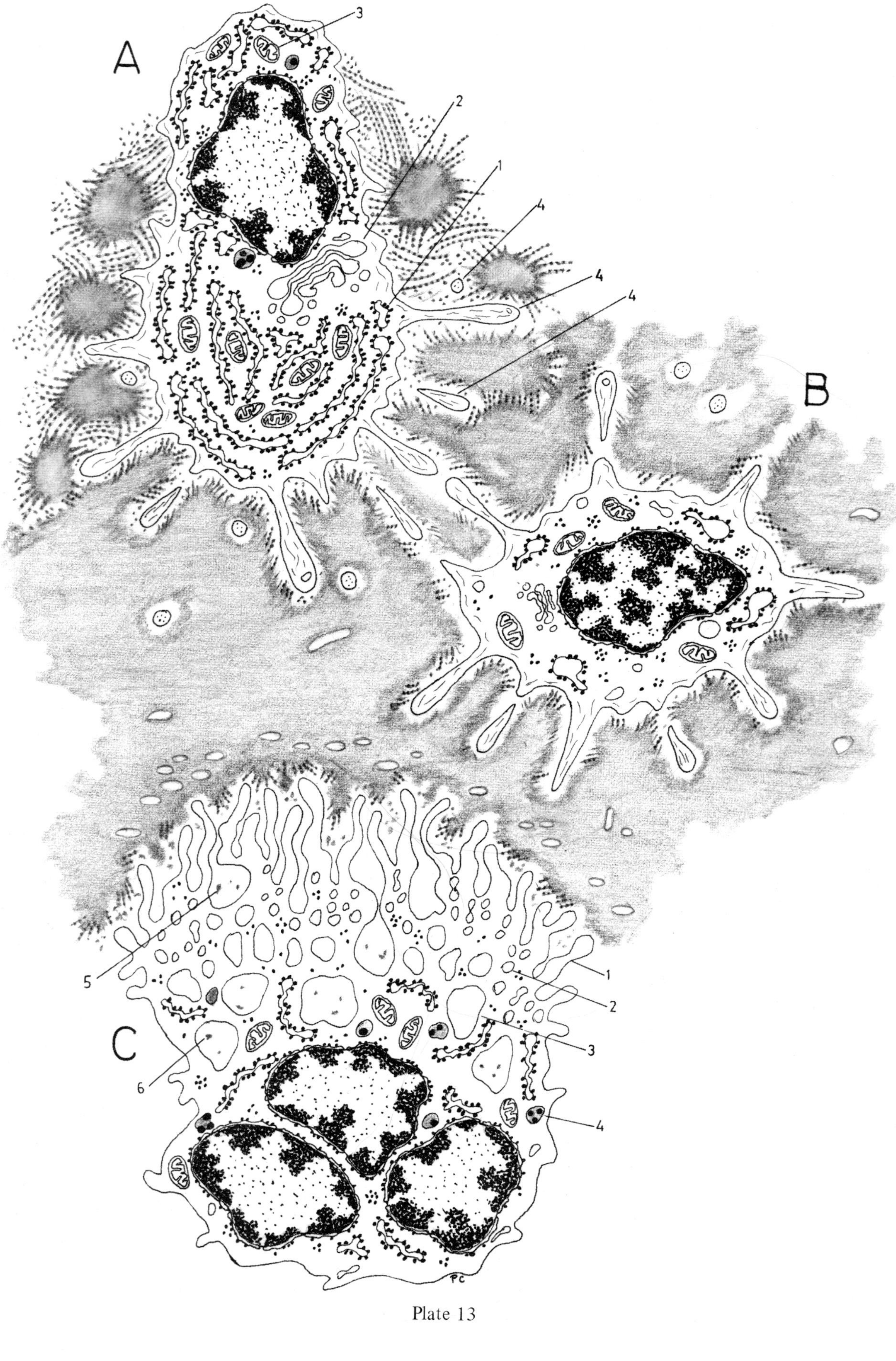

Plate 13

calcium–phosphate–carbonate salt), which, according to some observations, seem to attach to the surface of collagen fibrils and perhaps even form within some collagen fibrils. The crystals take the shape of tightly packed thin needles or rods of about 50 Å diameter.

This composition explains why bone structure is profoundly affected not only by changes in absorption, transport and metabolic control of minerals but also by changes in protein and collagen metabolism.

(3) Osteoblasts (Plate 13, Fig. A)

Since the osteoblasts produce the organic matrix component, they exhibit a prominent complement of the organelles involved in protein and polysaccharide synthesis, namely the rough endoplasmic reticulum (RER)[1] and the Golgi complex[2], as well as a fair amount of mitochondria[3]; in addition, they send out numerous thin and long cytoplasmic processes[4] which – when formation of mineralised matrix around them is completed – will come to occupy vital tunnels in the hard bone substances, the "canaliculi" that keep open the communication between cells and between cells and capillaries, the sources of oxygen and nutrients. Although these long processes are budding off the osteoblasts in all directions they are more often encountered in oblique and cross rather than longitudinal section.

According to all evidence, the osteoblasts manufacture the collagen and glucoprotein components of the bone matrix like fibroblasts and chondroblasts, respectively; in fact, like fibroblasts, osteoblasts require ascorbic acid for the proper manufacture of collagen: experimental scurvy in the guinea pig causes a reduction in the amount of ribosomes and RER cisternae and an accumulation of lipid in these cells and also diminishes collagen formation by them. Recent evidence suggests that collagen precursors are synthesized in the RER, move to the Golgi where they are assembled in *"procollagen"* filaments and then get out of the osteoblast through exocytosis of secretory visicles, the procollagen turning into collagen extracellularly. Mineralisation of the organic bone framework begins as soon as it is laid down, through the formation of hydroxyapatite crystals on the collagen fibrils, reportedly in regular relation to their striation. If this fascinating observation is confirmed by future research, it will suggest that certain repeating parts of the collagen molecule can induce crystallisation of hydroxyapatite either by a "seeding" effect of their molecule structure or by special enzymatic action. It is possible that osteoblasts contribute to the mineralisation process through their alkaline phosphatase activity, which may bring about a local rise of calcium and phosphate concentrations and thus promote their precipitation on the collagen fibrils. It should be emphasized that upon higher magnification the mineralised bone matrix does not appear as an amorphous mass (as shown in Plate 13), but as a pack of numerous, highly electron-dense, needle-shaped mineral crystals.

(4) Osteocytes (Plate 13, Fig. B)

Once the osteoblasts surround themselves completely with mineralised bone matrix (except for the canaliculi that lead to the next cell or capillary), there is no further need for massive organic matrix synthesis and consequently the large RER and Golgi are demobilised. Thus the bone-encased osteoblast changes to a somewhat smaller cell with less cytoplasm, little RER and a small Golgi, *i.e.* an osteocyte. That latter cell is not, however, inactive or at the end of the line, as evidenced by its appreciable ribosome content, which is presumably associated with continued activity related to the maintenance of bone matrix. That such an activity is not only going on but also vital is demonstrated by the fact that when osteocytes are killed (*e.g.* by infection, radiation, etc.) the bony substance around them is doomed to disintegrate.

(5) Osteoclasts (Plate 13, Fig. C)

Bone can be resorbed by the action of multinucleated giant cells called osteoclasts which are found on its surfaces. These cells develop many long villous processes[1] on their side that faces the bone surface they attack; they are further characterized by (a) appreciable numbers of polyribosomes and RER cisternae, (b) numerous small[2] and large[3] smooth vesicles, and (c) several lysosomes[4] in their cytoplasm; they have been reported to contain acid phosphatase and other lysosomal enzymes.

Osteoclasts are thought to erode bone by dissolving its mineral component through the local induction of a "microenvironment" of acid pH and the subsequent digestion of its organic component through the action of secreted lysosomal enzymes. The fact that tiny mineral particles are sometimes seen within the intervillous pockets[5] and within the cytoplasmic vesicles[6] suggests that bits of bone mineral may be also taken up by phagocytosis and dissolved intracellularly. The occasional finding of collagen fibrils between villous processes suggest that this material is depolymerised outside the osteoclast.

Osteoclasts can apparently originate from the fusion of either osteoblasts or ordinary macrophages (like the foreign body giant cells).

Several factors stimulate osteoclastic bone resorption, including parathyroid hormone; the latter seems to act by causing increased formation of osteoclasts (*i.e.* increased fusion of osteoblasts) and by changing the permeability of certain cell membranes for calcium and phosphate ions.

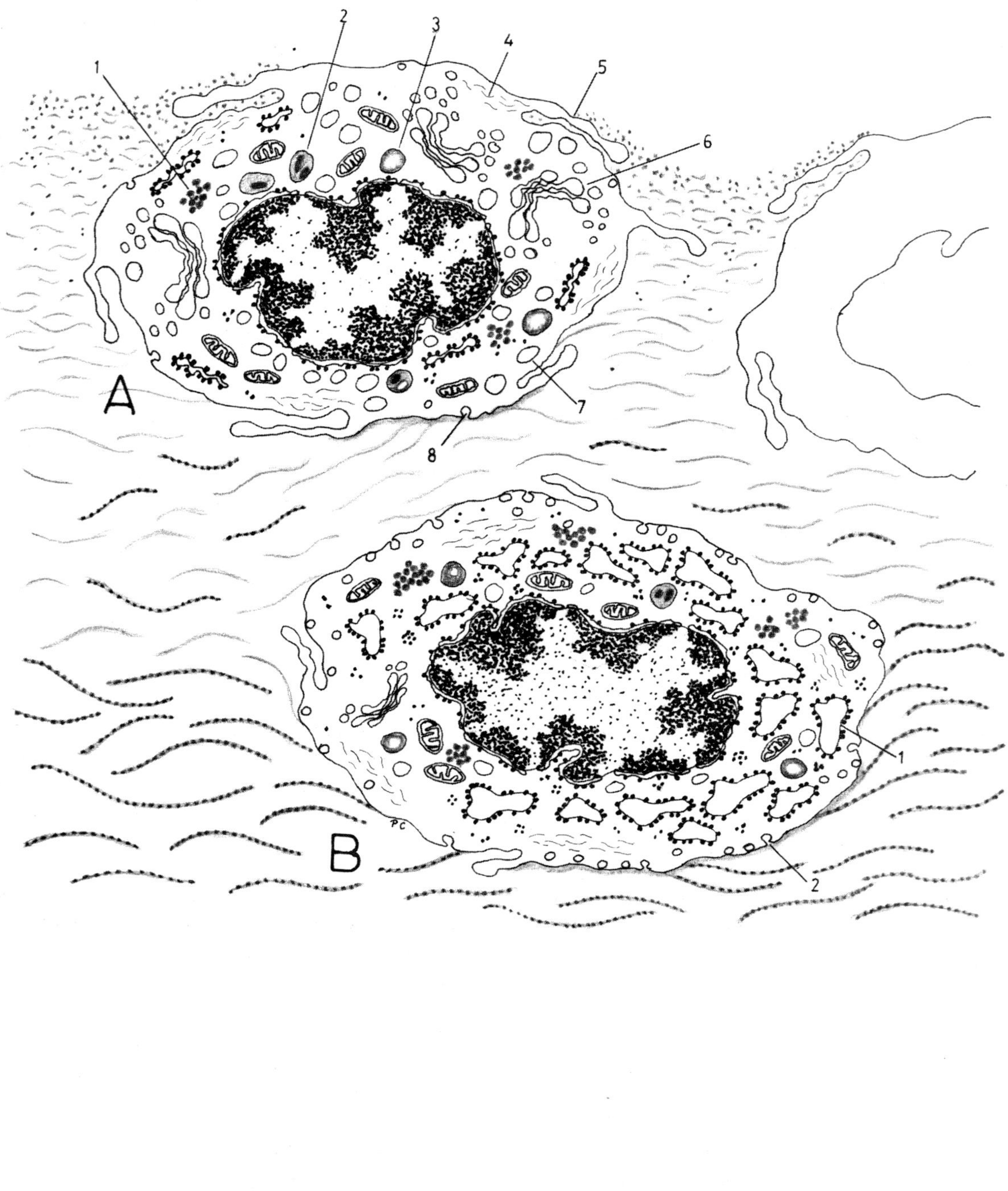

Plate 14

VI. JOINTS

(1) General and synovial

There are four types of joints: (a) syndesmosis (a joining of bones through dense fibrous tissue, (b) synchondrosis (a joining of bones through cartilage), (c) synostosis (a joining of bones through extensive interlocking), and (d) synovial joint (a joining with a cleft between the bones). Synovial joints merit a separate discussion because they have the most complex structure of all and they offer maximal mobility to the joining parts.

In a typical synovial joint the articulating bone ends are lined by hyaline cartilage, they are separated by a synovial space (cleft) which is filled with synovial fluid and they are joined by an articular capsule, plus, occasionally, intra-articular ligaments. The articular capsule consists, from inside outwards, of (a) a synovial lining or intima, (b) a subsynovial layer of areolar or adipose tissue (or a combination of the above) with numerous capillaries and lymphatics, some of which approach the synovial space very closely, and (c) an external dense fibrous layer. The synovial fluid represents a filtrate of plasma protein (from the subsynovial capillaries) mixed with hyaluronic acid (an unsulfated polysaccharide) which is largely present as a glycoprotein.

(2) Synovial lining (Plate 14, Figs. A and B)

In man, rabbit and guinea pig this consists of 2–3 layers of "synovial cells" which are loosely arranged and separated by a mostly collagenic matrix; the latter is exposed to the synovial fluid through gaps between the innermost synovial cells and gradually changes – from inside outwards – from a fine granular material to thin unbanded collagen fibrils and finally to thick banded collagen fibrils, several of them attached to the synovial cell surfaces. In the rat and certain other species, the synovial cells form a more compact epithelial layer, and are bound to one another through desmosomes and interlocking lateral membranes.

Two types of synovial cells are recognised in man: type A (Fig. A) and type B (Fig. B), the former being the more numerous. The two types probably represent different stages of activity of the same cell, type A possibly representing the secretion-release phase and type B the phase of resynthesis of secretory material. Both have the following features in common (Fig. A): (a) a fair number of mitochondria, (b) a few 500–700 Å thick, dense glycogen granules[1], lysosomes[2], lipid droplets[3] and fine (60–80 Å)filaments[4], (c) some thin processes[5] ("filopodia"), and (d) an only partial or no BM. *Type A* (Fig. A), however, is characterised by multiple Golgi systems[6], numerous large[7] and several micropinocytotic[8] vesicles and moderate numbers of ribosomes and RER cisternae, whereas *type B* (Fig. B) is distinguished by an extensive ribosome and RER system[1], only moderately developed Golgi and large vesicle systems, and numerous micropinocytotic vesicles[2]. The PM of both cell types exhibits ATP-ase activity.

The following three functions are discharged by the synovial cells: (a) the production of hyaluronic acid in the Golgi and its secretion through reverse pinocytosis (emiocytosis) into the matrix and the synovial space (supported by the histochemical identity of polysaccharide material within and outside synovial cells), (b) the phagocytic removal of debris and injected particles from synovial cavities (erythrocytes and fragments after hemorrhages, ferritin, thorium and carbon), and (c) the production of the unbanded and banded collagen of the matrix, which has been shown to occur in synovial cell cultures and to be inhibitable by hydrocortisone. Thus, synovial cells seem to combine the characteristics of fibroblasts and macrophages.

(3) Capillaries of subsynovial tissue

These are of the closed (unperforated) type: their endothelial cells occasionally exhibit rod-like crystalloid cytoplasmic inclusions of uncertain – possibly procoagulant – function.

VII. HEMOPOIETIC SYSTEM

(1) General

The hemopoietic system comprises two liquid tissues, blood and lymph, as well as several solid tissues (the bone marrow and the lymphatic tissues) that produce the cells and some of the chemicals contained in blood and lymph. Blood consists of a fluid, plasma, in which there are suspended (a) red cells, (b) two kinds of white cells (granular leukocytes and lymphoid cells), and (c) platelets, whereas lymph consists of a fluid with only one kind of cells (lymphocytes) suspended in it. Both blood and lymph run in a network of pipes of various calibers, the vessels.

The function of blood is (a) to transport thousands of chemicals (which are dissolved in its plasma) and oxygen (which is attached to its red cells) from one part of the body to another, (b) to provide a defence against invading foreign (antigenic) particles or living entities (bacteria, viruses, transplanted cells) through neutralizing chemicals (antibodies), the phagocytic action of its granular leukocytes or a direct cell-killing effect of its suitably activated lymphocytes, and (c) to seal breaks that might arise in vessel walls through the formation of plugs (thrombi), a process initiated by its platelets. The function of lymph is to transport certain chemicals and lym-

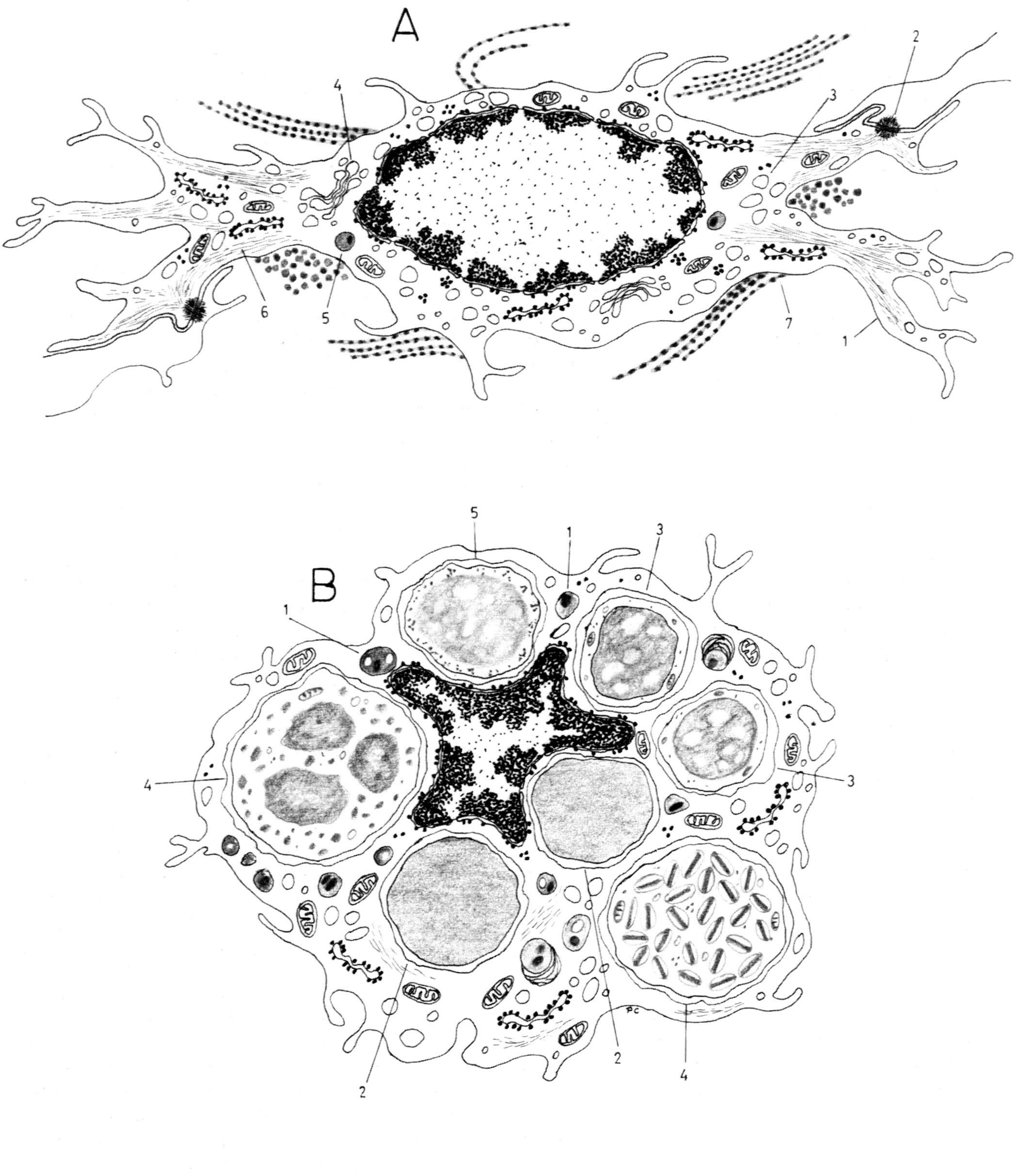

Plate 15

phocytes from the intestine and other tissues into the blood.

Red cells, granular leukocytes and platelets are produced primarily in the bone marrow but can also arise elsewhere; lymphoid cells arise mainly in "lymphatic" tissues, *i.e.* lymph nodes, spleen, thymus, tonsils and Peyer's patches, but are also generated in bone marrow.

Until recently, it was thought that the above cell species are rigidly specialized, that they do not interconvert or dedifferentiate and that each arises in only certain special sites of the hemopoietic system. As a result of much sophisticated research, involving the infusion of labelled blood cells into irradiated animals among other things, it is now believed, however, that the various blood cell species can arise practically anywhere in the hemopoietic system, and that under proper stimulation they can interconvert or dedifferentiate extensively.

Associated with the broad concept of the hemopoietic system is the functional concept of the "Reticuloendothelial" System (RES). The RES, in its original definition, comprised all those widely scattered cells in the body that rapidly remove from the blood any injected large foreign particles (*e.g.* carbon particles) by engulfing them. Such phagocytic properties turned out to be possessed not only by tissue macrophages and certain undifferentiated mesenchymal cells in hemopoietic tissues ("reticulum cells") but also by the lining (endothelial) cells of the sinusoids in all hemopoietic tissues and also in the liver and the endocrine organs.

In the bone marrow, the ordinary capillary and venule endothelium is unperforated and non-phagocytic but the endothelium of sinusoids or very wide capillaries (which is continuous and often only 500–1000 Å thick), is lysosome-rich and phagocytic – intravenously injected 150 Å particles land in its pinocytotic vesicles and are "embraced" by its flaps. Mature hemopoietic cells cross the interendothelial junctions of bone marrow sinusoids very easily – but through an unknown mechanism – to reach the bloodstream. In the spleen and the lymphnodes the sinusoids and capillaries, respectively, are perforated, allowing particularly rapid entry of lymphocytes into blood.

(2) Reticulum cells (Plate 15, Figs. A and B)

The concept of reticulum cells stems from the L/M observation that, underlying all hemopoietic tissues, is a network (reticulum) of fine collagen fibers to which are attached certain irregularly shaped large cells with a clear nucleus and a cytoplasm of vague boundaries; these cells which were often filled with phagocytised debris (dead red cells and lymphocytes or their fragments), and whose appearance was quite different from that of all other hemopoietic cells, were called "reticulum cells". It was thought that reticulum cells represent undifferentiated mesenchymal cells which (a) produce the collagenic framework of hemopoietic tissue, (b) phagocytise and remove all dead hemopoietic cells and other particles, and (c) can detach from the network and differentiate into specific hemopoietic cells, thus functioning as stem cells. Recent E/M studies, however, have revealed that all reticulum cells do not have the same structure and that they can be divided into two types: non-phagocytic and phagocytic.

The *non-phagocytic* reticulum cells (Fig. A), as studied in the thymus are star-shaped cells with numerous long, dividing branches[1] and are mostly connected to one another through desmosomes[2]; they average 10 μ in size and are characterised by (a) a concentration of chromatin at the nuclear periphery, (b) an extensive SER[3] of large and small vesicles, (c) multiple Golgi systems[4], (d) moderate numbers of ribosomes, RER cisternae and mitochondria, (e) a few lysosomes[5], (f) several bundles of tonofilaments[6], (g) surface attachment to several of the surrounding collagen fibrils[7], and (h) an occasional BM. Their function seems to be (a) to produce the collagenic structural framwork in which the hemopoietic cells are contained, (b) to add structural support to hemopoetic tissues through the desmosomal connections between their processes, (c) to adsorb antigens on their surfaces, and (d) perhaps to produce a humoral factor that stimulates lymphocyte development in their own as well as other hemopoietic organs. In the thymus, these cells are considered to be of epithelial (entodermal) origin and they form not only a loose network but also pericapillary sheaths, and concentric, onion-like clusters in which they may keratinize (Hassall's corpuscles).

The *phagocytic* reticulum cells (Fig. B) are distinguished from the non-phagocytic ones by the following main differences: (a) they are much larger (20 μ or more), ranking among the largest cells of the body, (b) they have a greater cytoplasm/nucleus ratio, (c) they are free, *i.e.* they are not attached to other cells or to collagen fibrils, (d) they have few or no microfilaments and (e) they contain many more lysosomes[1] and numerous phagosomes[2–5]. Their function is to phagocytise any living or dead foreign particles that come their way (*e.g.* bacteria or carbon) as well as the cellular debris that results from the normal turnover of hemopoietic cells (mainly dead erythrocytes and lymphocytes or fragments thereof); they apparently salvage some valuable materials from the dead cells (*e.g.* iron and possibly nucleic acid building blocks) and transmit them through an as yet unsettled mechanism to hemopoietic stem cells (such as erythroblasts) for re-utilisation; since they are more resistant to radiation than the other hemopoetic tissue elements, their cytoplasm can become filled with half a dozen or more erythrocyte[2], lymphocyte[3], polymorph[4] and "blast"[5] cell cadavers within a few hours of a suitable whole body irradiation. These cells represent

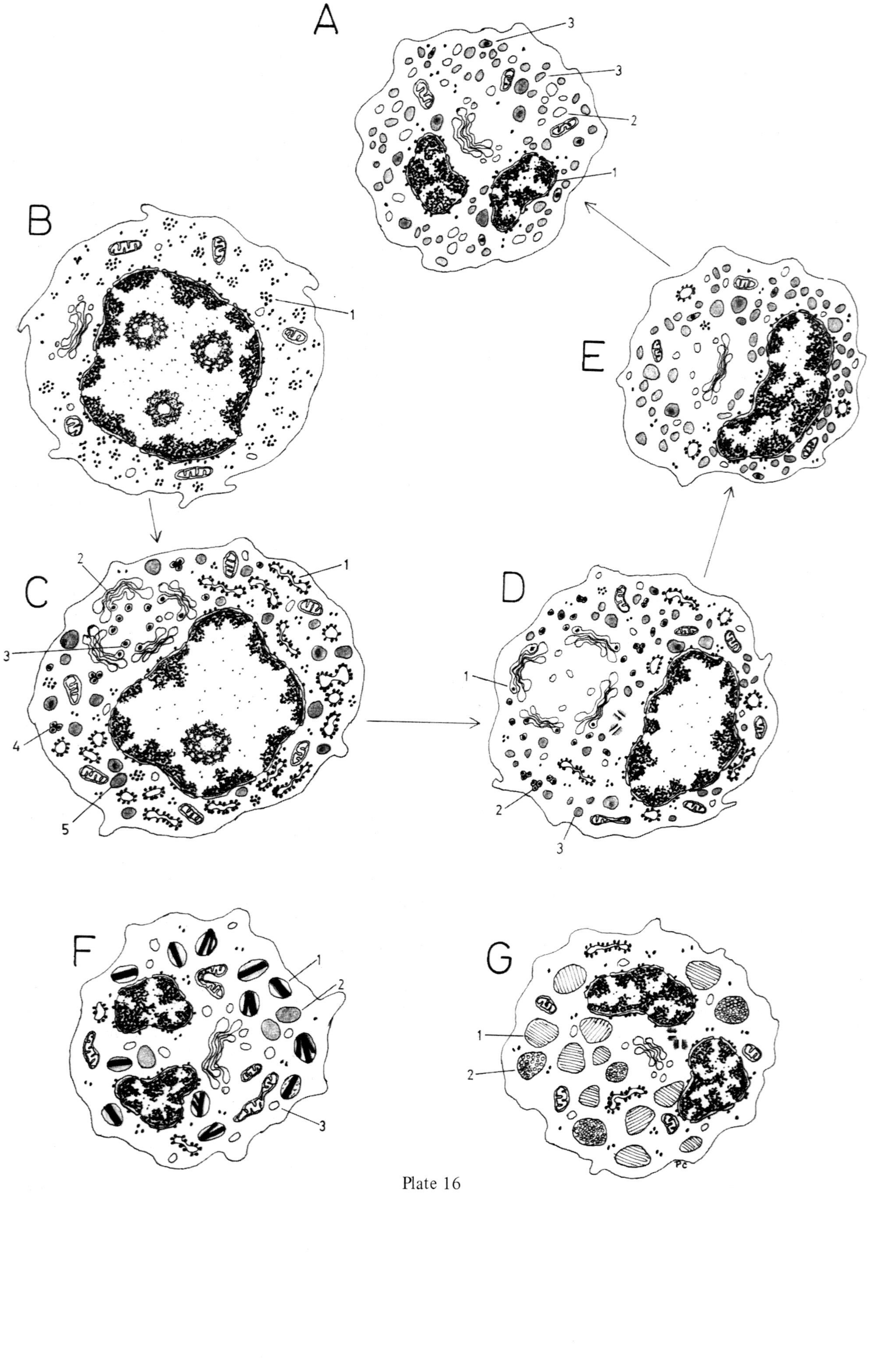

Plate 16

the indigenous macrophages or histiocytes of hemopoietic tissue and they are indistinguishable from the monocyte-derived macrophages that can immigrate into any tissue from the blood. Their relationship to the non-phagocytic ("epithelial") reticulum cells is unsettled.

It is, at the moment, uncertain whether either type of reticulum cell can, under proper stimulation, turn into a hemopoietic stem cell and thus ultimately into red cells, white cells or platelets; future kinetic studies in embryos and tissue cultures will settle such cell convertibility problems.

(3) Granular leukocytes (Plate 16)

(A) General

There are three structurally well defined types of mature granular leukocytes in the blood: the neutrophils (approx. 70% of all white cells), the eosinophils (approx. 2–8% of all white cells) and the basophils (approx. 0.5–1% of all white cells). All three types have a multilobed (segmented) nucleus and roughly similar standard organelle complements, but they each possess specific cytoplasmic granules of unique structure, in their mature stage.

(B) Neutrophils

Structure (Plate 16, Fig. A). The prominent features of these cells are (a) the lobulation of the nucleus which creates the appearance of multiple nuclei[1] because the connecting bridges between the lobes are usually missed in ultra-thin sections, (b) the very rudimentary or absent RER but fairly well developed SER[2], whose smooth vesicles exhibit acid phosphatase activity, and (c) the specific cytoplasmic granules[3], which constitute a spectrum of membrane-bound round or oval bodies of mostly moderate density, variable size (0.1–1.0 μ) and mainly microgranular substructure. These granules represent unusual lysosomes and lysosome-like bodies and they yield the following two fractions: (a) a minority of large "azurophilic" or "primary" granules, which contain acid hydrolases, large amounts of peroxidase ("myeloperoxidase") and some lysozyme and bactericidal cationic proteins, and (b) a majority of smaller "secondary" granules, most of which contain lysozyme and cationic proteins but no acid hydrolases or peroxidase. Both types of granules are rich in sodium ions.

Function. There are at least three presently known functions of these cells:

(i) They can phagocytise bacteria, debris, antigen–antibody complexes, etc., in a manner similar to that already described for the macrophages. The phagocytised microorganisms are apparently killed through the cooperation of several bactericidal agents (peroxidase, hydrolases, lysozyme, cationic proteins) that are discharged from the various granules into the phagosomal sacs; among these agents, peroxidase seems to play a prominent role and it acts by releasing oxygen from hydrogen peroxide (which is produced by another enzyme) in the presence of halides such as iodide or chlorides; inherited absence of either enzyme from neutrophils greatly diminishes their ability to kill ingested bacteria. Phagocytic activity leads to the disappearance of many granules (since the latter fuse with the phagosomes) and it is accompanied by a marked increment of oxygen and glucose uptake, CO_2 production and phospholipid turnover; the increased phospholipid synthesis presumably reflects the increased manufacture of new granule membranes and enzymes to replace those already consumed.

(ii) They can contribute certain chemical components to the formation of antigen–antibody complexes and the expedition of inflammatory processes.

(iii) By discharging certain of their enzymes after disintegrating they can contribute to the destruction of invading microorganisms, and the lysis of certain materials extracellularly. These cells are capable of ameboid movement, and it has been suggested that their smooth vesicles facilitate the formation of pseudopods by "building into" their plasma membrane and thus contibuting to its local expansion. The mechanism through which neutrophil leukocytes squeeze through the interendothelial junctions of venules to enter tissues where they are needed is still unknown; it may involve the enzymatic loosening of the junctions in addition to active ameboid movements.

Ancestry and granule biogenesis (Plate 16, Figs. B–E). The first cell in the lineage that leads to the mature (segmented) neutrophil is the *myeloblast* (Fig. B). This cell is distinguished by a large nucleus/cytoplasm ratio, multiple nucleoli, numerous free ribosomes[1] and an absent RER. The myeloblast is transformed into a *promyelocyte* (Fig. C), a cell that suddenly develops a luxuriant RER[1] and a prominent Golgi[2] from the concave aspect of which bud off tiny cored vesicles[3] that aggregate and coalesce[4] into large, approximately 1 μ granules, the so called "primary" or "azurophilic" granules[5]. These granules are the forerunners of the mature specific granules and, unlike the latter, show a tubular substructure and contain peroxidase and arylsulfatase as well as phosphatase. The promyelocyte, in turn, gives rise to a *myelocyte* (Fig. D), the cell in which production of primary granules ceases and is largely (but not entirely) supplanted by the development of a new generation of so called "secondary" granules from the convex aspect of the Golgi. These latter arise through the budding of tiny granules[1] with a microgranular substructure and phosphatase but no peroxidase activity; several such secondary granules coalesce[2] to form the mature specific granules of the neutrophil line[3], structures of lower

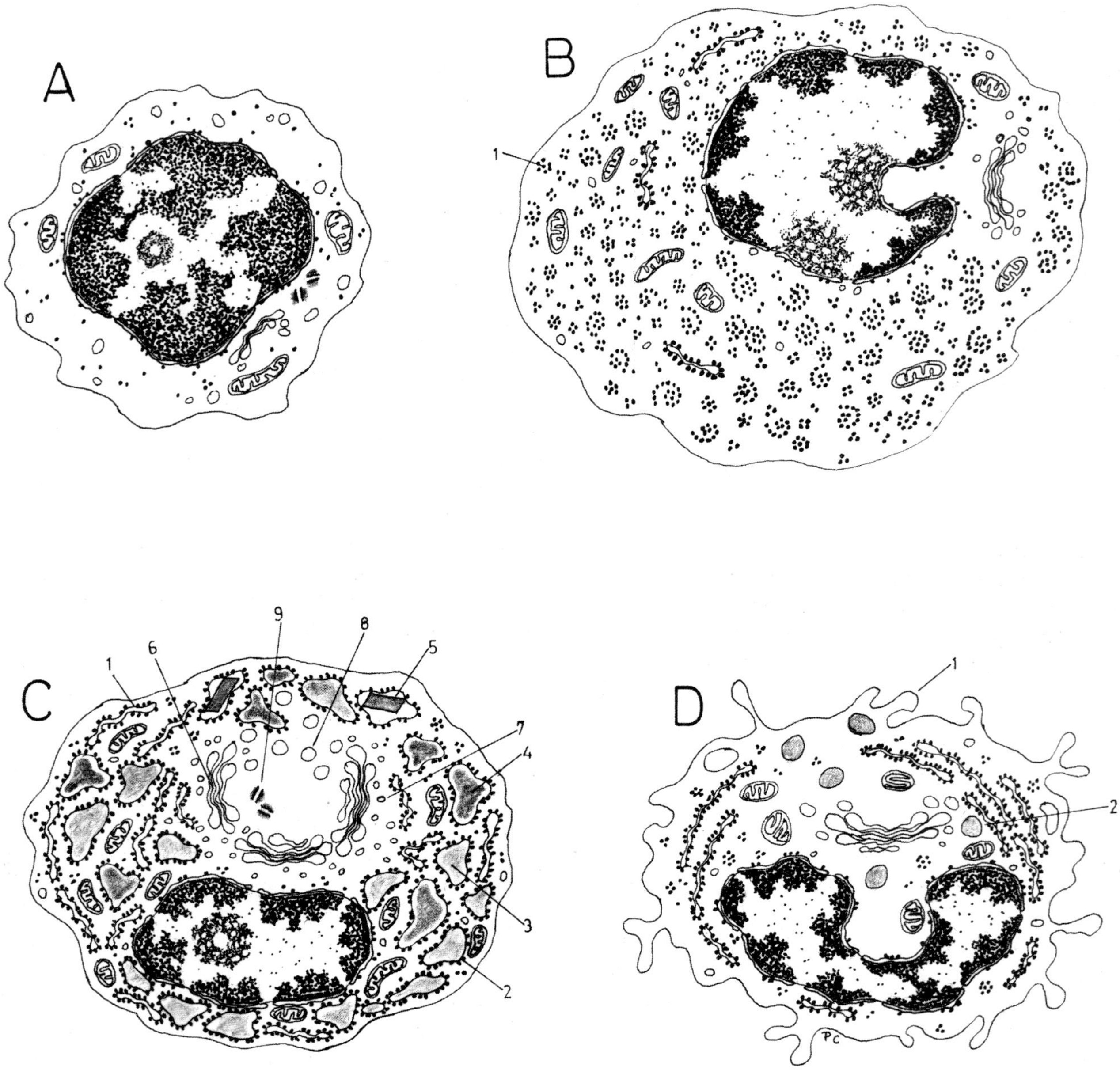

Plate 17

density and smaller size than their temporary "azurophilic" forerunners; the role of the Golgi system in the elaboration of the secondary specific granules is also shown by the finding that, upon its injection into the bone marrow, [^{3}H]lysine appears first in the Golgi and later in the specific granules of neutrophil and eosinophil myelocytes. The next stage, the immediate precursor of the mature neutrophil, is the *metamyelocyte* (Fig. E), a cell in which the nucleus begins to elongate, and most organelles, particularly the RER and the ribosomes, begin to regress or wither away. By further elongation and lobulation of its nucleus, the metamyelocyte finally turns into the mature, *segmented neutrophil leukocyte* already discussed (Fig. A). It should be noted that even at this last stage several large azurophilic granules survive, so that 80–90% of all granules are of the small, "secondary" type and 10–20% are of the large, "primary" type. The above process of maturation from myeloblast to mature leukocyte seems to be accompanied by cell divisions at most stages and is characterized by progressive shrinkage of cell size, nucleus/cytoplasm ratio, total nucleolar, ribosomal and mitochondrial mass, with a temporary blooming of the RER–Golgi systems at the promyelocyte–myelocyte stages for the elaboration of the two granule generations.

(C) Eosinophils

Structure (Plate 16, Fig. F). The most prominent features of these cells, besides the lobulated nucleus, are (a) the mature specific cytoplasmic granules[1] which are 0.5–1 μ large, round membrane-bound bodies containing one or more highly dense crystalline disc-shaped cores of rectangular profile (in man and other species) within a less dense homogeneous matrix, (b) occasional granules without crystalline cores[2], which appear to be immediate precursors of the mature ones, and (c) the very rudimentary or absent RER but fairly well developed smooth vesicle system[3].

Function. The specific granules of eosinophils contain acid phosphatase in their matrix and probably peroxidase in their crystalline cores, which have the substructure of a cubic lattice with a repeat unit of 40 Å in man. They thus seem to be quite different from the mature neutrophil granules. The function of these cells is still not entirely clear, but they seem to play a role in certain immune events since (a) they are attracted by and phagocytise antigen-antibody complexes, (b) their numbers in blood and tissues significantly increase in allergic conditions, and (c) they contain histamin in certain species. They also show a marked sensitivity to adrenocortical steroids, since they can almost disappear from the blood after cortisone treatment.

Ancestry and biogenesis of granules. The eosinophils originate from the same stem cell as the neutrophils, namely the myeloblast, and their genealogy parallels that of the neutrophils, stage by stage, as already described. The specific eosinophil granules first arise in the myelocyte stage through the pinching off of vesicles with a floccular-fine granular content from the Golgi, their coalescence to larger granules with at first homogeneous contents and finally the development of dense crystalline cores in them.

(D) Basophils

Structure (Plate 16, Fig. G). The basic cytoplasmic organelles of these cells are the same as those of the neutrophils and eosinophils. Their distinguishing characteristic is the specific granules which are up to 1.7 μ large, membrane-bound globules of a very dense content with a crystalline substructure (a regular hexagonal lattice showing either lamellar[1] or honeycomb[2] profiles).

Function. The function of the basophils, like that of the eosinophils, is not entirely elucidated yet, but seems to be related to immune processes: The production of basophils is increased after repeated injections of foreign serum and their concentration in the blood drops after cortisone treatment. These cells may also be somehow related to mast cells since they have been claimed to contain a major part of the blood histamine and since their granules show certain ultrastructural and light microscopic similarities to those of the mast cells. Recently basophils have been found to degranulate by exocytosis in response to anaphylactic shock (when antigen is injected into sensitized animals).

Ancestry and biogenesis of granules. The basophils develop from the same stem cell as the other two types of granular leukocytes, namely the myeloblast, and through the same stages. Their specific granules arise in the myelocyte stage through the budding of approximately 0.15 μ large vesicles of fine granular content from the Golgi, their coalescence to much larger mature granules and the development of a crystalline structure in them (through microfilamentous intermediaries).

(4) Lymphoid cells (non-granular leukocytes)

(A) General

Traditionally, the following two cell species should be grouped under the above heading: the lymphocyte (with a medium sized "resting" form, and a large "activated" or pyroninophilic form) and the plasma cell; according to some workers a third cell type also belongs here, *i.e.* the monocyte. All three types are distinguished from the granular leukocytes by the absence of mature neutrophil, eosinophil or basophil granules. All three types are found in tissues (*i.e.* in lymphatic, myeloid and areolar tissue) but normally only lymphocytes and monocytes travel in the blood; the latter two cells migrate extensively from the blood into the tissues but only the former returns to the blood through the lymph.

Masses of lymphoid cells (primarily lymphocytes and variously plasma cells) are the characteristic component of the "lymphatic" organs of the body (thymus, tonsils, Peyer's patches, spleen and lymphnodes), where they are concerned with defense against chemical and cellular intruders. The thymus is vital for the proper functioning of all the other lymphatic organs of mammals because, at an early stage of post-natal life, it colonises them with lymphocytes and possibly even controls their development through a humoral factor.

(B) Lymphocyte

Structure (Plate 17). Under normal conditions, the most common form of a lymphocyte is the medium sized (7–8 μ large) relatively quiescent lymphocyte (Fig. A). The most prominent features of this cell are (a) a high nucleus/cytoplasm ratio, (b) a single "resting" nucleolus in a heterochromatin-rich nucleus, and (c) the absence of rough endoplasmic reticulum (RER). Apart from the RER, all other standard organelles are present but in moderate amounts, and ribosomes exist as single units rather than as polysomal aggregates. The presence of a centriole attests to the mitotic potential of lymphocytes.

Function (Plate 17). Despite the absence of drama from its fine structure, this is a cell of great potentialities and important defence functions. Once it has reached a certain stage of development or "competence", it can recognize the presence of foreign macromolecules and cells (antigens) in the body and it will react to them by (a) enlarging its cytoplasm to a diameter of 12–15 μ or more (Fig. B), (b) producing much RNA mostly in the form of polyribosomes[1], (c) developing multiple prominent nucleoli that migrate to the nuclear membrane, and (d) proliferating energetically; thus it turns into a large cell packed with polyribosomes and containing even a few RER cisternae, a cell with strong affinity for the RNA-stain pyronine, the "pyroninophilic" cell (or "immunoblast" or "germinoblast", or "basophilic stem cell" of light microscopy) (Fig. B). The RNA that accumulates in these cells is apparently catalysing the synthesis of certain defensive protein molecules (antibodies) that are directed specifically against the foreign proteins (antigens) that aroused them. Under certain conditions, as when the antigens are cells (*e.g.* grafts of foreign tissue), the large pyroninophilic cells apparently revert to lymphocytes that look like the original smaller cells but are now "sensitized", and they attach bodily to the antigenic cells ("cyto-adherence") destroying the latter through the antibodies they have manufactured and carry on their cell surface. Under other conditions, the pyroninophilic cells seem to turn into plasma cells and to secrete large quantities of antibodies into the extracellular fluids. According to current views, the lymphocytes that attach bodily to antigenic cells and destroy them through their surface antibodies (the "killer cells" or effectors of "cell-mediated immunity") are produced in the thymus and are designated as "T-cells"; mutant rats that lack a thymus also lack T-cells and are congenitally unable to reject any foreign transplanted tissues – one can grow chickens' wings on them! By contrast, the lymphocytes that turn into plasma cells and secrete large quantities of antibodies into extracellular fluids (the effectors of "humoral immunity") are produced in the bone marrow in mammals (or in the tonsil-like bursa of Fabricius in birds) and are designated as "B-cells". Small B-cells migrate continuously from the bone marrow to the lymphnodes where they populate the germinal centres of the cortex and become the plasma cells of the medulla; T-cells also migrate from thymus to lymphnodes, where they populate the deep cortical zone. In the blood, the majority of all lymphocytes (*ca.* 70%) are thought to be of the T- and the remainder of the B-type.

It is presently believed that B-cells can respond to foreign antigens either directly or indirectly through a chain reaction that involves the help of T-cells and macrophages or reticular cells: the antigens are captured by the antibodies on the T-cell surfaces, some of the resulting antigen-antibody complexes are then picked up by the macrophages or reticular cells and "presented" to the B-cells which react to the antigen part of these complexes. In either case the B-cells respond to antigens by proliferating, turning into plasma cells and secreting specific antibodies.

Reactions between antigens and antibodies trigger a chain reaction in complement (a complex of mostly β-globulin proteins) that activates several of its components which, in turn, (a) cause lysis of cell membranes that happen to be in the neighbourhood, (b) provoke proliferation and transformation of neighboring lymphocytes, (c) induce histamine release, and thus increased capillary permeability (inflammation), (d) attract phagocytic cells to the scene and facilitate phagocytosis and (e) stimulate the production of a substance that inhibits virus proliferation (interferon). All above reactions contribute to the further destruction of foreign invaders even though some of them may also, on occasion, have host-damaging side effects. It is now being realised that complement can be activated not only by Antigen–Antibody complexes but also by many other complexes and macromolecules such as properdin, protamin–heparin complexes, dextran, inulin, bacterial lipopolysaccharides, and various plant substances.

One of the most interesting facts recognised lately through the study of the fate of thymidine-labelled cells has been that some lymphocytes live for only a few weeks while others can live for many months or even years. Although the genetic knowledge of even the most shortlived cells can be perpetuated by repeated mitosis, the presence of very long living "Methuselah" lymphocytes most probably contributes substantially to the "immunological memory" of higher organisms, *i.e.* to their readiness to deal promptly with invaders to whom they have been already exposed in the past.

(C) Plasma cell (plasmacyte)

Structure (Plate 17, Fig. C). This ovoid cell of about 10 μ diameter is distinguished by (a) much cytoplasm (low nucleus/cytoplasm ratio), (b) a luxuriant RER which may consist of either flattened[1] or dilated[2] cisternae that contain amorphous material of low[3] or high[4] density ("Russell bodies") or crystals[5], (c) abundant spirally arranged polyribosomes (cochleosomes) attached to the RER cisternae, and (d) a very large cup-shaped Golgi with evident components of stacked flattened smooth sacs[6], small "transfer" vesicles[7] and large secretion vesicles[8]. The centriole[9] usually seen in the Golgi area indicates that plasma cells can divide, a fact that has been already documented in L/M studies.

Function. The plasma cell synthesizes and secretes antibodies against antigens *i.e.* invading foreign macromolecules (including those on the surface of foreign microorganisms). Any macromolecule with a molecular weight of more than 10,000 and a "surface profile" different from that of all normal body macromolecules which invades the body after the production of its own macromolecules has been completed (*i.e.* after birth) is considered by plasma cells an antigen. According to present views, exposure of the body for the first time to a specific antigen seems to stimulate a certain group or "family" of plasma cells (a) to produce a specific antibody, and (b) to proliferate, and persist, thus perpetuating the production of this specific antibody throughout the body's life-span. When the body is exposed for a second time to the same antigen, the same watchdog "family" of plasma cells is alerted, increasing their production of antibody and undergoing another proliferation spurt. The above processes form the basis of "humoral" or "immediate" hypersensitivity.

Antibodies are glycoproteins with a globulin nucleus and a loose carbohydrate shell. The globulin nucleus consists of 4 polypeptide chains, of which 2 are "heavy" (MW *ca.* 50,000) and 2 are "light" (MW *ca.* 25,000); each heavy chain contains about 400 and each light chain about 200 aminoacids. The chains are bound to one another by strong covalent S–S (disulfide) bonds and by other weaker forces to form a large Y-shaped complex of roughly 100 Å overall diameter that can now, under certain conditions, be visualised with the electron microscope. Antigens attach to the tips of the 2 divergent branches of the Y, whose terminal structure varies to exactly fit the specific antigen that provoked its synthesis. The polypeptide backbones of antibodies are synthesized in the RER and transferred from there by means of transfer vesicles into the flattened Golgi sacs where they incorporate most of their carbohydrate components, as shown autoradiographically with labelled aminoacids and hexoses; they then move towards the PM and are released from the cell through an as yet unsettled mechanism. Once outside, they travel through the lymph to the blood stream so that they can interact with antigens in the immediate neighbourhood as well as at a great distance from their production site. Antibodies within cells are in monomeric form, but in the serum they can form large pentameric complexes that are visible with the E/M. The finding that reticulum cells in bone marrow are often surrounded by plasma cells has been thought to indicate transmission of antigenic information from the former to the latter.

Plasma cells seem to develop from large cells of a diameter greater than 12 μ with extremely abundant polyribosomes and only very few RER cisternae, *i.e.* from cells that are identical with pyroninophilic cells. These immature "*plasmablasts*" develop much RER and turn into plasma cells (*plasmacytes*) through intermediate "*proplasmacytes*".

(D) Monocyte

Structure (Plate 17, Fig. D). The prominent features of this cell are (a) numerous pseudopods and folds of the surface membrane[1], (b) a horse-shoe shaped nucleus, (c) several round or oblong dense bodies of probably lysosomal nature[2], that are similar to the large azurophilic granules of promyelocytes and contain peroxidase, (d) a fair number fo ribosomes and RER cisternae, (e) several mitochondria, and (f) a distinct Golgi. Under certain circumstances these cells also exhibit membrane-enclosed crystalloid packs of tubules with a periodicity of 90–100 Å and an uncertain function, the "Auer bodies".

Function. The monocyte, a cell of the blood, not only looks like the macrophage of areolar connective tissue but it also functions like the latter. It phagocytises particles through a mechanism similar to that already described for macrophages. When it crosses from the blood into the tissues it becomes a macrophage, *i.e.* it becomes indistinguishable from the macrophages already resident there. Thus it could be said that many macrophages of areolar tissue come from the blood (the others possibly originating by differentiation of local connective tissue stem cells into phagocytes).

The origin of the monocyte is not yet settled. It has been assumed for some time to develop from lymphocytes, but recent evidence from the labeling of bone marrow cells indicates that it can arise from bone marrow stem cells just like the lymphocytes – and perhaps from the same stem cells as the latter. Whatever its origin, its life-span has been reported to be short, of the order of perhaps three days.

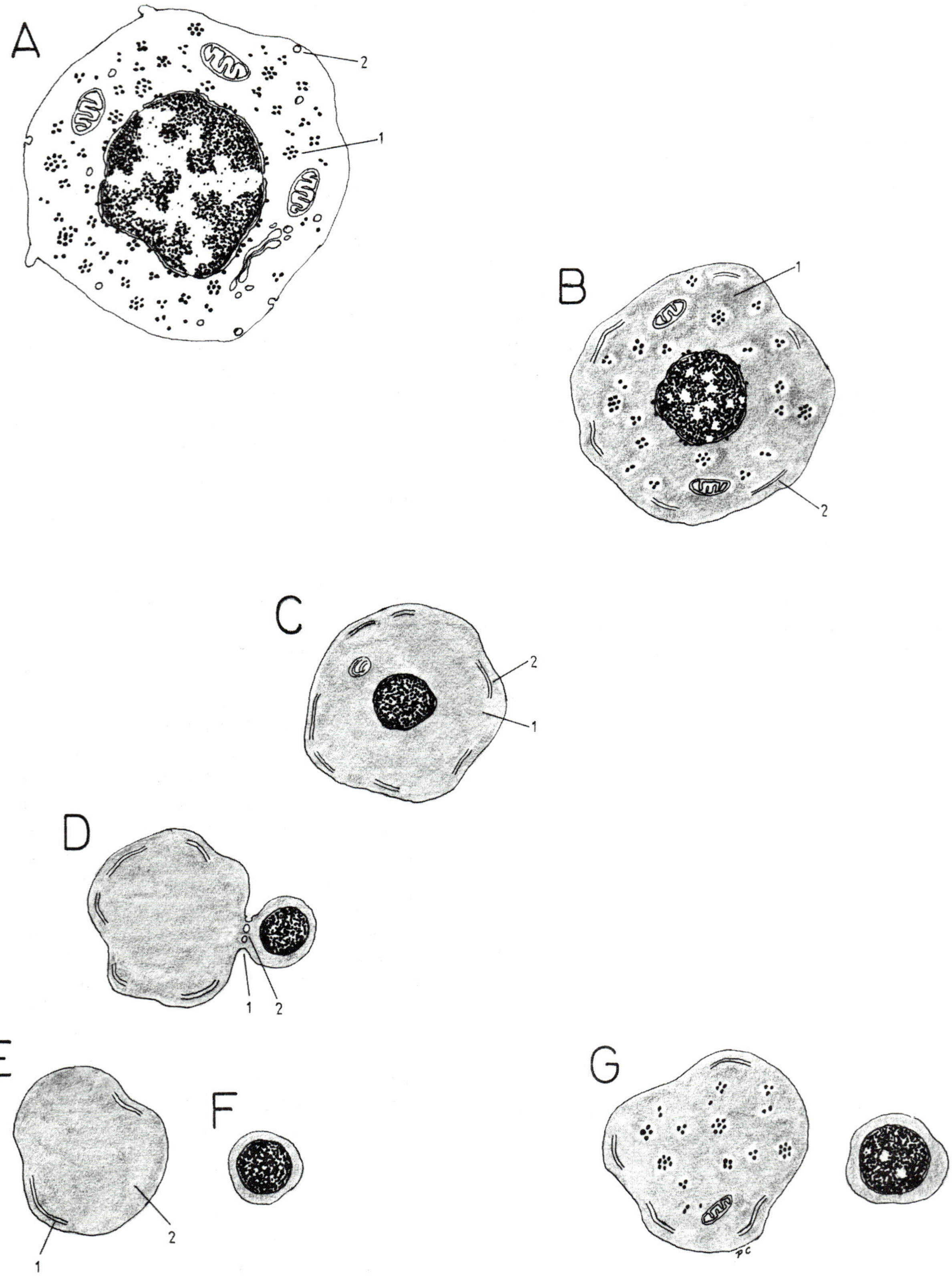

Plate 18

(5) Red blood cells (erythrocytes)

(A) General – erythropoiesis

Erythrocytes normally develop from stem cells in the bone marrow (proerythroblasts) that give rise to the following successive sequence of cells: basophilic erythroblasts, polychromatophilic erythroblasts, and normoblasts, the latter extruding their nucleus to become mature erythrocytes and enter the bloodstream. This sequence starts with cells possessing a large nucleus and rich in RNA, which is needed for the synthesis of hemoglobin, a metalloprotein. As the cells mature, their size and nucleus shrinks and hemoglobin appears in increasing amounts in their cytoplasm, while RNA and the other organelles gradually disappear, until they reach the final erythrocyte stage in which the cytoplasm contains little else besides hemoglobin. Sometimes, particularly when there is an urgent need for them, erythrocytes are thrown into the bloodstream before their maturation is completed, *i.e.* their nucleus is extruded before all RNA and other organelles have disappeared; such hastily formed red cells are called reticulocytes.

(B) Erythrocyte

Structure (Plate 18, Fig. E). The erythrocyte is a cell without a nucleus or organelles except for a few peripheral microtubule hoops[1] in some species, which presumably give it structural support, *i.e.* prevent it from collapsing. Its cytoplasm is filled with hemoglobin which represents a homogeneous mass, highly dense because of its iron content[2]. Dissolved in the cytoplasmic matrix, in addition to hemoglobin are various enzymes, including carbonic anhydrase, and ATPase (which has been demonstrated on the inner surface of the plasma membrane). Finally, the presence of blood-group specific antigens in the plasma membrane has been shown through the attachment of ferritin-conjugated specific antibodies on its external surface. These surface antigens are presumably identical with the polysaccharide-containing cell coat (glycocalyx) of erythrocytes, which can be demonstrated with colloidal iron and destroyed by neuraminidase.

Function. Erythrocytes carry oxygen from the lungs to the various body tissues and carry back some of the oxidation product, CO_2, from the tissues to the lungs. Oxygen is transported bound physically to the iron of hemoglobin. A drop in the oxygen supply to body tissues (hypoxia) – as *e.g.* after significant loss of blood due to hemorrhage – will stimulate increased production of erythrocytes in the bone marrow, which is evidently aimed at removing the state of hypoxia that caused it. In this feedback process, hypoxia seems to be sensed in the kidney where it increases the production of erythropoietin, an erythropoiesis stimulating hormone; renal erythropoietin will then stimulate red cell formation in the bone marrow. Erythropoiesis itself requires vitamin B_{12}, a coenzyme necessary for the formation of DNA and RNA, *i.e.* for the proliferation and maturation of the red cell ancestors. Vitamin B_{12} is absorbed from the food with the help of a mucopolysaccharide manufactured by the stomach wall; when either the vitamin or the mucopolysaccharide are absent, erythrocyte formation is greatly slowed down in the bone marrow and the new red cells produced are abnormally large and hemoglobin-rich, perhaps in an attempt to compensate with size and high hemoglobin content for what has been lost in numbers.

Ancestry and re-utilisation of salvaged iron (Plate 18). The stem cell of the erythrocyte-forming line, the *proerythroblast* is the largest cell of the series and is characterised by (a) a very high nucleus/cytoplasm ratio, (b) euchromatin-rich nucleus, (c) extremely abundant ribosomes, and (d) very sparse cisternae of rough endoplasmic reticulum. This cell gives rise to the slightly smaller *basophilic erythroblast* (Fig. A), a cell distinguished by (a) a somewhat smaller nucleus/cytoplasm ratio, (b) more heterochromatin, (c) still very numerous ribosomes, mostly as polyribosome clusters[1], (d) *no* rough endoplasmic reticulum, (e) large mitochondria, (f) pinocytotic vesicles[2] and (g) like its predecessor, *no* hemoglobin in the cytoplasm yet. The next stage is that of the *polychromatophilic erythroblast* (Fig. B) in which, in addition to the previous components, hemoglobin[1] makes its appearance in the form of flakes of dense material scattered between the ribosomes, and some peripheral microtubules[2] materialise, whereas nuclear size, mitochondrial size and ribosome numbers begin to decrease. The polychromatophilic erythroblast is next transformed into a *normoblast* (Fig. C), a cell with (a) a low nucleus/cytoplasm ratio, (b) dense chromatin and, (c) a cytoplasm full of hemoglobin[1] but only a few residual organelles, including some microtubules[2]. The normoblast extrudes its nucleus (Fig. D) by migration of the latter to the cell surface, constriction between the area containing it and the rest of the normoblast[1] and separation by the formation and confluence of a chain of small vesicles[2] across the constriction. The completion of this process leads to a mature erythrocyte (Fig. E) and an extruded nucleus covered by a thin rim of cytoplasm (Fig. F). The extruded nucleus disintegrates in the bloodstream or is picked up and phagocytized by reticuloendothelial cells which perhaps recognize it by its reduced surface charge. When the nucleus is extruded before all RNA and organelles disappear from the cytoplasm, the result is a *reticulocyte* (Fig. G), a cell which is apparently capable of active movement and passage through the endothelial junctions of bone marrow sinusoids. Reticulocytes apparently extrude their degenerating mitochondria by surrounding them with a chain of vesicles which coalesce to form a double-walled cyto-

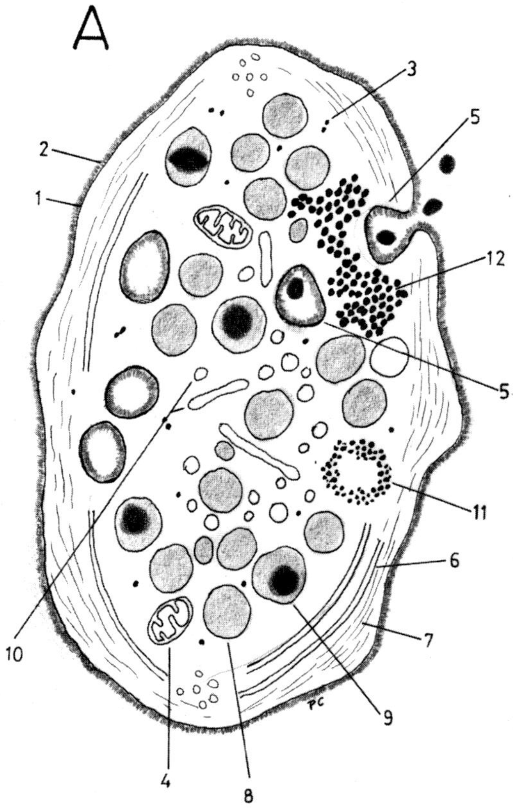

Plate 19

segresomal envelope around them; the outer sac of this cytosegresome then fuses with the reticulocyte PM and breaks at the point of fusion to release the mitochondrion (still wrapped in an inner sac) into the blood plasma.

Erythrocytes normally live for several weeks. When they die they are phagocytized by the large macrophage-like "reticulum cells" in the bone marrow and other hemopoietic tissues. The reticulum cells digest the erythrocytes, extract the iron from their hemoglobin, and seem to pass it on (through an as yet obscure mechanism) to erythroblasts for the manufacture of new hemoglobin. Reticulum cells surrounded be several closely adhering basophilic erythroblasts ("blood islands") have been seen in the bone marrow and interpreted as indicating direct iron transmission from reticulum cell to erythroblasts, but there is as yet no definitive evidence that such a process really takes place. While reticulum cells store the digested erythrocyte iron in the form of visible ferritin molecules (scattered free in the cytoplasm or collected in clusters within "siderosome" sacs), the coated pinocytic vesicles of erythroblasts do not, as a rule, contain ferritin. It is, therefore, considered possible that reticulum cells may transmit their iron to erythroblasts via the plasma transferrin system.

(6) Platelets, megacaryocytes and fibrin

(A) General

Platelets are miniature cells without a nucleus. They represent membrane-bound fragments breaking off the cytoplasm of certain giant cells, the megacaryocytes; they are normally produced in the bone marrow and they are primarily concerned with the sealing of breaks in the continuity of vessel walls, *i.e.* they initiate the formation of thrombi over sites of vascular injury.

(B) Platelet

Structure (Plate 19, Fig. A). This 2–5 μ long oval miniature cell is bounded by an ordinary trilaminar plasma membrane[1] which exhibits ATPase activity and whose outer dense leaflet is described as being thicker than its inner dense leaflet; the plasma membrane is covered by a 150–200 Å thick "fuzzy coat"[2] of low density which apparently consists of negatively charged acid polysaccharides, notably sialic acid. In its cytoplasm, apart from ribosomes[3] and mitochondria ("β"-granules)[4], the platelet contains the following special organelles and inclusions: (a) invaginations of the surface leading to crypts and partly intercommunicating vacuoles or "canaliculi" lined with fuzzy coat[5] which are concerned with phagocytosis or pinocytosis of materials and solutions from outside the cell, (b) hoops of 200–400 Å thick microtubules[6] running parallel to the surface, each composed of 10–14 35 Å subfilaments and presumably contributing to the structural support of the platelet shape, (c) sub-surface 50 Å thick microfilaments[7] which probably consist of "thrombosthenin", an actomyosin-like contractile protein that has been isolated from microfilament-rich platelet species, (d) numerous membrane-bound granules of moderate density ("α"-granules) without[8] or with[9] dense nucleoids, the former apparently containing acid phosphatase and phospholipid, the latter acid phosphatase, serotonin and other amines – the platelet serotonin content having been claimed to parallel its content of cored α-granules, (e) small vesicles and tubules[10] ("γ"-granules), (f) occasional ferritin-containing phagosomes with a clear center and often no apparent bounding membrane, the so called "siderosomes"[11] or "δ"-granules, and (g) glycogen[12] grains ("ϵ"-granules). There is no rough endoplasmic reticulum, or regular Golgi apparatus – the "γ"-vesicles and tubules are considered to originate from the Golgi of the megacaryocytes, the platelet ancestors. The microfilament- and microtubule-containing periphery of the platelet constitutes the "hyalomere", the rest the "granulomere" of this cell. Like the microtubules of mitotic spindles, the microtubules of platelets are destroyed by colchicin and Vinca alkaloids.

Function in initiation of thrombosis (Plate 20). Platelets detect and plug breaks in the continuity of the endothelial lining of vessels and thus help to prevent fatal hemorrhages.

When the endothelium and the vessel wall is normal, platelets keep their distance from it and do not adhere to it (Fig. A). This is probably due to several factors, among them (a) the fact that both normal platelets[1] and normal endothelium[2] are negatively charged and thus tend to repel each other, (b) the fact that normal endothelium represents a smooth surface, and (c) the tendency of cells and particles to move closer to the central axis of the blood stream, creating a relatively cell-free peripheral zone under conditions of non-turbulent "laminar flow".

When, however, the vessel wall is injured as a result of mechanical trauma, inflammation or many other factors, then breaks develop in the endothelium due to injury and sloughing off of endothelial cells or opening of the interendothelial junctions (Fig. B). Such breaks immediately attract platelets, through a mechanism which is not yet entirely clear but probably includes the following: (a) the breaks expose subendothelial materials to the bloodstream, notably collagen[1], which the platelets would never encounter under normal conditions, (b) they create a rough surface which is bound to cause eddies and disrupt the smooth laminar flow, thus moving cells right up to the vessel lining, (c) they cause the local disappearance of the negatively charged endothelial surface, and (d) they cause the local leakage of various

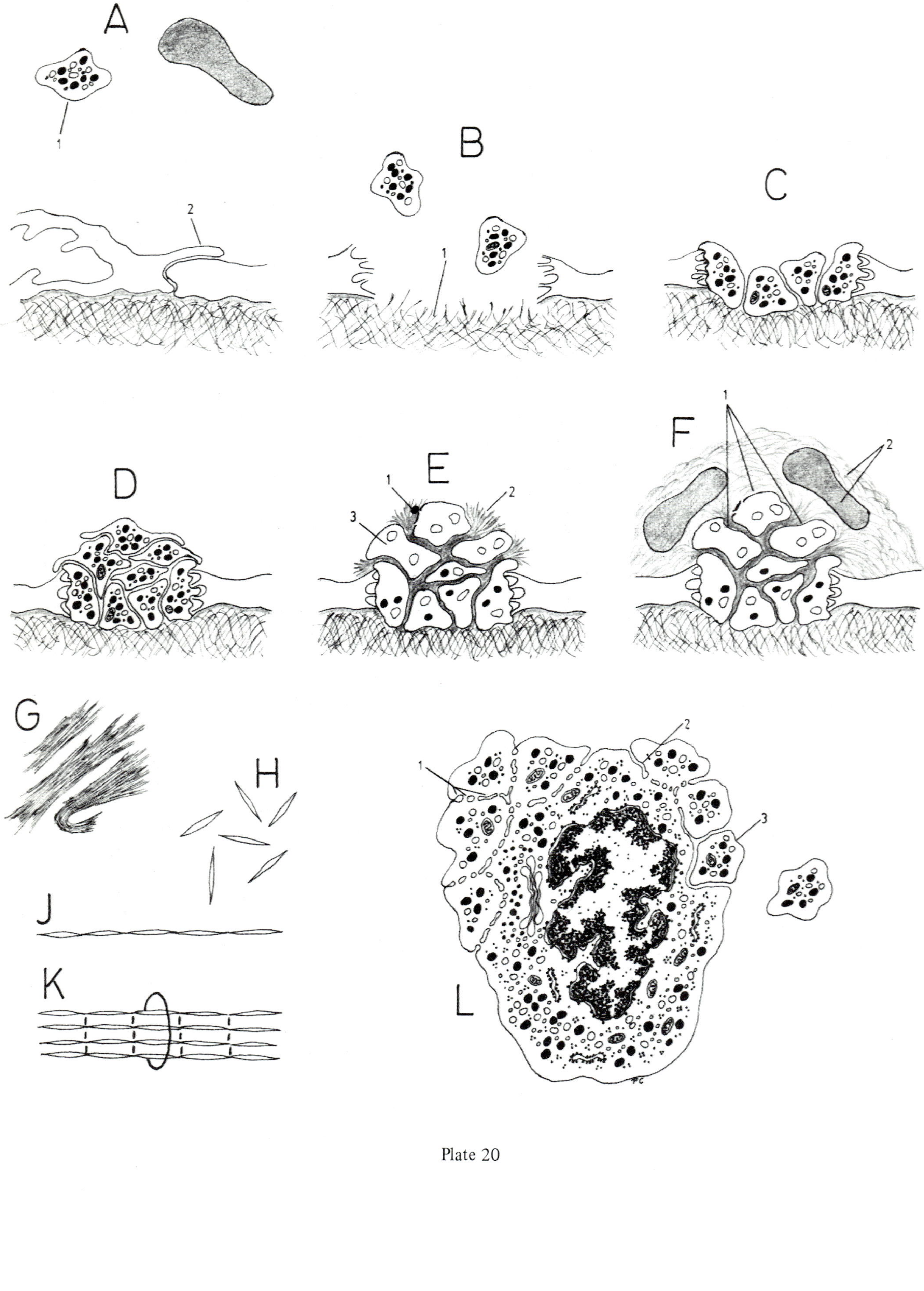

Plate 20

intracellular chemicals, notably adenosine diphosphate (ADP), from injured cells into the bloodstream.

The following sequence of events is then triggered by the local vascular injury: *First,* some platelets home for the injury area and *adhere* to it (Fig. C). *Next,* more platelets arrive, develop pseudopods and adhere to those already lining the injury area as well as to each other, building up a pile of tightly packed thrombocytes (Fig. D). This platelet *"aggregation"* is believed to be caused by ADP that leaks from the injured vascular cells and from the platelets themselves under the catalytic action of collagen which acts like an ATPase, splitting a phosphate off platelet ATP and turning it into ADP; the role of this compound in inducing platelet aggregation is supported by the fact that ADP produces whereas its analogues inhibit (competitively) platelet aggregation *in vitro* and *in vivo* – even though the mechanism of these effects is still a matter of speculation. Up to this point, the platelet plug is a fairly unstable structure. In the *next stage*, however, the platelets *degranulate* (Fig. E), *i.e.* they discharge most of their granules, including the phospholipid-rich α-granules, some of which can be seen lying outside the thrombocytes for a while[1]; it is believed that platelet phospholipid (originating from the granules or membranes of the platelets) then activates plasma thromboplastin and initiates a chain reaction in the surrounding plasma which leads to the formation of thrombin from prothrombin, and finally to the *precipitation of fibrin*[2] from fibrinogen through the catalytic action of thrombin. Simultaneous with their degranulation and the beginning of fibrin formation around them, the platelets undergo an edematous, balloon-like change[3], some of them disintegrate and their vacuoles increase in size. Finally, fibrin formation increases to the point where it generates a thick shell of this substance (permeated with trapped blood cells) over the platelet plug (Fig. F), protecting the latter from premature detachment. A thrombus has now been created, with a "white"[1] (platelets) and a "red"[2] (fibrin plus blood cells) component. The above description has been based for didactic purposes on an artificial separation of platelet-induced thrombogenesis into several sharply defined stages, when in reality these stages overlap widely.

Fibrin, an insoluble protein, can under certain conditions also develop in the body by activation of blood clotting factors in the absence of prior platelet aggregation. Whether preceded or not by platelet aggregation, fibrin (Fig. G) consists of flake-like bundles of tightly packed striped filaments with a (often not evident) periodicity of approximately 220 Å. It originates from the soluble plasma protein fibrinogen, whose molecules are *ca.* 2000 Å long, thin needles containing negatively charged arginine at both ends and therefore, probably, repel one another (Fig. H). Under the action of the proteolytic enzyme thrombin, these negative ends are chopped off, allowing the fibrinogen molecules to link end-to-end to form chain polymers (Fig. J). Several such chains are then bound together by lateral cross-linkages to form bundles (Fig. K), each bundle constituting a single fibrin filament visible with the E/M.

Fibrin can be dissolved by fibrinolysin, an enzyme that breaks its lateral cross-linkages and depolymerises its chains into soluble fragments. Fibrinolysin accompanies fibrinogen in the bloodstream and, therefore, some of it becomes trapped in thrombi, contributing to their dissolution when they have a small mass.

Function in phagocytosis. Apart from their main function of initiating thrombosis, platelets are also capable of absorbing extensively various particles from the blood (chylomicrons, viruses, ferritin, latex particles, thorotrast, SiO_2, etc.) into their vesicles. This uptake seems to occur through pinocytosis or through passive entry of the particles into the channels that lead from the platelets surface to its sponge-like interior. It is not clear at the moment what the role of this phagocytic activity is in the overall defense of the body against foreign particles.

(C) Megacaryocytes (Plate 20, Fig. L)

These gigantic cells exhibit in their cytoplasm the same organelles as platelets but contain more ribosomes and prominent Golgi areas since they continuously synthesize new cytoplasm and specific platelet granules (which originate in their Golgi system); the peripheral cytoplasm of these cells (the "ectoplasm") differs from the rest in that it contains only ribosomes. Platelets develop by the demarcation of certain territories in the megacaryocyte cytoplasm through chains of smooth, glycoprotein-containing vesicles[1] and sacs that fuse to form demarcating clefts[2]; the latter fuse all around a given territory, clothing it with unit membrane and separating it from the rest of the megacaryocyte to transform it into a platelet[3]. These platelet-producing cells are evidently very active protein and membrane-manufacturing factories since they keep turning out platelets to replace those continuously lost from the circulation. Immature megacaryocytes are termed by some "promegacaryocytes" before the appearance of demarcating clefts and "megacaryoblasts" before the development of the specific platelet granules.

Survival studies with labelled platelets indicate that the average life span of a platelet in man is about 7–10 days; at the end of this interval, platelets appear to be phagocytised by reticuloendothelial cells and by circulating blood monocytes.

Platelets appear to be released into the sinusoids as follows: Pseudopods of megacaryocytes move through endothelial junctions into the sinusoid lumen and split off platelets into the bloodstream, after the specific platelet organelles have flowed into these processes.

Chapter 5

Muscle

I. GENERAL

Muscle is a tissue that contracts actively and thus causes movement of the body in relation to its external environment or movements of its internal parts in relation to one another. There are three types of muscle: (a) skeletal, (b) cardiac, and (c) smooth. *Skeletal muscle* consists of multinucleated long fibers that show a regular striation when seen under the L/M and are under voluntary control; it connects and moves skeletal parts by attaching to them directly or through collagen fibers (tendons). *Cardiac muscle* consists of striated single branched cells that attach firmly to one another, forming chains in the wall of the heart; its contraction is involuntary and propels blood. *Smooth muscle* consists of spindle-shaped unstriated cells that attach to one another through short collagen fibrils; they form ring-like chains within the walls of tubular organs (such as the vessels and the intestinal tube) or sac-like organs (such as the uterus and the gallbladder); their contraction shortens the diameter of the above organs and thus regulates the flow of liquids in them or propels (peristalsis), expels (detrusor function) and prevents the expulsion (sphincteric function) of their contents. All muscle cells are derived from the middle embryonic layer (mesoderm).

II. SKELETAL MUSCLE

(1) Structure (Plate 21)

The structural unit of skeletal muscle is a cylindrical multinucleated structure resulting from the fusion of several embryonic muscle cells, the "muscle fiber" or "myotube" (the left half of Fig. A shows a longitudinal section of a segment of it). The plasma membrane (PM)[1] of the muscle fiber is covered by a basement membrane-like polysaccharide-containing coat[2] in which several collagen fibrils can be embedded; the PM together with its external coat constitutes the "sarcolemma" of light microscopy. Situated at various intervals directly under the PM are the numerous nuclei[3] of a fiber. The prevailing organelles within the cytoplasm ("sarcoplasm") are long myofibrils[4] and a unique system of channels and sacs wrapped around the myofibrils that consist of two components: (a) ring-like, transversely running channels that open onto the fiber surface, the so-called "T-tubules"[5], and (b) collar-like longitudinally oriented networks of flattened sacs that do not communicate with the fiber surface or the T-tubules (but seem to get very close to the latter (within 100 Å or less), the so-called "sarcoplasmic reticulum" (SR)[6]; the development of this sac system seems to parallel the speed of muscle contraction since in an ultra-fast lobster antenna muscle it comprises about 75% of the muscle fiber volume. When sodium ions or ferritin molecules are introduced into the fluid bathing myotubes they find their way into the T-tubules[5] but not the SR-sacs[6] (see right half of Fig. A for demonstration of the T and SR-system in relief). Filling in the spaces between the sac-wrapped myofibrils are glycogen granules[7], and the periphery of the fiber is occupied by numerous mitochondria[8] with abundant cristae – the smaller the animal the greater the mitochondrial population. There are extremely few ribosomes and no rough endoplasmic reticulum or Golgi apparatus in a mature muscle fiber; the fiber ends, however, always contain some ribosomes.

The myofibrils show an alternation of translucent "I"[9]- and dense "A"[10]-segments. The center of each I-segment is occupied by a dense disc, the "Z"-band[11], while the center of each A-segment is occupied by a relatively translucent "H"-band[12] which in turn contains a relatively dense "M"-disc[13]. The segments between two successive Z-bands are the functional units of myofibrils and are termed "sarcomeres".

Under high magnification, each sarcomere of a *relaxed myofibril* (Fig. B) is seen to consist of a bundle of interlocking thin[1] and thick[2] "myofilaments". The thin filaments are free at one end[3] but attached at the other to the "Z"-line[4], which seems to be nothing else but a series of junctions or interlocking loops between the frayed ends of the thin filaments of two neighbouring sarcomeres; they have a diameter of 50–60 Å, a length of 2 μ and are made of actin, a protein. The thick filaments are free at both ends and possess numerous short

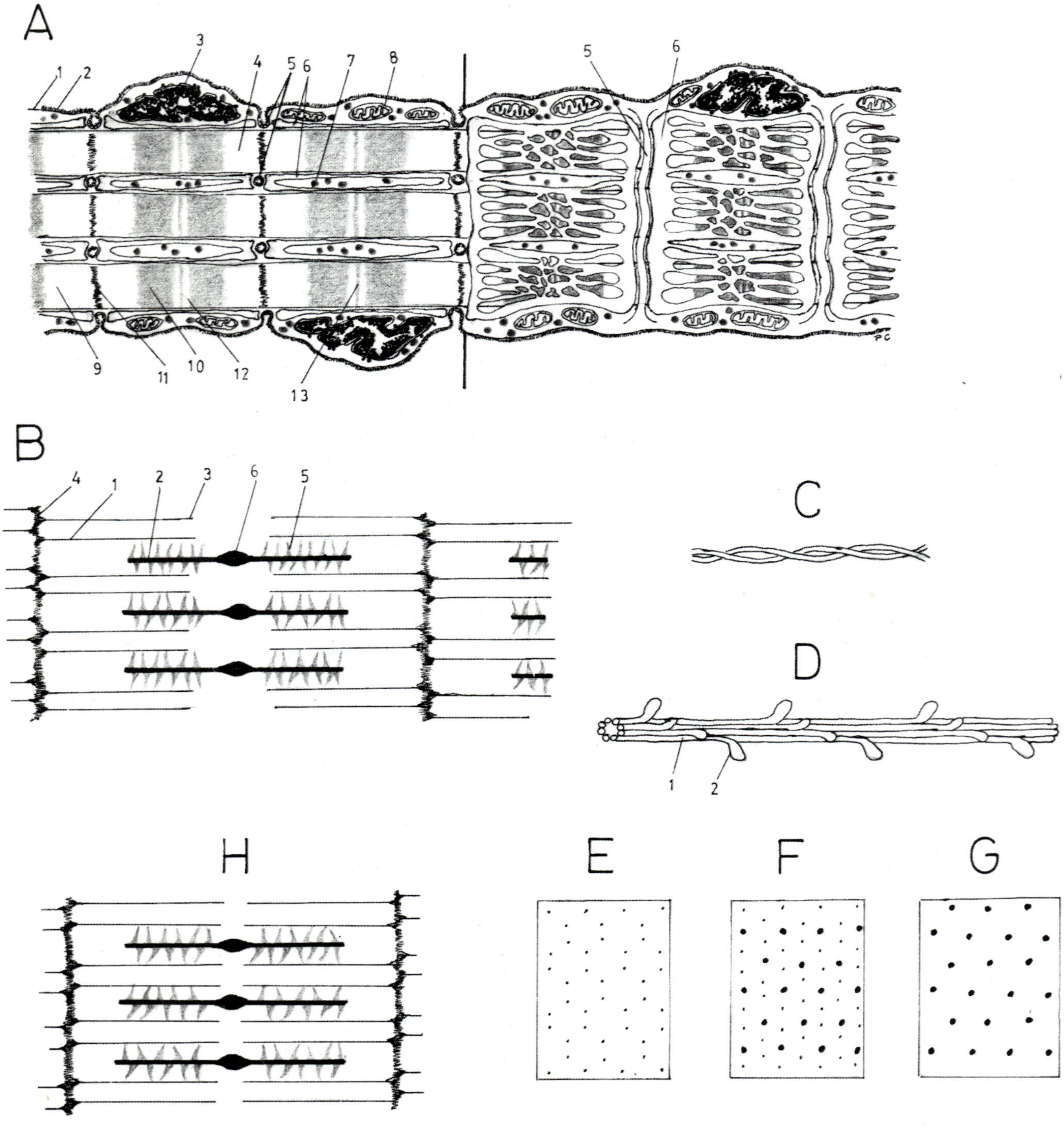

Plate 21

lateral projections, the "cross bridges"[5] through which they brush against the adjacent actin filaments. They have a knob-like thickening of uncertain composition in their center[6] which is responsible for the "M"-disc, a diameter of 100 Å, a length of 1.5 μ and are made primarily of myosin, another protein. Each actin filament represents a pair of spirally intertwined threads with globular subunits (Fig. C). By contrast, every myosin filament is a bundle of golf-stick-like myosin molecules (Fig. D) that consist of slender long stems[1], the "L-meromyosin" parts, and stubby bent ends[2], the "H-meromyosin" parts which possess ATP-ase activity and represent the laterally projecting cross-bridges of the thick filaments; within each thick filament, the myosin molecules are arranged in such a regular manner that their protruding H-meromyosin ends follow a spiral line around the filament.

Inspection of Fig. B and of cross-sections of myofibrils at various levels show that the translucent I-segments of the myofibrils consist of thin filaments only (Fig. E), the dense A-segments of thin and thick filaments mostly (Fig. F), and the H-zones in the centers of the A-segments of thick filaments only (Fig. G). The cross-sections also show the extremely regular stacking of the myofilaments within the myofibrils, each myosin filament being surrounded by six actin filaments in the dense (mixed) segments of mammalian sarcomeres (Fig. F).

In the sarcomere of the *contracted myofibril* (Fig. H) the free ends of the thin actin filaments of both sides have slid past the thick myosin filaments towards the sarcomere center and each other and the distance between the two bounding Z-lines has consequently shortened. As a result, the translucent I-segments have shortened and the H-zones have disappeared. In "supercontraction", where the sarcomere shortens to less than the length of the myosin filaments, *e.g.* to 1.4 or 1.3 μ, the latter seem to either bend back (as in chicks) or to perforate the Z-bands (as in barnacles).

At their ends, the muscle fibers develop several invaginations. Attached to the plasma membrane of the bottoms and sides of these pouches are the collagen fibrils that connect muscle to bone; attached to the same sites of the plasma membrane from inside are the ends of the myofibrils.

(2) Function

Contraction occurs as follows: The surface of the relaxed (unexcited) muscle fiber presents a negative electric potential of −70 mV, *i.e.* it is "polarised".

When the fiber is excited to contract by the arrival of a nervous impulse the following chain reaction is initiated: (1) the local permeability for Na^+ ions of the fiber's plasma membrane (PM) at the site of the neuromuscular junction increases as a result of the firing of acetylcholine against the PM by the nerve ending; (2) the locally increased Na^+ permeability allows a local "invasion" of the fiber by Na^+ ions from outside and at the same time a local leakage of some K^+ out of the fiber; (3) the influx of Na^+ ions causes a local loss of electronegative surface potential of the fiber, and a change from −70 mV to +40 mV at that site, *i.e.* a "depolarisation"; (4) the above event causes a tiny current to flow between the depolarised (*i.e.* no longer negative) excited surface site and the neighbouring still polarised (*i.e.* still negative) non-excited surface site; (5) as a result of the current flow, the neighbouring site rapidly loses electrons and becomes less and less electronegative; when its surface potential drops from −70 mV to −50 mV, its permeability for outside Na^+ ions suddenly increases, allowing a local influx of Na^+ ions which depolarise it; (6) as the above process is repeated over and over again, a wave of depolarisation sweeps over the surface of the muscle fiber; (7) the depolarisation reaches the T-tubules and spreads along the latter into the fiber interior where it is transmitted to the adjacent sarcoplasmic reticulum (SR) systems; (8) depolarisation of the SR systems causes a release of Ca^{++} ions from the SR sacs on to the myofibril surfaces; added to these endogenous (SR-derived) Ca^{++} ions are apparently also some exogenous Ca^{++} ions that reach the myofibrils from outside the muscle fiber through the T-tubules and through the depolarised surface membrane (along with the inflowing Na^+ ions); (9) the Ca^{++} ions reach the thick myofilaments and activate the ATP-ase in the protruding H-meromyosin parts of the myosin molecules; (10) the activated ATP-ase in the thick myofilaments splits ATP into ADP + Phosphate, releasing energy for the sliding of the myosin between the actin filaments, *i.e.* for the contraction of the sarcomeres; the actual mechanism of sliding is still unknown, but the spiral arrangement of the "cross bridges" along the thick filaments suggests the possibility of a screw-like rotation and propulsion of the latter along the surrounding thin filaments.

After contraction has occurred, "cation pumps" located in the membranes of the muscle fiber will pump out the Na^+ and exogenous Ca^{++} ions that entered the fiber and will pump in the K^+ ions that were lost from the fiber during contraction, thus re-establishing the original status quo; simultaneously the endogenous Ca^{++} ions are returned to the SR sacs from which they were extruded. Since these ion movements have to take place against osmotic concentration gradients, they require energy, which is apparently provided through the splitting of ATP by ATPases such as those that have been localised in the membrane of the SR close to the plasma membrane of the fiber. At the same time, ATP is resynthesized from ADP + Phosphate presumably in the mitochondria through energy released from the oxidation of carbohydrate (the glycogen next to the myofibrils). Dur-

A

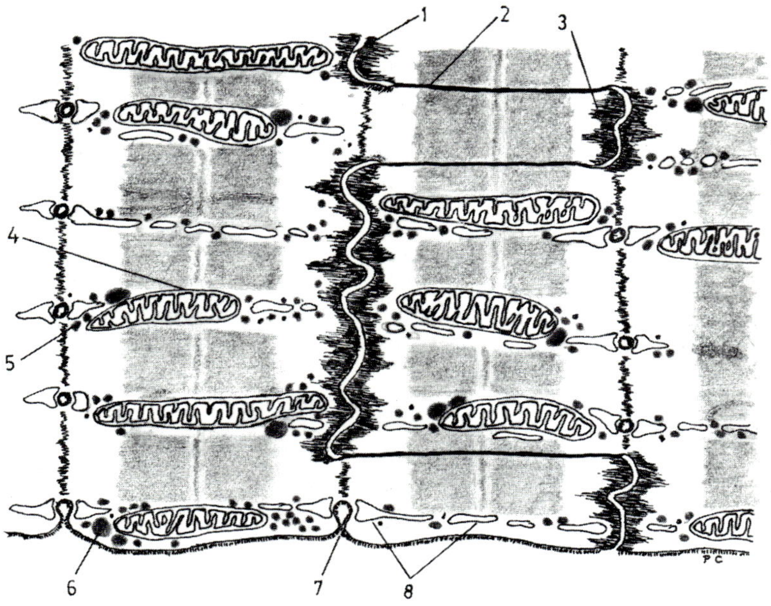

B

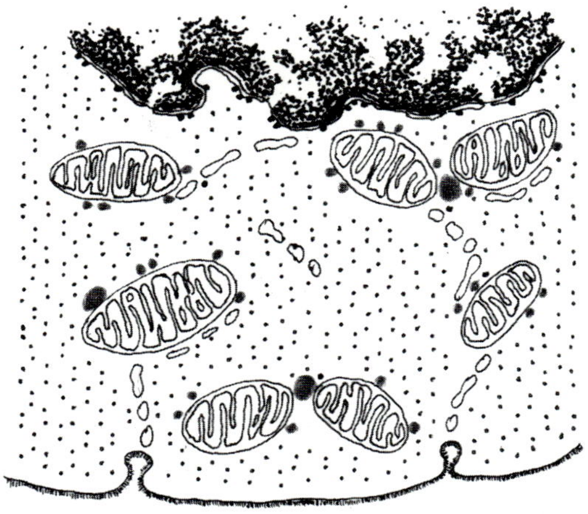

C

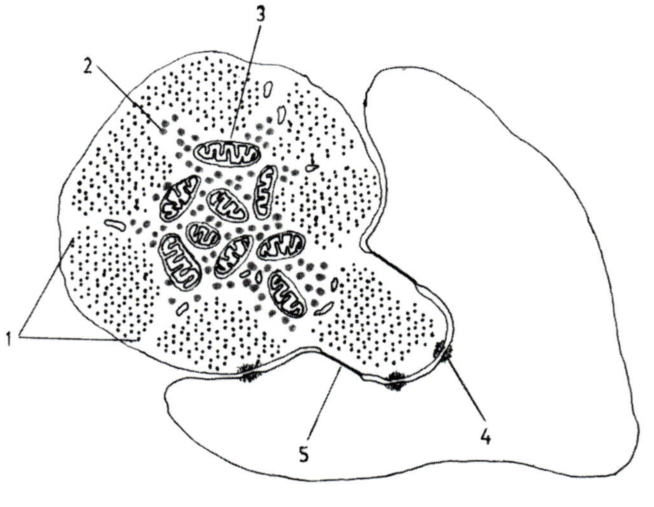

Plate 22

ing the above ionic reconstitution period, which lasts about 10 msec, the muscle fiber is refractory to renewed excitation and contraction.

Origin. The muscle fiber is really a multinucleated giant cell arising from the fusion of several spindle-shaped ribosome-rich embryonic cells, the "myoblasts". The newly created muscle fibers acquire myofilaments gradually, as a result of synthetic activity by ribosomes which are situated mostly in their terminal sarcoplasm; as the number of myofilaments increases, the number of ribosomes decreases. Postnatally, muscle seems to grow in size not so much by the creation of new muscle fibers but by the widening and lengthening (hypertrophy) of those already laid down prenatally. Both types of growth seem to originate at the ends of the fiber. Muscle fibers grow wider by the formation and lateral apposition of more myofibrils, and they grow longer by the generation of new sarcomeres at the ends of the myofibrils. They hook up to tendons by the generation of collagen fibrils within narrow pockets at the fiber ends; it is quite possible, though not yet proven, that some of the collagen fibrils that appear within such pockets are synthesized by the ribosomes of the muscle fiber itself.

In *regeneration* following destruction of skeletal muscle, embryonic myoblasts reappear seemingly "out of nowhere" and divide repeatedly by mitosis to form long chains of new cells which then fuse to create new myotubes. The origin of these myoblasts is not yet entirely elucidated. There is evidence that under certain circumstances some of them develop from surviving nuclei that "pinch off" the injured muscle fiber, but it appears that very commonly the dividing nuclei may belong to hidden "reserve" myoblasts which are pressed against the muscle fiber and masquerade as parts of its own nuclear complement, the "satellite" cells. The latter also seem to mitose and fuse with the myotube, thus providing it with more nuclei, during its period of postnatal growth.

Some types of injury (*e.g.* limb amputation) cause *dedifferentiation* of muscle fibers in amphibia, with concomitant loss of all myofilaments, vigorous ribosome production, and separation into single cells; this is soon followed by proliferation and redifferentiation with polyribosomal synthesis of new myofilaments.

The *denervation* of skeletal muscle fibers leads to their severe atrophy through a series of changes involving first the appearance of lysosomes and autophagosomes, then the development of multilamellar packs of smooth cisternae, and finally the gradual dissolution of their myofibrils. Similar atrophy changes develop in certain sex-dependent muscles after *castration.*

Muscle fibers appear to pick up *fatty acids* (through an unknown mechanism) and use them as fuel for energy; prolonged infusions of *norepinephrine* induce the development of appreciable numbers of lipid bodies without envelopes in muscle fibers, probably because by raising the plasma concentration of fatty acids they cause increased entry of these molecules into the muscle fibers and thus increased synthesis of triglycerides within the latter.

III. CARDIAC MUSCLE – ORDINARY

(1) Structure (Plate 22, Fig. A)

The structure is similar to that of skeletal muscle with the following differences: The units of cardiac muscle are not multinucleated giant fibers (as in skeletal muscle) but mononuclear elongated and branched fibers, each corresponding to one cell and each attached firmly to the other end-to-end through desmosomes[1] and tight junctions[2]. The desmosomes serve to create mechanical cohesion between the joined cells (a function enhanced by their winding, suture-like profiles), while the tight junctions serve to transmit the contraction impulse from one cell to the next. At the desmosomes, the terminal membranes of the joined cells are separated by a gap of about 200 Å while their myofilaments seem to attach to the terminal membranes embedded in an abundant dense material[3] – which is responsible for the appearance of the "intercalated discs" of the L/M. The desmosomal gaps are bisected by central plates that connect through many small side arms with the plasma membranes of the cells on either side, thus increasing intercellular cohesion at these sites. While the desmosomes always occupy a transverse position in relation to the length axis of the unicellular muscle fibers, the tight junctions are oriented longitudinally, *i.e.* they represent side contacts between the terminal processes of neighbouring fibers.

As in skeletal muscle, the contractile elements are thin actin and thick myosin myofilaments organized in typical sarcomeres with A- and I-segments and Z-lines as already described, but, unlike skeletal muscle, the myofilaments are *not* packed in discrete bundles (*i.e.* myofibrils); instead, they form a continuous pool of filaments, all in register from one side of the fiber to the other. Scattered *throughout* this pool of filaments (not just at its periphery) is an enormous number of mitochondria[4] (much greater than in skeletal muscle) which are intimately surrounded by glycogen granules[5] and lipid globules[6] and can be of giant size in animals with very rapid heart beat. Traversing the sarcoplasm also are T-tubules[7] lined by surface coat and SR system; this consists of a simple network of thin tubules[8] scattered among the myofilaments and coming into close contact with the Z-discs of myofilament bundles (to which they reportedly attach with short threads), T-tubules and intercalated discs at many sites. The nucleus is located deep in the cytoplasm as can be seen in a cross-section of a fiber at the level of an I-segment (Fig. B). It is very

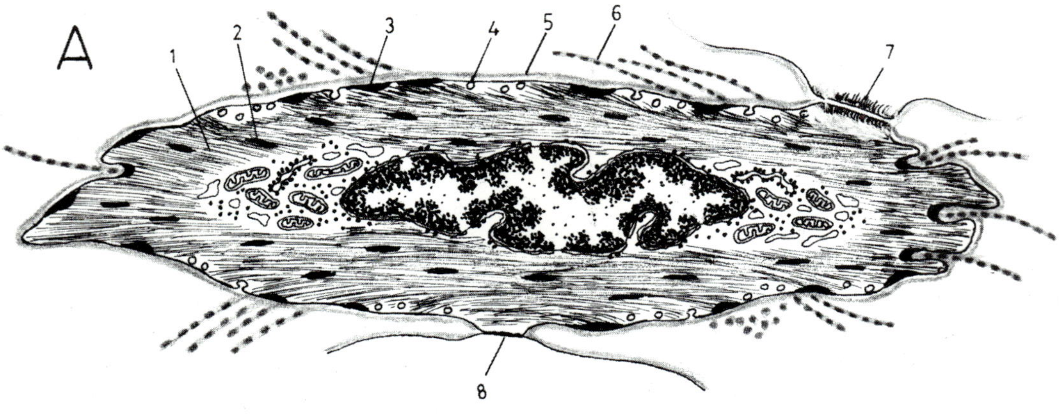

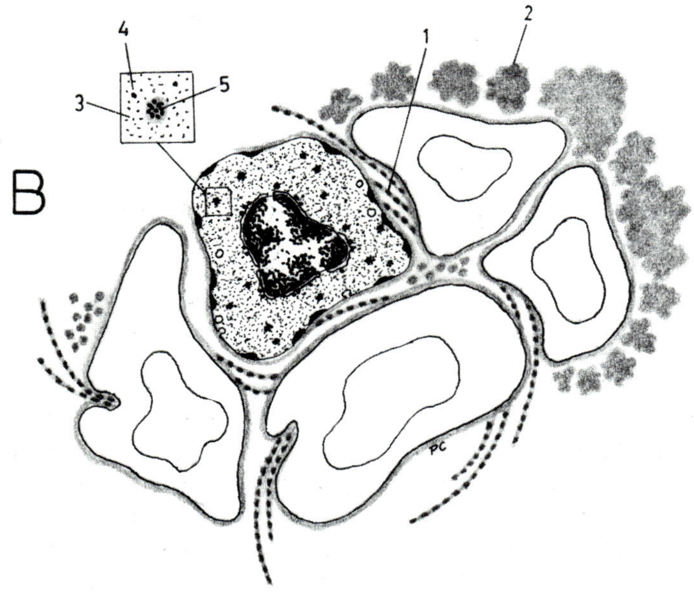

Plate 23

interesting that neuromuscular junctions have been seen in the myocardium and that granules of a catecholamine type are often found in the fibers of vertebrates, particularly in the atria. As cardiac muscle fibers age they accumulate lipofuscin bodies, certain cytosegresome-like structures that also accumulate in ageing neurons (see Ch. 6, Nervous Tissue, Sect. II, 1, Cytoplasm (perikaryon), p. 73).

(2) Function

Cardiac muscle *contracts* through the same mechanism as that operating in skeletal muscle. The much greater *mitochondrial population* of cardiac as compared to skeletal muscle probably reflects the much higher level of oxidative activity in the former in view of its continuous action 24 hours a day. The *lipid* globules close to the mitochondria represent stores of high energy fuel and appear to be synthesized in the SR and the mitochondria from fatty acids entering the muscle cell, as shown by autoradiographic studies with labeled oleic acid; thus, the great increment of mitochondrial size induced by polyunsaturated fatty acid deficiency may represent a compensatory organelle hypertrophy.

In vitro experiments indicate that calcium is essential to the integrity of the *zonulae adherentes* in the intercalated discs, since the latter will open when the calcium concentration of the perfusing fluid falls below a certain minimum level.

Myocardial hypertrophy induced by enhanced work is associated with an increased ribosome, myofilament, SR sac and mitochondrial population and a focal or uniform widening of the Z-zone which is probably due to the formation of new sarcomeres in this area of the fiber; similarly, digoxin (which enhances myocardial work) also causes increased mitochondrial numbers.

Under normal conditions, the nuclei of adult myocardial fibers only very rarely take up labelled thymidine, *i.e.* they exhibit a very low rate of DNA synthesis, but when a part of the myocardium becomes necrotic (as in infarction), the nuclei of all surrounding fibers start synthesizing new DNA intensively. Since they are incapable of mitosis, however, these nuclei merely enlarge into giant polyploid shapes and their fibers do not divide.

The function of the cored catecholamine-like *granules of atrial muscle* is still a mystery; perhaps they are secreted into the bloodstream to help regulate its pressure and are thus part of one of the "barostat" mechanisms of the body.

Among the changes of the chemical environment with the most dramatic effect on heart muscle are elevations of the ambient *potassium* concentration; perfusions of this tissue with solutions containing more than 12 mmoles/l K^+ cause irreversible disintegration of the thin myofilaments.

IV. CARDIAC MUSCLE – CONDUCTING STRUCTURE AND FUNCTION (Plate 22)

(1) The sinuatrial node, the A-V node and the proximal part of the common bundle

They consist of networks of slender striated fibers, similar in structure to but smaller in size than ordinary cardiac muscle fibers.

(2) The fibers of the distal part of the common bundle and the Purkinje fibers (Plate 22, Fig. C)

These fibers are distinguished from ordinary cardiac muscle fibers by (a) being larger than ordinary fibers, (b) having a cytoplasmic matrix of lower density, (c) having myofilaments which are sparse, bundled into discrete myofibrils[1] and located mostly in the fiber periphery, (d) having more glycogen[2], and having it concentrated along with the mitochondria[3] in the central area of the fiber, (e) often invaginating lateral processes into neighbouring fibers and attaching to them through desmosomes[4] and tight junctions[5], and (f) lacking T-tubules in many mammalian species. At their terminations the Purkinje fibers assume the structure of ordinary cardiac fibers.

V. SMOOTH MUSCLE

(1) Structure (Plate 23, Fig. A)

The smooth muscle unit is an elongated cell with a single central nucleus (myocyte) whose ultrastructure is unsettled but now under very active exploration. After routine processing, vertebrate smooth muscle (unlike vertebrate skeletal muscle) exhibits myofilaments of apparently only one, thin, type[1], but under special conditions, *e.g.* acid pH or rapid fixation in highly concentrated glutaraldehyde, it shows filaments of two types of diameter: 30–65 Å (the majority) and 80–200 Å (the remainder). Furthermore, recent studies of unfixed smooth muscle after ethylene dehydration (a procedure thought to preserve tropomyosin B, an easily lost soluble component of myosin) clearly demonstrate the existence of very thick myosin-like filaments in mammalian smooth muscle. Thus, the findings with specially fixed or unfixed smooth muscle suggest that thick myosin filaments are scattered among thin actin ones and slide relative to one another, as in skeletal muscle. It should be noted, however, that although both actin and myosin have been shown to exist in smooth muscle (the latter with immunohisto-chemical light microscopic as well as chemical extraction techniques), the chemical composition of the various types of filaments in terms of these two proteins, and their spatial relationships to one another are just beginning to be elucidated. Scattered (a) throughout the cytoplasm[2] and (b) along the plasma membrane (PM)[3] are elongated dense bodies which seem to represent mostly thick segments of myofilaments embedded in a dense material and either bundled together or attached to the PM; this interpretation is supported by the fact that (a) the dense bodies resemble the "Z"-line material of skeletal muscle and the dense material of desmosomes, and (b) that when smooth muscle cells contract, invaginations of the PM develop at PM sites occupied by dense bodies, as if the myofilaments were "pulling" on the PM at such sites.

The smooth muscle cell is further characterised by (a) local accumulations of abundant ribosomes, a few RER-cisternae, a few glycogen granules and some smooth endoplasmic reticulum and mitochondria at both ends of the nucleus, (b) tiny invaginations and vesicles of the pinocytotic type[4] at the PM, (c) a polysaccharide coat (basement membrane)[5] around the PM, with collagen fibrils attached to it[6], and (d) occasional junctions of the "zonula adherens"[7] or the "zonula occludens"[8] type with other smooth muscle cells. Cross-sections (Fig. B) show to advantage how smooth muscle cells are harnessed to each other by collagen fibrils that take off and land on their surfaces[1], their close association with elastin[2] (in vessel walls), and – at high magnification under the proper conditions – the two types of myofilaments (thin[3] and thick[4]) as well as the substructure of the "dense bodies"[5].

(2) Function

The smooth muscle cells are less specialised than skeletal or cardiac muscle. These relatively undifferentiated cells are apparently capable not only of contraction but also of impulse transmission, collagen and elastin production and of intensive proliferation after proper stimulation – notably after injury of some myocytes.

The mechanism of *contraction* of myocytes, like the structural organisation and the chemical composition of their filaments, is still obscure, but structural changes during contraction begin to be described. Thus, evidence has been presented that under certain conditions relaxed fixed myocytes exhibit only thin (30 Å) filaments, whereas in contracted myocytes both thin (30 Å) and thick (80 Å) filaments materialise.

Impulse transmission from one myocyte to the next is apparently occurring at the tight junctions (zonulae occludentes or "nexuses") which represent low resistance pathways. Impulse transmission seems to be blocked when the junctions are ruptured by certain agents. The ability of myocytes to transmit the contraction stimulus to one another explains how all the cells in the muscle coat of a given vessel or intestinal wall segment can contract even though only some of them are stimulated by nerves, and it also explains automatic (peristaltic) movements of hollow muscular organs in the absence of nervous stimulation.

The ability of smooth muscle cells in certain organs (*e.g.* in vessel walls) to produce *collagen and elastin* is demonstrated, among other things, by the fact that (a) in the media of normal artery walls the only cells present are myocytes, therefore no other cells could produce the collagen fibrils and elastin lamellae scattered between (and attached to) the smooth muscle cells, and (b) when the artery walls are injured, their muscular component proliferates giving visibly rise to new collagen and new elastic masses among the regenerating smooth muscle cells. This view is further reinforced by the finding that estrogen increases both the ribosome-rough endoplasmic reticulum system within and collagen formation around uterine smooth muscle myocytes.

Smooth muscle cells in reproductive organs are very sensitive to and display marked E/M changes under *hormonal growth stimulation*. Thus, both estrogen and pregnancy cause marked proliferation and an enormous increment in the ribosome population of uterine myocytes (as expected in view of the greatly increased need for new organelle synthesis in these rapidly growing cells); furthermore, pregnancy appreciably increases the number of glycogen granules in uterine myocytes, presumably in anticipation of the need for this material during the contractions of delivery.

Embryonic myocytes are extremely rich in ribosomes but the numbers of the latter greatly diminish when the myofilaments appear. Finally, as myocytes *age* they tend to accumulate phospholipid, a change possibly related to the increasing accumulation of lipofuscin granules in their cytoplasm.

Chapter 6

Nervous Tissue

I. GENERAL

Nervous tissue consists of *neurons* and their processes, the *dendrites* and *axons*, through which they receive and emit impulses. Specialized contacts between neuronal processes or between neuronal processes and neuronal or other cell bodies (*synapses*) make possible the transmission of impulses between neurons and between neurons and other cells. The neurons and their processes are surrounded and enveloped by *glia cells*; the latter insulate neurons, produce *myelin sheaths* for many of their axons and probably service them in several as yet unexplored ways.

The central nervous system (brain and spinal cord) contains communicating, fluid-filled *central cavities, i.e.* the ventricles and the spinal canal; these cavities are lined by a single layer of *ependymal cells* which produce the cerebrospinal fluid in them. Of the two components that can be distinguished by naked eye inspection in brain and spinal cord, the *grey substance* is made of neurons, glia cells and mainly unmyelinated neuronal processes, whereas the *white substance* consists of glia cells and mainly myelinated axons.

In the peripheral nervous system, *nerves* are composed of (a) bundles of axons, (b) peri-axonal peripheral glia cells (Schwann cells) with or without myelin production, and (c) connective tissue between axons (endoneurium), around axon bundles (perineurium), and around the whole nerve (epineurium); *ganglions* are composed of (a) neurons and their processes, (b) peri-neuronal glia cells (satellite cells), and (c) connective tissue.

All cells of nervous tissue are derived from the outer embryonic layer (ectoderm).

II. NEURON – STRUCTURE

(1) Cytoplasm (perikaryon) (Plate 24, Fig. A)

The most prominent features are (a) groups of *cisternae*[1] of rough endoplasmic reticulum (RER) with numerous *polyribosomes*[2] between them (the "Nissl bodies" of light microscopy), (b) mostly elongated *mitochondria*[3] with remarkably rare matrix granules and frequently longitudinal cristae, (c) *microtubules*[4] with a diameter of 200–260 Å, a 60 Å thick wall apparently made of 12–13 stacked filaments, and sometimes a visible central thin core that appears as a central dot in cross-sections (inset A_1), (d) *neurofilaments*[5] of a 100 Å diameter, which at high resolution prove to be tubules with a 30 Å thick wall of globular substructure and radiating spoke-like processes (cross-section in inset A_2), and (e) multiple *Golgi areas*[6] often associated with coated ("alveolate") vesicles, multivesicular bodies and – in some neurons – cored neurosecretory vesicles.

The coated vesicles seem to be of two kinds: (a) *small coated vesicles*[7] (500–600 Å) that contain acid phosphatase and have an external honeycombed coat which in sections creates the appearance of numerous bristles attached to the outer vesicle surface; they seem to arise from the Golgi cisternae since the dilated ends of the latter often exhibit a coat of bristles; (b) *large coated vesicles*[8] (1000 Å) which do not contain acid phosphatase and appear to arise from the cell surface by pinocytosis-like invagination[9]. The *multivesicular bodies*[10] sometimes show a partial coat of bristles and have been seen to store marker proteins (ferritin, peroxidase) presented to neurons in culture; they seem to arise from the coalescence of small and large coated vesicles; they are considered the functional equivalent of "secondary lysosomes" resulting from the union of "primary lysosome" equivalents (small coated vesicles) with "phagosome" equivalents (large coated vesicles). The *neurosecretory cored vesicles*[11] (1200–1500 Å) occur in hypothalamic neurons, where they develop in the Golgi region.

Other structures commonly seen in adult neuron cytoplasm are (a) *lysosomes*[12] with dense matrix (of the classical type that occurs in macrophages and other cells), (b) *lipofuscin granules*[13], which are membrane-bound granules with a dense matrix and a variable number of low density inclusions, seem to arise from lysosomes that incorporate phospholipids (notably phosphatidylethanolamine), and greatly increase in numbers with ageing. Arguments for an autophagosome or cyto-

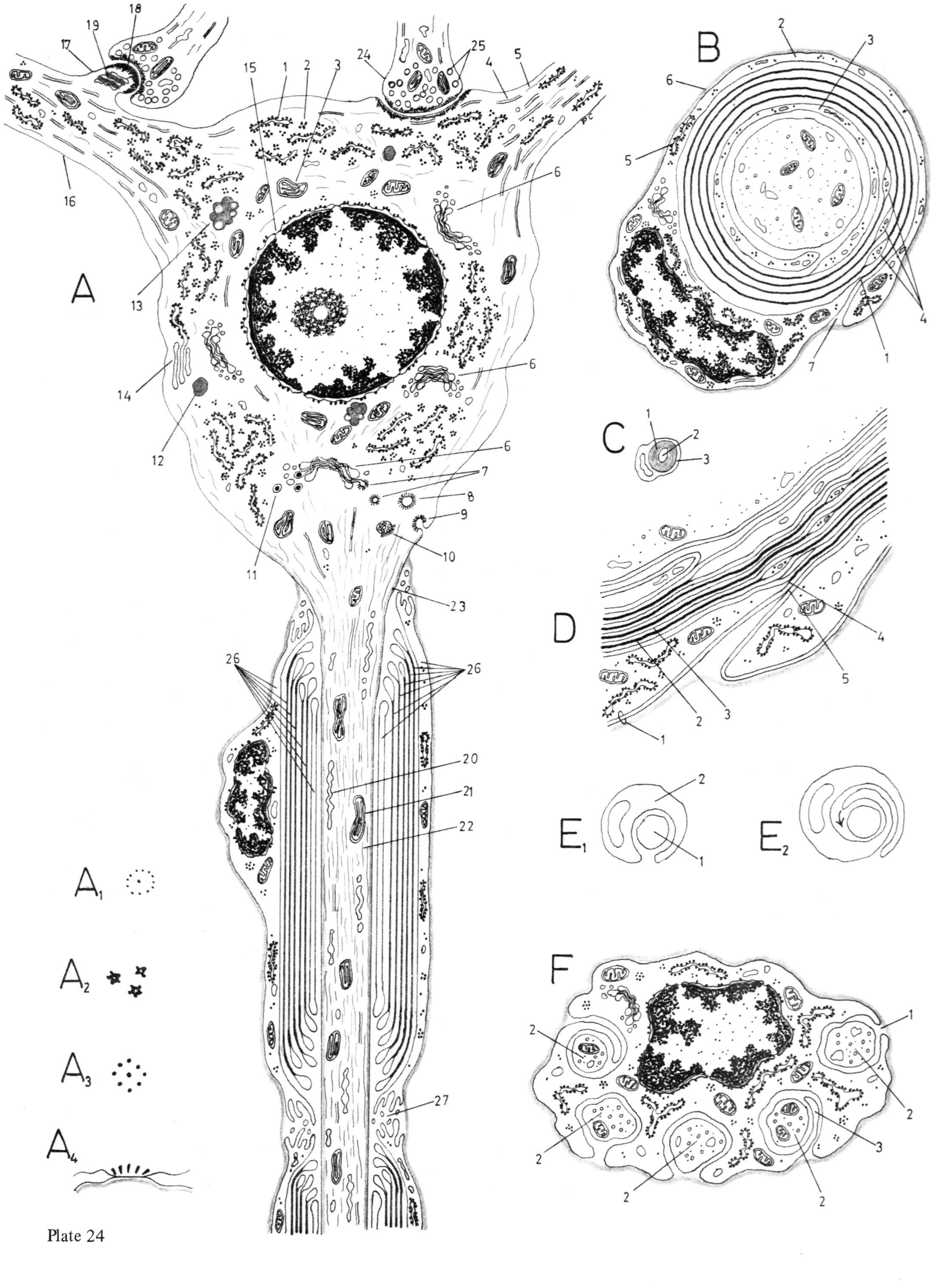

Plate 24

segresome role of the lipofuscin bodies include their display of some hydrolytic enzyme activity, their structural similarity to cytosegresomes of other cells, and their experimental production by prolonged, severe hypoxia.

Finally, the following structures occasionally materialise in neurons of various mammals: (a) small stacks of smooth *sub-surface cisternae*[14], apparently in communication with the closest RER-systems, (b) *modified cilia* with a core of only 9 microtubule pairs ("9 + 0" type) and a centrosome often attached at a right angle to their basal body, (c) *inclusions* of a laminated (fingerprint-like) or fibrillary knot type, (d) membrane-enclosed *"cylindroid bodies" i.e.* spiral rolls of pentalaminar membrane apparently originating from the fusion of 2 unit membranes and seemingly representing residual autophagosomes, and (e) *"neuromelanin"* pigment granules which are structurally similar to lipofuscin granules and abound in the neurons of the Substantia Nigra and the Locus Cœruleus.

(2) Nucleus (Plate 24, Fig. A)

The nuclear envelope is characterised by round 700 Å "pores"[15] that are closed by thin diaphragms which show a central density in "en face" views (inset A_3) and a crown of stamen-like rodlets growing outwards from their margins in profile views (inset A_4). On its inner aspect, the envelope is lined by a fibrous lamina (inset A_4).

In the nucleus interior, focal tangles of 200 Å *chromatin* (DNA) strands are separated by a cotton-like *interchromatin matrix* constituted of even finer filaments and containing scattered "interchromatinic" or "perichromatinic" granules 200–350 Å thick (see Ch. 2, The Cell, Sect. I, General ultrastructure, p. 9).

The nucleolus consists of a *granular* (150–200 Å granules) and a fibrillar (amorphous) part, both containing RNA. The fact that it is always prominent in neurons indicates that a very intensive protein synthesis is going on constantly in these cells. In neurons of female animals, the XX-chromosome (sex chromatin) may be visible as a *paranucleolar satellite.*

(3) Dendrites (Plate 24, Fig. A)

Dendrites[16] contain (a) most of the *standard cytoplasmic organelles* (although their numbers decrease with increasing distance from the cell body), (b) *numerous microtubules* (their most characteristic component), and (c) *a few neurofilaments*. They form numerous processes called *"spines"*[17] which often show a bulbous terminal supported by a thin neck, and rapidly increase in numbers with increasing distance from the cell body, reaching a total number of up to 4,000/neuron and representing more than 40% of the total neuronal surface in some instances. Since most synapses of a neuron occur at the spines[18] and the stems of its dendrites, spines possibly represent an increment of the neuronal surface which is available for synaptic contact. Spines often contain packs of 2–3 smooth cisternae alternating with dense laminae and called "spine apparatuses"[19]. At their terminations, dendrites sometimes form enlargements packed with enormous numbers of mitochondria with longitudinal cristae, the so called "growing terminals".

(4) Axons (Plate 24, Fig. A)

The cytoplasm within an axon is also termed "axoplasm". Large axons are distinguished from dendrites in containing (a) only smooth endoplasmic reticulum (*i.e. vesicles and "varicose" tubes*)[20] and elongated *mitochondria*[21], no RER or ribosomes, (b) *numerous neurofilaments*[22] (their main component), and (c) only *a few microtubules* (*i.e.* the reverse composition of that of dendrites). As their diameter decreases, however, the number of neurofilaments decreases to the point where the smallest unmyelinated axon twigs contain only a few microtubules and are therefore difficult to differentiate from small dendrite branches. Running directly underneath the plasma membrane (axolemma) of the proximal (initial) segment of axons is a 100 Å thick dense *undercoat*[23]. At their synapsing ends, the *axon terminals* enlarge somewhat to form a bulbous expansion (the "bouton")[24] which is filled with *synaptic vesicles* of various types[25]. The synaptic vesicles contain impulse-transmitting chemicals which somehow move out of the axon terminals to reach and stimulate the neurons with which the axons synapse (see Sect. IV on synapses for details, p. 78).

Embryonic neuron processes grow at their distal tips rather than their proximal parts, through the incorporation of new membrane that has at first very few or no intramembranous particles, but acquires more and more of the latter as it matures. It is probable that the new membrane material is built into the PM of the growing tips through the exocytosis of smooth vesicles that originate in Golgi elements of the pericaryon and travel down the processes – as has been found to be the case for growing processes of embryonal glial cells.

(5) Schwann cells and myelin sheaths of axons (Plate 24, Figs. A–E)

Axons can be either myelinated (Figs. A–D) or unmyelinated (Fig. E). *Myelinated axons* (Fig. A) are wrapped in a multilayered sheath made of the extremely attenuated sheet-like cytoplasm of Schwann cells[26] (a type of glia cells) that spirals and winds itself tightly around the axon (as shown in Fig. B, which is a cross-section of Fig. A at the level of a Schwann cell nucleus). The spiralling

Schwann cell sheet (Fig. B) has been reduced to a thin film consisting of the fusion of two plasma membranes [1] due to the squeezing-out of all cytoplasm between them. Only the first turn [2], the last turn [3] around the axon and certain spots in intermediate turns [4], the so called "Schmitt–Lanterman clefts" (SLC), contain sparse amounts of cytoplasm; the significance of the SLC is still obscure, but they may represent spiral streams of cytoplasm that connect the first with the last turn. Such a hypothesis is supported by the recent finding that the protein tracer peroxidase reaches the axon travelling via the SLC. Schwann cells contain moderate numbers of ribosomes, mitochondria and smooth vesicles and an appreciable number of rough endoplasmic reticulum (RER) cisternae [5]; the outermost surface of the cylindrical laminated sheath they form around the axon is covered by a glucoprotein-rich basement membrane [6] that also bridges over the narrow celft (the "mesaxon") [7] which marks the beginning of the potential space between the spiralling turns of the Schwann cell cytoplasm; finally collagen fibrils surround the Schwann cell sheaths in nerves, presumably produced by the "endoneurial" fibroblasts found within these structures.

The fact that the spiral sheath consists almost entirely of plasma membranes (PMs) makes it extraordinarily rich in lipids, especially phospholipids; when viewed under the light microscope (Fig. C) it, therefore, appears as a thick coat of lipid or a *"myelin sheath"* [1] around the axon [2], wrapped in a very thin film of Schwann cell cytoplasm [3] (the "neurilemma").

At high E/M magnification (Fig. D) capable of resolving the trilaminar structure of the unit membrane [1], the myelin sheath shows an extremely regular pattern of "major dense" lines [2] alternating with lighter "intraperiod lines" [3], with a periodicity of *ca.* 180 Å in peripheral and *ca.* 160 Å in central axons. The "major dense lines" are formed by the apposition of the inner leaflets of two PMs that belong to the same spiral turn [4], while the lighter "intraperiod lines" are formed by the apposition of the outer leaflets of two PMs that belong to neighbouring spiral turns [5].

It takes many Schwann cells to complete the myelin sheath of an axon. At the loose boundary between two neighbouring Schwann cells, the so called "node of Ranvier", the axon is briefly deprived of its myelin sheath and covered only by a thin glycoprotein film (see item 27 of Fig. A) while the Schwann cell ends break up into several villi.

The spiral sheaths (Fig. E_1) seem to be formed (a) by the incorporation of axons [1] in grooves of Schwann cells [2], and (b) by the continuous proliferation of one lip of the groove that forces it to slip between the other lip and the axon (Fig. E_2) and grow in a spiral direction. The myelin sheaths for the axons of the central nervous system (CNS) are provided by the oligodendroglia cells, apparently in the same manner as Schwann cells produce the myelin sheaths of axons in the peripheral nervous system.

In both CNS and nerves myelinisation is a slow process that starts late in fetal life and continues for many months after birth before it reaches completion.

Unmyelinated axons (Fig. F) are simply situated within grooves of Schwann cells [1], usually several axons [2] to one Schwann cell. Although some groove lips [3] attempt to grow around the axon, they never spiral around it nor do they lose the cytoplasm between their two limiting membranes. Acetylcholinesterase has been demonstrated in the cleft between axolemma and Schwann cell PM, in unmyelinated autonomic axons.

III. NEURON – FUNCTION

The unusually prominent *RER* and *Golgi* system of neurons is apparently the structural expression of an extremely active and continuous synthesis and secretion of protein derivatives or nitrogenous compounds by these cells. The materials in question are either secreted at synaptic sites on to the surface of other neurons, which they depolarise and thus stimulate (as in the case of the "transmitter" substances norepinephrine and acetylcholine), or they are secreted into the blood stream and they reach and stimulate distant cells (as in the case of the "neurosecretory" polypeptides oxytocin and vasopressin). "Neurosecretory" hormones are proven to condense in the Golgi from which they detach and travel down the axon as large vesicles with dense cores, but it is not certain yet where the smaller "transmitter" molecules are created and bottled into synaptic vesicles; it is quite possible that the latter are made at the axon terminal from polypeptides or amino acids that are manufactured in the RER and travel down the axon and that the axonal SER provides unit membrane for their enclosure into vesicles. There is actual autoradiographic evidence for the existence of such an "axon flow" since labeled amino acids (leucine and lysine) made available to neurons appeared first in the perinuclear cytoplasm and later travelled down into the axon. Recent studies indicate that different molecules travel with different speeds down the axon and that the axon flow rate of *e.g.* [^{3}H] fucose glucoprotein is of the order of 130 mm/day (from pericaryon to synapse.) The abundance of free *ribosomes* in the neuron probably expresses a high production rate of enzymes and internal unit membrane involved in synthesis, transport and wrapping of continuously consumed (secreted) transmitter substances and neurosecretory hormones. It is interesting that when the transmitter substance norepinephrine is depleted through the action of reserpine, the Golgi enlarges and the activity of dopamine-synthesizing enzymes increases, presumably in an attempt at compensation.

Of the neuronal processes, the *dendrites* usually receive impulses from other neurons, while the *axons* usually transmit impulses to other neurons through the release of the transmitter substances from the synaptic vesicles contained in their terminals (see Sect. IV on synapses for details).

Impulses are generated at synaptic sites on the surface of a neuron by the depolarising effect of transmitter substances released from the axon terminal of another. They are thought to spread along the length of unmyelinated neuronal processes as waves of depolarisation, in the manner already described for impulse transmission in muscle; in myelinated axons, however, the impulse is believed to jump from one Ranvier's node to the next, thus travelling much faster ("saltatory transmission").

It had been previously thought that microtubules (neurotubules) and neurofilaments are interconvertible, *i.e.* that they represent different aggregation states of the same elementary unit. This idea was based on the finding that treatments which cause disappearance of microtubules (*e.g.* colchicin, vinblastin, cold) induce at the same time a considerable increment of neurofilament numbers, both processes being reversed after cessation of treatment. However, recent findings of biochemical differences between microtubule and microfilament proteins challenge the above hypothesis.

The function of neurotubules is not yet established but some recent evidence indicates that they may be concerned with rapid transport of certain materials along axons: destruction of microtubules in retinal ganglion cells by vinblastin greatly retarded the transport of $[^3H]$ proline from the eye to the superior colliculi in the midbrain via the optic nerve axons.

Contrary to earlier beliefs, neurons have been shown capable of pinocytotic uptake of large protein molecules from their environment through large *coated vesicles* that form *multivesicular bodies*, as already described. No free particle exchange has been observed, however, to occur between cytoplasm and nucleus possibly because of the diaphragms that seal the nuclear pores.

Neurons also possess a very active lysosome system. Perhaps the most dramatic change that occurs in many of these cells (in man and animals) as they age – and one that has long puzzled histologists since the end of the previous century – is the gradual accumulation of huge masses of *lipofuscin* in their cytoplasm to the point where they fill up most of the neuron. It now seems possible that these growing deposits of lipofuscin represent nothing else but autophagosomes (residual bodies) resulting from the sequestration of used organelle membranes, and that they pile up either because they cannot be lysed by the lysosomes or because they cannot be extruded from the neuron. While the cause of the lysosomal or extrusion failure is not yet known, it has been found that large lipofuscin deposits can be induced in the neurons of young animals – where they normally do not occur – by protracted hypoxia (low oxygen air or acetanilid poisoning leading to Met-hemoglobin formation), or ascorbic acid deficiency.

The function of the *subsurface cisternae,* the *spine apparatus*, and the *laminated or fibrillary inclusions* is not known, while the occasional atypical *cilia* seem to be centrioles modified by unknown forces; the fact that the latter have been recently produced within neurons of experimental animals by amine oxidase inhibitors may help to explain the mechanism of their development. Regular *centrioles* tend to appear only in embryonic or neoplastic neurons – an expression of the fact that mature neurons do not divide.

The function of the *Schwann cells* is (a) to produce myelin sheaths for peripheral axons, (b) to possibly "nurse" axons metabolically, (c) to guide regeneration of severed or injured axons, and (d) to phagocytise part of the debris produced during axonal destruction. The function of *myelin* is evidently to promote speedy impulse transmission, because myelinated axons conduct impulses much faster than unmyelinated ones – and, furthermore, transmission speed is proportional to the diameter of the myelinated axons – but it is not entirely clear how myelin accomplishes that. It is thought at present that, by insulating large internodal segments of axons and exposing them only at the nodes of Ranvier, the myelin sheath promotes a very rapid "saltatory" travel of the impulses from node to node.

One of the most fascinating problems of contemporary neuron research is the question of the structural substrate of *memory*. Both RNA and protein molecules (with their infinite possible structural permutations) have been incriminated as the physical substrate of the information storage function we call memory; the finding that intracerebral injection of puromycin (an inhibitor of protein synthesis) will inhibit avoidance-discrimination learning in animals seems to support the role of neuronal protein synthesis in this function.

After *cutting, crushing* or other *destruction of a given axon site*, the following changes materialise: (a) the part of the axon distal to the interruption degenerates (as manifested by decreased axolemmal and increased axoplasmic density and swelling of its mitochondria with massive focal dilatations), disintegrates and is phagocytised by the enveloping astrocytes, oligodendrocytes or Schwann cells, (b) the lamellae of the myelin sheath distal to the interruption separate along the intraperiod lines and disintegrate into spiral segments that turn into droplets which seem to be phagocytised by Schwann cells (and by extraneous phagocytic cells as well, when sufficiently large numbers of myelin sheaths are involved), (c) the Schwann cells proliferate, enlarge and increase their nuclear surface through multiple indentations while also acquiring crystalloid cytoplasmic inclusions, (d) the proximal axon stump expands and becomes filled with large masses of tightly packed lysosomes, cytolysosomes (autophagosomes), mitochondria, microtubules and microvesicles (which develop from the microtubules by pinching off), (e) from the proximal axon expansions grow several finger-like buds which represent regenerating axons and are embraced by the newly proliferated Schwann cells but tend to vacuolate and become phagocytised within a few weeks, and (f) in the perikaryon of the neuron whose axon was cut many autophagic vacuoles develop and the central (though not the peripheral) rough endoplasmic reticulum (RER) disappears, but protein synthesis is greatly increased in the remaining ribosomal system, presumably in association with the attempted proximal axon stump regeneration.

IV. SYNAPSES – STRUCTURE AND FUNCTION

(1) General

Synapses in their broadest sense comprise all functional contacts between a neuron and another cell, *i.e.* all contacts between (a) neurons and other neurons, (b) neurons and muscle, and (c) neurons and epithelial (including glandular) cells. At a synapse, an impulse may originate in the neuron and be transmitted from it to another neuron, a muscle cell or an epithelial cell – and this is the type to be discussed here – or, conversely, the impulses may originate in the muscle or the epithelial cells and be transmitted from them to the neuron – a type to be discussed with the sensory organs.

Depending on the mechanism of impulse transmission there are two basic types of synapses: (a) chemical (by far the commonest in mammals) and (b) electric (prevalent mostly in lower vertebrates and invertebrates). In the *chemical synapse* the impulse is usually transmitted from the axon terminal of one neuron to the plasma membrane of another neuron or effector (muscle or gland) cell through the firing of a chemical transmitter substance (acetylcholine, norepinephrine) across a distance of a few hundred Å (synaptic gap); the transmitter substance is released from the axon terminal of the emitting neuron, travels across the synaptic gap and through some as yet unsettled mechanism "depolarizes" the plasma membrane of the receiving cell, initiating in it a wave of excitation that spreads out from the synapse site in a manner similar to that already summarized in the muscle chapter. An interesting variation of the above mechanism has developed in the case of the *neurosecretory neurons* where the transmitters released at the axon terminals (oxytocin, pitressin, pituitary-stimulating hormone) have to travel through the bloodstream before they reach the effector cells they are destined to excite, *i.e.* smooth muscle, renal epithelium and anterior pituitary cells.

The following four transmitters are known to be released during the function of various mammalian chemical synapses: norepinephrine, acetylcholine, serotonine and dopamine; additional transmitters seem to operate in some synapses of other vertebrates (γ-aminobutyric acid, glutamate, ATP). Norepinephrine appears to be "re-absorbed" by the axon terminal from the synaptic gap after firing and to be re-utilised many times; its reuptake by the axon terminal requires energy from ATP and is made possible through the function of an "amine pump" which is located in the pre-synaptic (axon terminal) PM; this amine pump is probably operated by a Na–K activated ATPase in the pre-synaptic membrane. A similar process of re-utilisation involving an amine pump has been proposed (but not yet proven) for serotonine and dopamine. Unlike norepinephrine, acetylcholine is degraded outside the axon terminal by acetylcholinesterase.

In the *electrical synapse* the plasma membranes of the two synapsing cells fuse or come so close to each other that the impulse passes directly from one to the other without the release of any transmitter substances. If one includes in the broadest definition of synapse the impulse-transmitting contact between any two excitable cells (not just neurons), then a typical example of an electrical synapse in mammals has been already encountered in the "tight junctions" of heart muscle, which transmit the contraction impulse from one cardiac muscle cell to another.

(2) Neuro-neuronal synapse, chemical

(A) Synapses with clear vesicles (Plate 25)

According to the nature of their two parts, synapses can occur between axons and parts of other neurons (axo-dendritic, axo-somatic, axo-axonic), between dendrites and parts of other neurons (dendro-dendritic, dendro-somatic) and between the bodies of two neurons (somato-somatic). The most common and most important ones are, however, the *axo-dendritic* and *axo-somatic* ones, most of which can be divided in two types: types "I" and "II".

A typical synapse of the so called *type I* (Fig. A), the most frequent of the two, consists of (a) a pre-synaptic component[1], (b) a post-synaptic component[2], and (c) a synaptic cleft[3] (gap) in between. The *presynaptic component* is usually an expansion at the tip ("bouton terminal") or along the stem ("bouton en passant") of an axon and is free of the myelin sheath; it contains (a) numerous clear mostly round 400 Å synaptic vesicles[4], (b) a small amount of filamentous (pre-synaptic) dense web[5] along the synapsing plasma membrane, (c) some mitochondria, (d) in some species – such as the cat – loops of neurofilaments, (e) in sensory organs "presynaptic ribbons", *i.e.* linear densities surrounded by rows of vesicles, and (f) in some cases, a hexagonal arrangement of 500 or 1000 Å particles along the synapsing membranes. The *synaptic cleft* is 300 Å wide, is bisected by a dense occasionally interrupted plate[6] and may be traversed by a few filaments[7]; it contains basic and acidic proteins but little or no calcium. The *post-synaptic component* contains (a) a greater and denser amount of filamentous web than the presynaptic component along its synapsing membrane, the so called *"sub-synaptic web"*[8], and (b) occasionally some mitochondria or ribosomes. Some mammalian synapses further show the following *specialized post-synaptic organelles*: (a) a *"spine apparatus"* (found in dendritic spines) consisting of 2–3 smooth cisternae separated by a dense material (Fig. A_1), or (b) a string of 200–250 Å particles lined up approximately 500 Å beneath the post-synaptic membrane, the *"post-synaptic bodies"* (Fig. A_2). Type I synapses are wide and often come in multiple sets.

Type II synapses (Fig. B) are similar to those already described, with the following differences: (a) the synaptic cleft is only 200 Å wide, (b) there is no plate or row of filaments in the cleft, and (c) the presynaptic web is not necessarily thinner than the post-synaptic one; it may be equal (as pictured in Fig. B) or even thicker.

Clear 400 Å presynaptic vesicles such as those described above are found throughout most synapses of the central nervous system, in some peripheral autonomic and in all neuromuscular synapses. They almost certainly contain acetylcholine since (a) this transmitter substance is found in homogenate fractions consisting of such vesicles, and (b) since inhibitors of acetylcholine synthesis greatly decrease the number and size of these clear vesicles. It is evident that the clear synaptic vesicles participate somehow in the impulse transmission process: Evidence from neuromuscular synapses show that repeated nerve stimulation leading to muscle contraction causes a dramatic drop in the number of synaptic vesicles, while recovery from stimulation brings about their numeric restitution. The mechanism, however, through which acetylcholine is fired into the synaptic cleft is uncertain. It is possible that acetylcholine is discharged from the vesicles into the cleft by emiocytosis (reverse pinocytosis), but unequivocal E/M evidence for this has not yet been provided; it is also possible that upon arrival of an impulse in the axon terminal some synaptic vesicles disintegrate (like grenades) releasing free acetylcholine into the cytoplasm which then diffuses out through the plasma membrane into the synaptic cleft – but this, too, has to be proven. Finally, a third possibility has arisen from recent freeze-etch studies which show that depolarisation causes the development of shallow depressions (*ca.* 200 Å deep) on the presynaptic PM, to which synaptic vesicles attach from inside; perhaps the contacts between the synaptic vesicles and the convex surface of these depressions represent leaky sites through which transmitters are fired into the cleft.

Recent cytochemical studies indicate that, in addition to acetylcholine, clear synaptic vesicles also contain appreciable amounts of inorganic cations such as sodium ions, but the significance of this interesting finding remains to be established.

Similarly unknown at the moment is the significance of a "membrane recycling" process that has been postulated on the basis of observations made on peroxidase-immersed sympathetic ganglia. It appears that stimulation of axon terminals in such preparations causes endocytic uptake of peroxidase into coated vesicles at the sides of the terminal and exocytic release of the same material into the synaptic cleft; thus PM is transferred from the sides to the front of the axon terminal.

It has been suggested that type I synapses are physiologically excitatory whereas type II are inhibitory. This hypothesis fits some but not all facts, since some known excitatory synapses exhibit type II structure and since many synapses show a structure which is intermediate between type I and type II.

Synapses mature structurally during the first few weeks after birth. In the rat, *e.g.*, synapses exhibit no synaptic vesicles or synaptic clefts during the first week but develop these features rapidly during the second week of post-natal life, under the accompaniment of a temporary upsurge in local ribosome populations; clear synaptic vesicles have been described but not yet proven to originate from dilatations of neurotubules.

Following sectioning of an axon or destruction or extirpation of its neuronal cell body, its synapsing terminal (the "presynaptic bag") degenerates and dies, going through the following sequence of changes: (a) within 24 hours the presynaptic bag shrinks and becomes very dense (dark) because its synaptic vesicles swell and clump together in one tight pack while its cytoplasmic matrix as well as the matrix of its mitochondria greatly increase their density, (b) within 2–3 weeks the synaptic vesicles and terminals are phagocytised by the astrocytes that envelop them. The development of changes of the above type in axon terminals of mesenteric ganglia following extirpation of viscera such as the gall bladder confirmed the existence of autonomic afferent axons with cell bodies in the visceral organs.

(B) Synapses with small cored (granular) vesicles (Plate 25, Fig. C)

Such synapses occur mainly in the peripheral autonomic system. Their synaptic vesicles are mostly round, with a diameter of 500 Å and an inner dense core of 300 Å. They seem to contain catecholamines (norepinephrine) since their numbers correlate well with the nerve catecholamine content: they disappear together with the norepinephrine content after reserpine or benzoquinolizine (RO4–1284) treatment. It is interesting that axon terminals with cored vesicles of this type do not

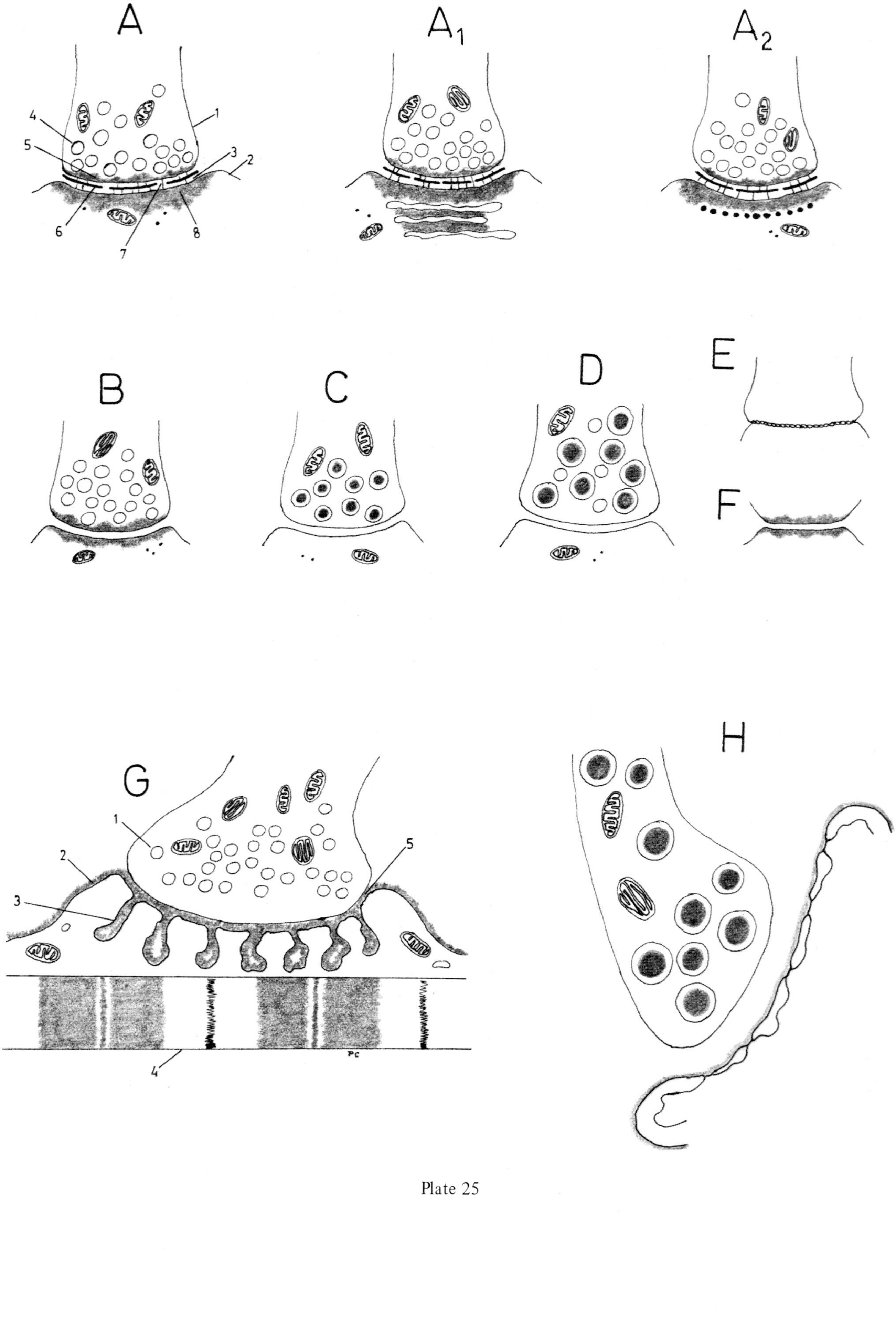

Plate 25

only seem to release endogenous catecholamines but they also appear capable of "absorbing" exogenous ones, *i.e.* they somehow pick up labeled catecholamines administered *in vivo*. At least in the case of certain axon terminals (*e.g.* in the olfactory bulbs of cebus monkeys), small cored vesicles seem to bud off the Golgi apparatus, like the much larger neurosecretory cored vesicles.

(C) Synapses with large cored (granular) vesicles (Plate 25, Fig. D)

Such synapses occur both in the peripheral autonomic and the central nervous system. Their synaptic vesicles are almost twice as large as those of the previous category, namely 900 Å wide with a 500 Å dense core, and they are usually accompanied by some 400 Å clear vesicles. Their transmitter substance is not known, but judging by morphochemical analogy it is probably an amine, perhaps serotonine or dopamine. Contrary to earlier views, such vesicles are not found exclusively in neurons of the sympathetic division of the autonomic nervous system.

(3) Neuro-neuronal synapse, electrical (Plate 25)

Electrical synapses can be either *"tight junctions"* involving fusion of the outer leaflets of the plasma membranes of the two synaptic components (as in the zonula occludens type junctions between adjacent cardiac muscle cells), or they may represent *extreme approximation* of the two synapsing membranes with *multiple focal fusions* of their outer leaflets (Fig. E). In the latter type, (which occurs in certain fishes), the synaptic cleft is reduced to a width of 20 Å but is still permeable to lanthanum salts. Tangential sections at the synaptic cleft level of such synapses reveal a polyhedral pattern which is presumably formed by the outer leaflets of their synapsing membranes. Electrical synapses may occur side by side with chemical ones.

(4) Mechanical attachments between neurons (Plate 25)

Mechanical joints attaching parts of different neurons to one another occur widely in the central nervous system. They are called *puncta adherentia* (Fig. F), resemble the desmosomes and zonulae adherentes of non-nervous tissues, and can be distinguished from synapses primarily by the absence of synaptic vesicles from both joining components and by the usually equal (symmetrical) development of dense web material along both apposed membranes – except when one of the two joined components is an axon, in which case web material is missing on the axonal side. A dense plate may or may not bisect (desmosome-like) the gap between the apposed membranes. The puncta adherentia seem to serve purely as mechanical attachment devices, not as sites of impulse transmission; they are often multiple and are often intermingled with true impulse-transmitting synapses.

(5) Neuro-muscular synapses in skeletal muscle
(Plate 25)

The best studied neuromuscular junctions are those in which the muscle is skeletal (Fig. G). In such junctions (a) the presynaptic component (axon terminal) contains clear 400 Å vesicles[1] and a variable number of mitochondria, (b) the postsynaptic component[2] (a lateral bulge of a skeletal muscle fiber with a depression to receive the bouton) is multiply invaginated to form plasma membrane pockets[3] (junctional folds) that dip down to reach the myofibrils[4], (c) the synaptic cleft is as wide as that in a type II chemical neuro-neuronal synapse, namely 200 Å, and (d) the post-synaptic (skeletal muscle) plasma membrane is covered by the continuation of the muscle basement membrane which thus fills the synaptic cleft[5]. The myelin sheath peters out at the sides of the bouton. Cholinesterase, the enzyme that inactivates the transmitter acetylcholine has been demonstrated histochemically on both the pre- and post-synaptic membranes and within the synaptic cleft. Autoradiographic studies with labeled difluorophosphate, a chemical that binds (and inhibits)acetylcholinesterase at a 1 : 1 molecular ratio, indicates that a typical neuro-muscular junction in skeletal muscle contains 10,000,000–30,000,000 molecules of this enzyme.

Recently neuro-muscular synapses have also been found in cardiac muscle (*e.g.* in the right atrium of the heart) and consist of vesiculated axon terminals that approach the heart muscle cells very closely (to within 200 Å of their surface).

(6) Neuro-muscular synapses in smooth muscle

Present data indicate that these synapses are operated through vesicle-laden terminal or lateral axon bulges (boutons) but that the synaptic gap (*i.e.*, the neuromuscular distance), is very much greater than in the case of nerve-skeletal muscle synapses. The neuro-muscular distance here appears to range from 500 Å (as in visceral smooth muscle) to 3000–4000 Å (as in vascular smooth muscle) and the transmitter is believed to diffuse across this distance in active form. Usually, a patch of acetylcholinesterase activity can be demonstrated cytochemically on the PM of the smooth muscle cell at the point where it faces the vesiculated axon process.

(7) Neuro-epithelial synapses

Little is known about their fine structure at present.

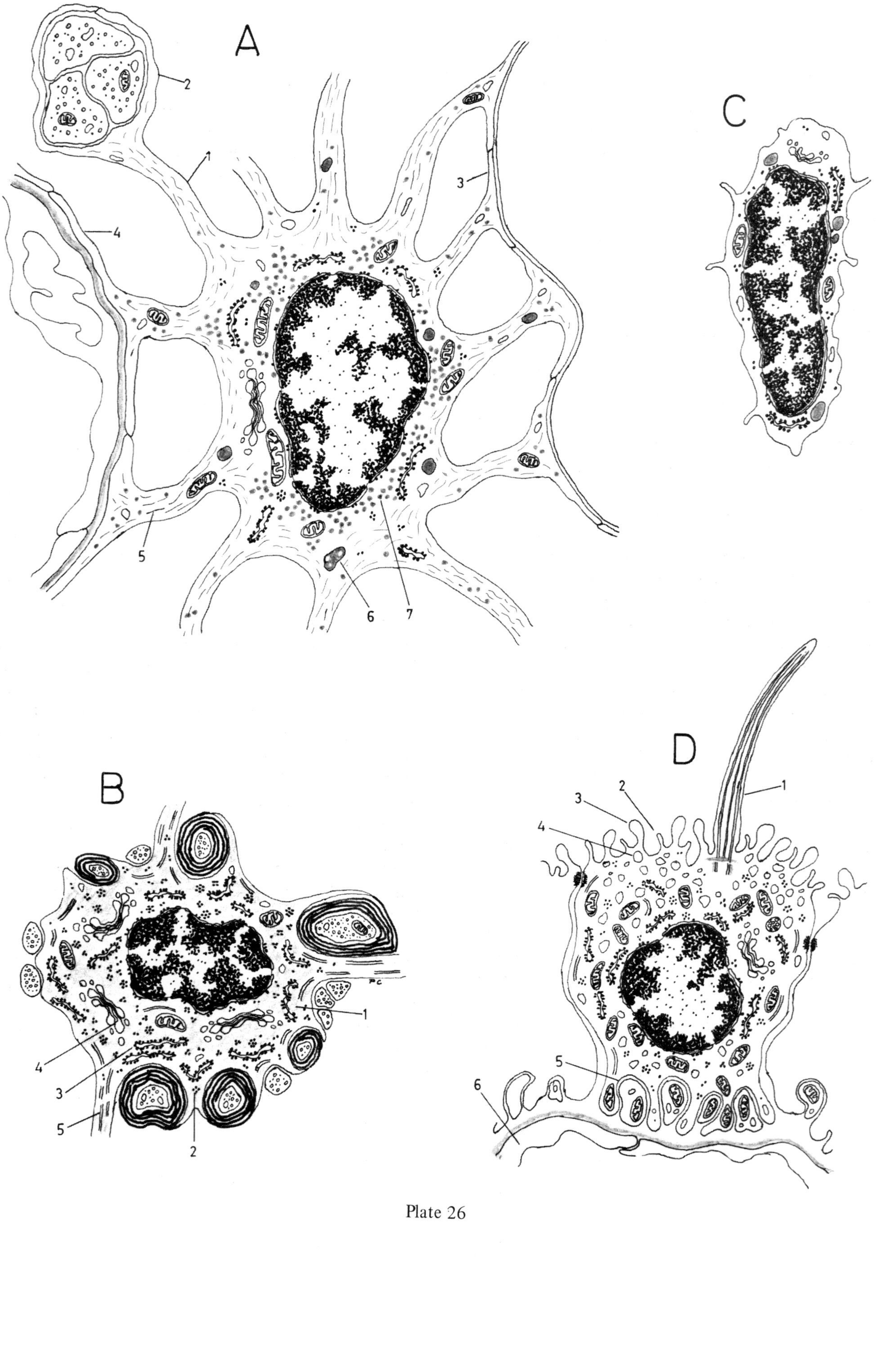

Plate 26

(8) Neuro-secretion (Plate 25)

There are at least two well recognised neurosecretory systems in mammals: (a) the system of hypothalamic neurons (supraoptic and paraventricular) whose axons terminate around the capillaries of the posterior pituitary gland (Fig. H) and secrete vasopressin and oxytocin into the blood stream at these sites, and (b) the system of arcuate nucleus neurons whose axons terminate around the hypophyseal portal capillaries and secrete into the blood a factor that releases anterior pituitary hormones. The perikarya, axons and axon terminals of the neurons of both systems contain numerous large cored vesicles which represent the hormones they elaborate and secrete into the blood stream. The cored vesicles of the axons that secrete into the capillaries of the posterior pituitary are 1200–1500 Å wide and are nearly filled by large dense cores; evidence that these 1200–1600 Å cored vesicles contain vasopressin and oxytocin rests on the facts that (a) the above two hormones are found in isolated fractions of such vesicles, and (b) after appropriate physiological stimulation (*e.g.* dehydration) both the cored vesicles and the hormones are lost from the posterior pituitary (because they are discharged into the blood stream). On the other hand, the cored vesicles of the axons that secrete into the hypophyseal portal capillaries are 1000 Å wide and represent anterior pituitary release factor (*i.e.* a factor that causes release of anterior pituitary hormones). Non-specific stress greatly increases the number of 1000 Å cored vesicles in axon terminals of the latter type.

A third neurosecretory system of yet obscure function, the "subfornical organ" is now under study in the cat. It appears that neurons of this organ send axons with neurosecretory vesicles to the ependymal lining of brain ventricles as well as to capillaries; they may therefore "secrete" into the cerebrospinal fluid as well as into the blood.

The production of neurosecretory materials can be not only under metabolic but also under hormonal and environmental control. Thus, castration increases whereas sex hormone treatment diminishes nucleolar size and ribosome and cored vesicle numbers in hypothalamic neurons, indicating the existence of a negative feedback effect of peripheral sex hormones on the synthesis of the neurosecretory materials that promote their own production (by stimulating gonadotrophin production). Furthermore, the RER of arcuate nucleus neurons greatly expands during every diestrus phase of the estrous cycle. On the other hand, nuclear volume and neurosecretory material synthesis show a definite relationship to light and darkness (and therefore to day-night and summer-winter rhythms) in neurons of lower vertebrates and invertebrates.

V. GLIA

(1) General

There are three types of glia cells in the central nervous system: astrocytes, oligodendrocytes and microglia; all three occur in the grey as well as the white substance of the brain and spinal cord. The glia of the peripheral nervous system consists of (a) the Schwann cells of nerves (oligodendrocyte-like cells that ensheath axons, already discussed in the section on neurons), and (b) the satellite cells of ganglia (oligodendrocyte-like cells that ensheath neurons at such sites).

(2) Astrocytes

(A) Structure (Plate 26, Fig. A)

Astrocytes represent roughly 20% of all glia cells. They send out numerous processes[1], some of which flatten out to form extremely *thin sheets* around bundles of neighbouring axons[2] or around neighbouring neurons[3], while others attach to the basement membrane of neighbouring capillaries, ensheathing the latter with their flattened *pericapillary end feet*[4]. The *extracellular space* between the thin astrocytic sheaths and the neuronal structures they envelop is, like that between the tightly packed neuronal structures, very narrow, varying reportedly between 35 and 200 Å, depending on the type of fixative used and on whether fixation was immediate or followed several minutes of asphyxia; it seems to be filled with a lucent anionic material, probably an acid mucopolysaccharide. Astrocytic processes of the same or different cells are joined to one another mechanically by means of *puncta adherentia* or variants of *tight junctions* such as those already described in the section on electrical neuro-neuronal synapses. The segments of astrocytic plasma membrane that are closely apposed to neuronal or capillary surfaces have been found to exhibit strong ATPase activity.

Internally, the astrocyte is characterised by (a) numerous *fibrils*[5] (which, like neurofilaments, are hollow tubes but are thinner, with a total diameter of only 60–80 Å, (b) lysosomes[6], (c) glycogen granules[7] and (d) a moderate development of the standard organelles of protein synthesis and oxidative energy production. The type of cell shown in Fig. A normally prevails in grey matter and is called a "*fibrous astrocyte*"; another variant with relatively more cytoplasm, less fibrils and some microtubules is normally found in the white matter and is called a "*protoplasmic astrocyte*". All astrocytes tend to have an unusually lucent ("watery") cytoplasmic matrix.

(B) Function

The following four functions of astrocytes seem established: (a) the provision of a *structural skeleton* for nervous tissue through the mechanical attachment of astrocytes to each other and to the vascular framework of the nervous system, (b) the *repair* of injuries to nerve tissue by proliferation and formation of astrocytic scars, (c) the *insulation* of the excitable surfaces of neurons and their processes through the extensive system of astrocytic sheaths which prevent straying and scattering of impulses and (d) the ability to *phagocytise* dead neuron parts and large molecules such as ferritin. The theory of a fifth *"nurse cell"* function has not yet been proven: According to the nurse cell concept astrocytes absorb nutrients and other metabolites from capillaries through their "end feet" and transmit them to the neurons through their sheet-like enveloping processes; this hypothesis is based (a) on the great narrowness of the extracellular spaces between the tightly packed cells of nervous tissue which has been thought to prevent significant large-molecular traffic between the blood of the capillaries and the distant neurons, (b) on the bridge-like position of astrocytes between capillaries and neurons, and (c) on the marked ATPase activity of the astrocyte plasma membranes at both the capillary and neuronal contact areas which was thought to indicate marked capacity for molecular transport processes at both these sites. A strike against the first of the arguments mentioned has been the finding that when introduced directly into the ventricles of the brain, certain fairly large molecules such as peroxidase and ferritin have travelled for appreciable distances into the narrow extracellular spaces of the neuropil. On the other hand, the recent histochemical finding that almost half of the brain chloride space is located within glia cells tends to support the notion of unusual fluid traffic through the cytoplasm of these cells.

(3) Oligodendroglia

(A) Structure (Plate 26, Fig. B)

Oligodendrocytes constitute the majority (about 75%) of all glia cells. They lie between axons and around neurons, approaching the latter very closely so that their plasma membrane is often separated from the neuronal plasma membrane by a gap of only about 200 Å; sometimes a thin astrocytic sheet intervenes between oligodendrocyte and neuron.

They are characterised by (a) fewer processes than astrocytes, (b) abundant cytoplasm, with often eccentric nucleus and clumped chromatin, (c) appreciably denser cytoplasmic matrix[1] than astocytes because of the presence of numerous tiny matrix granules that fill the spaces between organelles, (d) numerous ribosomes[2] and marked development of the rough endoplasmic reticulum[3], (e) prominent Golgi vesicles[4], (f) almost no fibrils or glycogen, and (g) appreciable microtubule[5] numbers so that oligodendrocyte processes may be difficult to differentiate from dendrites.

(B) Function

Oligodendrocytes appear to produce the myelin sheaths of the axons in the central nervous system (at least in the baby) because (a) they proliferate intensely and line up along axons just before myelinisation begins in early post natal life, and (b) connections between them and the myelin sheath of CNS axons have been demonstrated in both the developing and the adult CNS. In addition, these cells have been found capable of phagocytosis of dead neurons and of ferritin molecules. It has also been postulated that oligodendrocytes play a role in the nutrition of neurons but this possibility is at the moment as much lacking in proof as the analogous theory of a "neuron-nursing role" of astrocytes.

Finally, in peripheral ganglia, dark oligodendrocyte-like "satellite" cells wrap around neurons, enveloping them in spiralling or overlapping thin cytoplasmic sheets; the finding of intense pinocytic activity on the side of their cytoplasm that faces the neurons indicates that a very active metabolic exchange takes place between glia cells and neurons at these peripheral sites.

(4) Microglia

(A) Structure (Plate 26, Fig. C)

The electron microscopic identification of the cells which with the light microscope are labelled "microglia" in the normal CNS is not quite settled yet. It appears probable, however, that certain small cells which constitute about 5% of all CNS glia cells and which contain no fibrils, glycogen or microtubules but only a few microvilli and standard organelles and some dense bodies in their sparse cytoplasm correspond to the resting microglia of light microscopy.

(B) Function

Microglia cells have been traditionally regarded as the potential phagocytes of the CNS, *i.e.* the cells which scavenge debris from necrotic neurons in cases of CNS injury, and proliferate as well as enlarge in the process to form the foamy lipid-filled "gitter cells" or "compound granular corpuscles". There are some doubts, however, at the present time as to whether the large round lipid-filled scavenger cells that appear in damaged CNS tissue represent transformed microglia cells in the traditional sense; it is now considered probable that they really represent monocytes attracted to the injury site from the blood.

VI. EPENDYMAL CELL

(A) Structure (Plate 26, Fig. D)

The ependymal cells form a single or in some species a double cell layer that lines the ventricles of the CNS. They are characterised by (a) luminal cilia[1], thin[2] and bulbous[3] microvilli, (b) numerous smooth vesicles[4] of 500–1000 Å diameter, (c) moderate presence of ribosomes, rough endoplasmic reticulum and apical microtubules (d) appreciable numbers of mitochondria, (e) frequent basal infoldings[5] and processes which get into close contact with capillaries[6], particularly in the case of the so called "ependymal tanycytes", and (f) apical intercellular junctions of the zonula occludens or adherens type.

(B) Function

Ependymal cells are involved in the production of cerebrospinal fluid (CSF) from the blood that runs in the capillaries directly underneath them. The mechanism of CSF production is not yet completely elucidated but it is likely that fluid is actively tranported from the capillaries through the ependymal cytoplasm into the ventricles, in a manner similar to the production of sweat in the sweat glands; it probably enters the base and sides of the ependymal cells and is carried (perhaps through microvesicular transport) towards the apical surface from where it is released into the ventricle with the cooperation of the microvilli. Stimulation of CSF elaboration (caused by removing CSF from ventricles) induces swelling of the apical microvilli and widening of the interependymal clefts.

Since the size of the apical bulbous projections apparently varies with the phases of the menstrual cycle in the female monkey (it is reportedly maximal in mid-cycle) but is constant in the male animal, the manufacture of CSF may depend on hormones, among other things.

One of the most intriguing discoveries of recent years has been the finding that in several mammals and lower vertebrates axons often penetrate through the ependymal lining and dip into the fluid of brain ventricles where their terminals either lie free (often sending out cilia) or synapse with the apical surface of ependymal cells. The functional significance of this occurrence is as yet unknown but it is possible that the intra-ventricular axons act as sensors, picking up information on the composition of the cerebrospinal fluid, and (or) that they stimulate secretory or absorptive activity in the ependymal cells.

Chapter 7

Circulatory System

I. GENERAL

This system provides a major network of channels (blood vessels) and the motor force (the heart pump) through which blood is brought into close contact with all cells of the body to sustain them with vital materials as well as to carry away their wastes and metabolites; it also provides a minor channel network (lymphatic vessels) through which tissue fluid (lymph) is carried from the tissues into the blood vessel network.

The *heart* is essentially a very thick contractile tube whose main substance consists of cardiac muscle (the myocardium); it is lined by the endocardium internally and the epicardium externally and it lies in the pericardial sac. In the *blood vessel circuit* of the circulatory system, blood moves out of the arterial end of the heart into elastic arteries and from there through muscular arteries, arterioles, terminal arterioles and metarterioles into capillaries; after it exchanges materials with the various tissues at the capillary level, blood returns through venules and veins to the venous end of the heart. In the *lymphatic circuit* of the circulatory system, tissue fluid (lymph) drains out of the body tissues first into small then into large lymphatic vessels and through the latter into veins. In the following sections, the vascular tree is discussed starting with the capillaries and moving up from there to progressively larger channels, for purposes of didactic convenience.

II. CAPILLARIES

(1) Capillaries with continuous endothelium

(A) Continuous endothelium with zonulae adherentes

Structure (Plate 27, Fig. A). This is the type of capillary that prevails in muscle (skeletal, cardiac and smooth). In addition to sparse amounts of the standard organelles, the endothelial cells are characterised by (a) a thin "fuzzy" feltwork-like coat[1] on the surface of the luminal plasma membrane (visible only at high magnification and with special techniques), (b) numerous pinocytotic vesicles[2] (caveolae) of 600–750 Å diameter throughout their cytoplasm, (c) bundles of 40–90 Å thick microfilaments[3], which on rare occasions show striations and (d) variable numbers of mostly longitudinally oriented thicker microtubules[4]. A roughly 500 Å thick basement membrane[5] underlies the basal plasma membrane. The endothelial cells of this type of capillary are joined to one another primarily by zonulae adherentes[6], which are distinguished by (a) an interendothelial cleft about 40–250 Å wide, which is occupied by a very low density material (apparently a glucoprotein), and whose bordering plasma membranes seem to be lined by the continuation of the thin fuzzy coat that lines the luminal endothelial surface, and (b) an apron-like cytoplasmic "flap"[7] that projects over the junction from one of the two neighbouring endothelial cells. In certain organs such as the heart, where rapid blood–tissue exchange is vital, the endothelium becomes extremely thin, consisting of only two plasma membranes and a thin film of intervening cytoplasm.

Attached to some capillaries and enveloped in their basement membranes are occasionally certain relatively undifferentiated cells, the "pericytes"[8].

Function. The "fuzzy" surface coat that lines the luminal endothelial membrane – and may continue over the junctional part of the cell membrane – apparently consists of acid polysaccharide that binds ruthenium red. Being electronegative, this polysaccharide coat may normally repel platelets and red blood cells (whose surfaces are likewise negatively charged) and thus prevent the formation of thrombi and red cell sludges over the intact capillary endothelium.

Transport of material from the blood through this type of endothelium into the pericapillary space apparently takes place through at least the following four mechanisms:

(a) The *pinocytotic vesicles* apparently pick up various molecules from the blood, carry them across the cytoplasm and discharge them on to the basal surface of the endothelial cells. Such pinocytotic vesicle transport has been shown to account for most of the transendothelial crossing of certain relatively large molecules such

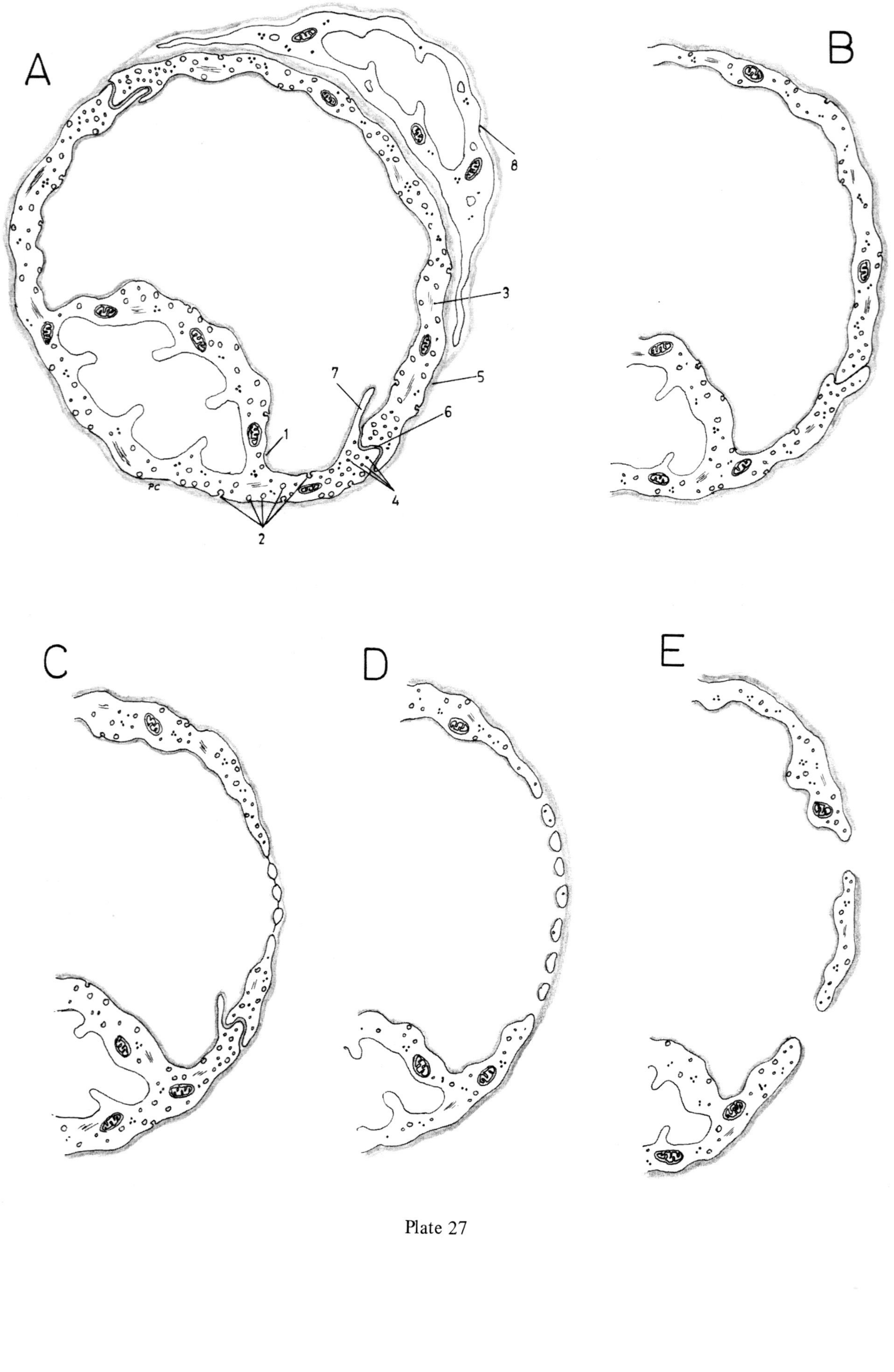

Plate 27

as ferritin (diameter *ca.* 110 Å) in intravenous infusion experiments; it is also possibly the mechanism for the transport of fatty acid–albumin complexes. This "vesicular transport" seems to represent the structural equivalent of the "large pore system" postulated by physiologists several decades ago.

(b) The *junctions* between the endothelial cells apparently allow certain relatively small molecules such as lanthanum salts or peroxidase (diameter *ca.* 40 Å) to squeeze through. They seem to represent the "small pore system" postulated by physiologists for the passage of small non-lipid molecules.

(c) A third mechanism, not yet sufficiently studied, is the "diffusion" of certain molecules right through the two plasma membranes and the cytoplasmic matrix of endothelial cells, such as occurs in the case of lipid solvents (e.g. ether, chloroform) and possibly in the case of several lipid and other compounds.

(d) Finally a fourth mechanism, equally unexplored, is the active, energy-consuming transport of certain compounds across the endothelium involving their capture, partial chemical change and transfer by means of PM and matrix enzymes.

Unfortunately, the specific transport mechanism for each of the *physiologically important* molecules that cross this kind of capillary endothelium continuously and in both directions is largely unexplored as yet. We still do not know how *e.g.* sugars, amines, polypeptides, and the various proteins, glucoproteins, lipoproteins, lipids, and metabolic wastes cross the endothelial lining.

Almost all endothelial permeability research is currently undertaken with dense markers of different particle sizes which are usually injected intravenously in overwhelming amounts; with the exception of the proteins ferritin and peroxidase, most of these markers are inorganic and especially metallic particles that are not normally involved in the body economy such as colloidal gold, carbon, thorotrast, lanthanum, or ruthenium. Experiments with the above markers, several of which are toxic, tell us something about the transendothelial transport of the markers tested, but they do not automatically elucidate the specific transport mechanisms of all the other physiological molecules of interest. Particle size is not the only factor that determines the transport mechanism of a given molecule – its shape, electrical charge, hydro- or lipo-solubility and specific chemical effects are also important determinants; furthermore, several of the dense markers commonly used (ferritin, thorotrast, peroxidase) have been shown to have biological effects of their own on endothelial permeability. It, therefore, appears that different molecules cross the endothelium in different ways, and that one cannot conclude about the transport mechanism of materials other than those one has studied. For these reasons, the methods of the future in this area appear to be fine grain autoradiography and immunocytochemistry.

There is also increasing evidence that different segments of the vascular tree are lined by functionally different endothelium, with different permeability characteristics. Thus, the continuous, unperforated endothelium of normal capillaries has recently been found to be much more permeable to lipids than the endothelium of normal arteries.

Although it has the appearance of a barrier, the *basement membrane* is permeable to all the molecular traffic that occurs between the capillary lumen and the pericapillary space; it does, however, seem to retard the exit of large particles such as ferritin or carbon particles.

Apart from the continuous peristaltic movements of certain endothelial tubes (*e.g.* the simple ascidian heart), there are several indications that endothelial cells are capable of *contraction* under proper stimulation, *e.g.* in response to certain amines or kinins such as histamine, serotonin and bradykinin. Such contractility could well account for the "opening" of the endothelial junctions in certain pathological circumstances and the consequent leakage of plasma into the pericapillary space; it would also relate the endothelial cells to the underlying smooth muscle cells – an assumption supported by the embryological kinship of the two types of cells. The microfilaments probably represent contractile protein of an as yet undetermined nature, perhaps myosin in finer aggregation than in skeletal muscle, while the microtubules seem to provide structural support. Myosin has been identified in endothelial cytoplasm with fluorescent antimyosin at the L/M level, but its ultrastructural localisation has not yet been established.

The function of the *pericytes* which in the L/M era were thought to be contractile (myocyte-like) cells is not yet quite clear. The absence of specific smooth muscle organelles such as myofilaments and dense bodies suggests that these cells are undifferentiated reserve elements.

Among the most dramatic nutritional influences on the endothelium is that of *ascorbic acid deficiency*: it has been found to cause opening of the junctions, and loss of basement membrane and pericapillary collagen, thus leading to capillary hemorrhages.

(B) Continuous endothelium with zonulae occludentes (Plate 27, Fig. B)

These capillaries have the same structure as those just described but their endothelial cells are joined to each other by means of "tight junctions" (zonulae occludentes) in which there is no junctional cleft because of the fusion of the outer leaflets of the two bordering cell membranes. As a result, the movement of certain molecules and particles across this type of endothelium

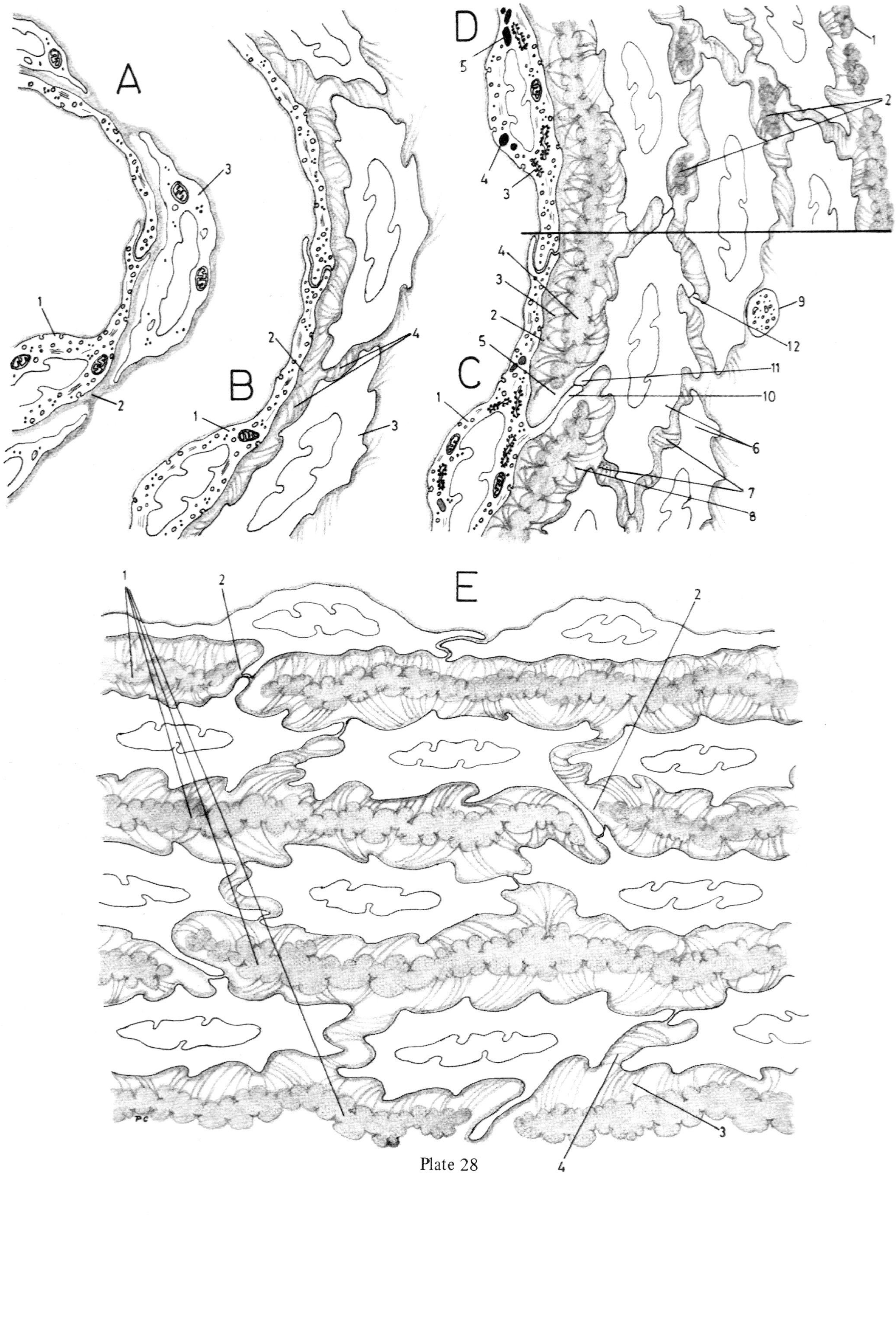

Plate 28

is slowed down or completely stopped. This very tight-walled type of capillary prevails in most of the brain and the retina and explains the long known phenomenon of the "blood–brain barrier". Following intravenous injection, Evans Blue, ferritin and peroxidase do not cross into the bulk of the brain tissue, not even after prolonged intervals, except at a few small areas which have been found to be supplied by normally permeable capillaries of the type found in muscle (with zonulae adherentes), or even by perforated capillaries: the neurohypophysis, pineal, area postrema and intercolumnar tubercle.

(C) Continuous endothelium with mixed junctions

It seems that some capillaries (and arteries) may possess both zonulae adherentes and zonulae occludentes. The "mapping" of the body's capillary regions with respect to the frequency of these two junction types has yet to be done.

(2) Capillaries with discontinuous endothelium

These capillaries are all distinguished by very thin walls and they can be classified into the following three types, listed in order of increasing discontinuity (and permeability) of their wall:

(A) Perforated endothelium with diaphragms and basement membranes (Plate 27, Fig. C)

This type shows chains of multiple perforations of the endothelial cytoplasm or "pores", around 1000 Å wide, which are sealed by very thin membranes or "diaphragms", thinner than a single plasma membrane; the spotwise sieve-like endothelium is surrounded by a basement membrane. Such capillaries prevail in the intestinal villi, in endocrine glands and in the hemopoietic tissues where they probably allow a more rapid molecular traffic between the intra- and extra-capillary spaces than would be possible with capillaries of the continuous endothelium type. A high degree of capillary permeability would of course favour rapid absorption into the blood of vital materials from the intestinal lumen and of urgently needed hormones from endocrine glands. The extra thin diaphragms of these capillaries have proven permeable to intravenously injected fine carbon particles.

The perforations of this and the next two capillary types are thought to be structures in a flux, appearing and disappearing continuously.

(B) Perforated endothelium without diaphragms but with basement membranes (Plate 27, Fig. D)

The endothelial pores of this type of capillary are not sealed by diaphragms, but the endothelial lining is surrounded by a thick (about 1500 Å wide) basement membrane. This variant prevails in the glomeruli of the kidney where it allows the rapid filtration of all constituents of blood plasma except the largest molecules (proteins) out of the capillary lumen.

(C) Perforated endothelium without diaphragms and without basement membranes (Plate 27, Fig. E)

These are the capillaries with the highest permeability since their wall shows complete wide gaps (0.1–3 μ wide) that are not sealed by diaphragms or basement membrane; the latter is limited to fragments underlying the solid parts of the endothelium. Thus the whole plasma of the blood moves freely out of these capillaries and continuously bathes the cells outside them. They prevail in the liver and the spleen where they ensure the maximum possible contact between plasma and the largest metabolic factory and the largest reticuloendothelial organ, respectively. The endothelial cytoplasm of these wide-lumen capillaries tends to contain more organelles than that of other capillary types, notably ribosomes and lysosomes, indicating more active enzyme-production and phagocytic potential than is found in the endothelium of other capillary types. In the spleen, however, the phagocytic ability of the endothelial cells is greatly surpassed by that of the macrophages in the parenchyma.

III. ARTERIOLES AND ARTERIES

(1) Metarteriole (Plate 28, Fig. A)

The wall of a metarteriole (a vessel less than 15 μ wide) consists of endothelium[1] and basement membrane[2] which splits to envelop pericytes[3] that form a discontinuous periendothelial layer. The endothelium is of the type found in muscle capillaries, with often fibrillar cytoplasmic matrix; the pericytes, as in capillary walls, are undifferentiated cells.

(2) Terminal arteriole (Plate 28, Fig. B)

The wall of a terminal arteriole (a vessel less than 50 μ wide) consists of endothelium[1] similar to that of metarterioles, basement membrane[2] (BM) and a single continuous layer of smooth muscle cells[3] (myocytes). The latter are attached to the endothelial BM and to one another by means of collagen fibrils[4] which they produce along with translucent glycoprotein. The fibrils are thin and unstriated close to the endothelium but thicker and striated further away from it.

(3) Arteriole proper (Plate 28, Fig. C)

The wall of an arteriole proper consists of (a) an endothelium[1] similar to that found in the previous two vessels, (b) a basement membrane[2] (BM), (c) collagen fibrils[3] attaching the BM to (d) an "internal" elastic lamella[4] with large pores[5] (fenestrae), (e) at least two layers of smooth muscle cells[6] (myocytes), (f) collagen fibrils connecting the myocytes to one another[7] and to the elastic lamella[8], and (g) occasional axon terminals[9] synapsing with one of the outer myocytes. The endothelial cells (a) show prominent bundles of microfilaments, and (b) send occasional processes[10] through the "fenestrae" of the internal elastic lamella to "synapse" with inner myocyte processes[11] through "myo-endothelial junctions" that have a 50 Å intrajunctional cleft. The myocytes also communicate with one another by means of tight junctions[12] (zonulae occludentes or "nexuses") between their processes. The extracellular solid materials of the arteriolar wall (collagen and elastin) are apparently produced by the indigenous wall cells, while the origin of the translucent glycoprotein that permeates collagen is uncertain (it may be derived from the plasma).

It is thought that *contraction* of the arteriolar wall may be elicited in two ways: *from outside* (through arrival of an impulse in an innervating axon terminal) or *from inside* (in response to chemicals or a pressure drop in the luminal blood).

When contraction is elicited by nervous stimulation, the impulse is transmitted from an axon terminal to an outer myocyte through a neuro-muscular synapse and from that myocyte to all the other smooth muscle cells by means of the tight junctions between them.

When contraction is elicited in response to chemical or hemodynamic stimuli operating from the lumen, the endothelial cells are thought to serve as "sensors" for the above stimuli and to transmit them through the myo-endothelial junctions to some inner myocytes from where the stimuli are propagated to the rest of the smooth muscle cells through the tight junctions between them.

(4) Muscular artery (Plate 28, Fig. D)

The wall of a muscular artery is essentially the same as that of an arteriole, with the following differences, which materialise gradually as the vessel grows bigger and as its wall thickness increases: (a) the arterial wall acquires more myocyte layers which, in their entirety, form the "media", (b) it develops first a fenestrated thin "external" elastic lamina[1] and then increasing numbers of short "intermediate" elastic laminar segments[2], and (c) a condensation of areolar connective tissue all around the vessel (the "adventitia") containing fibroblasts, arterioles, capillaries and venules (the "vasa vasorum") and axons (the "nervi vasorum"). Furthermore, the endothelial cells of most vertebrates arteries often exhibit a more substantial and more active rough endoplasmic reticulum[3] than is usually found in arterioles, as well as oval[4] or rod-shaped[5] membrane-bound dense bodies with crystalline substructure, particularly in the large vessels. Some of these dense inclusions seem to represent the thromboplastic materials which are known to exist in arterial intima, since they resemble the α-granules of platelets and are apparently released into the blood along with thromboplastins under certain experimental conditions. An interesting possibility that also merits exploration is that certain dense endothelial bodies may represent pressor or depressor substances secreted by the endothelium into the bloodstream in response to sensed hemodynamic changes and contributing to the homeostasis of blood pressure.

Recently, it has been found that the intercellular junctions of the arterial endothelium can open in response to a great variety of agents such as high and low concentrations of angiotensin, hypertension, high concentrations of catecholamines, calcium-removal through chelation, extreme or very prolonged hyperlipemia, very alkaline pH, cyanide, and mitosis following endothelial injury. Some of these agents work by causing contraction or degenerative changes in endothelial cells, others by destroying the cementing materials in the intercellular junctions, and mitosis can apparently produce small gaps between the two daughter cells which are later replaced by a new junction. Temporary gaps in the endothelium are caused not only by opened junctions but also by the sloughing off of individual endothelial cells following all kinds of severe injury. Finally, several agents have been reported to increase pinocytosis by endothelial cells (*e.g.* hypertension, prostaglandins, low concentrations of catecholamines). Since the most important arterial disease results from the entry and accumulation in the arterial wall of materials that come from the blood (lipids), it is evident that any agent which can "open doors" in the endothelium for these materials can be pathogenic.

(5) Elastic artery, neonatal structure (Plate 28, Fig. E)

Its wall has the same basic structure as that of a muscular artery, with the addition of several elastic laminae[1] (several dozen in the human aorta) which are alternating with myocyte layers. All elastic laminae have multiple fenestrae[2] through which cells of different layers establish contacts with one another (myoendothelial junctions and nexuses). These fenestrae frequently contain small islands of elastin which are often connected to the surrounding rims through elastin bridges and thus plug most of the lumen of the apertures in which they are lodged. The myocytes are attached to the elastic laminae[3] and to one another[4] by means of collagen fibrils embedded in translucent glycoprotein.

During embryonic life, elastic laminae are produced mainly by the smooth muscle cells that make up the bulk of the arterial media, by their undifferentiated mesenchymal precursors, and by the fibroblasts that border the outer media. Autoradiographic studies with labeled amino acids suggest that these cells produce first soluble proelastin in their RER and that this is later incorporated into the definitive extracellular elastin.

Copper seems to be essential for the structural integrity of elastic lamellae, particularly during youth: nutritional deficiency of this metal in young swine or chicks leads to defective, fragmented elastic laminae and therefore to weakening and rupture of arterial walls. The main chemical defect here seems to be a failure of transformation of soluble proelastin into definitive elastin.

(6) Carotid and aortic body (glomus)

Attached to the common carotid and the aorta are certain clusters (glomuses) of aterioles and perforated capillaries. Scattered between the capillaries and closely adhering to their thin wall are chemoreceptor cells (also called "type I" or "enclosed" cells) that contain dense granules, *i.e.* 350–1900 Å thick cored vesicles of the monoamine type; they are apparently contacted by both afferent and efferent axons and, along with the latter, they are surrounded by supporting cells (also called "type II" or "enclosing" cells). The chemoreceptor cells seem to respond to rises of blood CO_2 (and drops of pH or O_2) by firing impulses into the sympathetic nervous system and (b) by releasing catecholamines from their cored vesicles into the blood stream. They pick up labeled catecholamine and indolamine precursors (like adrenergic axon terminals) and the density of their granules is appreciably diminished – but not abolished – by reserpin.

IV. VENULES AND VEINS

(1) Venules (Plate 29, Fig. A)

As in arterioles, the wall of venules rapidly changes structure with increasing vessel size but its thickness always lags behind that of arterioles of corresponding diameter. Thus, at a diameter of about 20 μ, venules are mere endothelial tubes surrounded by a basement membrane, like muscle capillaries; at about 50 μ they acquire a discontinuous sheath of pericytes, like metarterioles (Fig. A), while at 200 μ this sheath turns into a continuous single myocyte layer, as in terminal arterioles. The venular endothelial cells (a) are characterised by a remarkably low frequency of pinocytotic vesicles, (b) contain a fair number of lysosomes[1], more than are found in the endothelium of any other segment of the terminal vascular bed, and (c) are joined to one another through junctions of the zonula adherens type[2] mainly, with a cleft of about 150 Å or more.

Venules represent the most permeable segment of the blood-containing vascular tree and are the prime actors in the inflammatory response of vessels to injury, when they dilate and leak abundant plasma and leucocytes into the injured tissues. Their endothelial junctions readily open in response to histamine, bradykinine, serotonine, leucocytic materials, etc., probably as a result of endothelial cell contractions induced by the above substances. Both granular leucocytes and lymphocytes leave venules by passing through their loosened endothelial junctions.

(2) Veins (Plate 29, Fig. B)

The wall of a large vein is generally similar to that of a large muscular artery of corresponding diameter with the following differences: (a) its media is much thinner, (b) its media contains much more collagen and also some fibroblasts[1] and (c) its adventitia is often thicker than the media and may contain longitudinally or spirally running myocytes[2] which are thought to help propel the blood towards the heart through a peristaltic or "wringing" action. Venous valves are folds of endothelium with a core of collagen.

V. LYMPHATIC VESSELS

(1) Lymphatic capillaries (Plate 29, Fig. C)

These represent simple endothelial canals that apparently begin as blind (closed-end) tubes, without any open communication with the tissue spaces. Their endothelium is generally similar to that of the blood-carrying capillaries, with the following differences: (a) it is thinner than in blood capillaries, (b) it is *not* enveloped by a basement membrane and (c) *no* pericytes are attached to it; its junctions are mixed and often open.

The above structural features make lymphatic capillaries more permeable to macromolecules than blood capillaries and make the former eminently suitable for their function which is to drain tissue fluid with any macromolecules and particles it may contain.

(2) Larger lymphatic vessels

With increasing caliber, the wall of lymphatic vessels acquires first pericytes and finally myocytes, imitating the structure of veins but always lagging behind the latter in thickness. The largest lymphatic vessel of all, the thoracic duct, has even more muscle in its media than the largest vein (the vena cava).

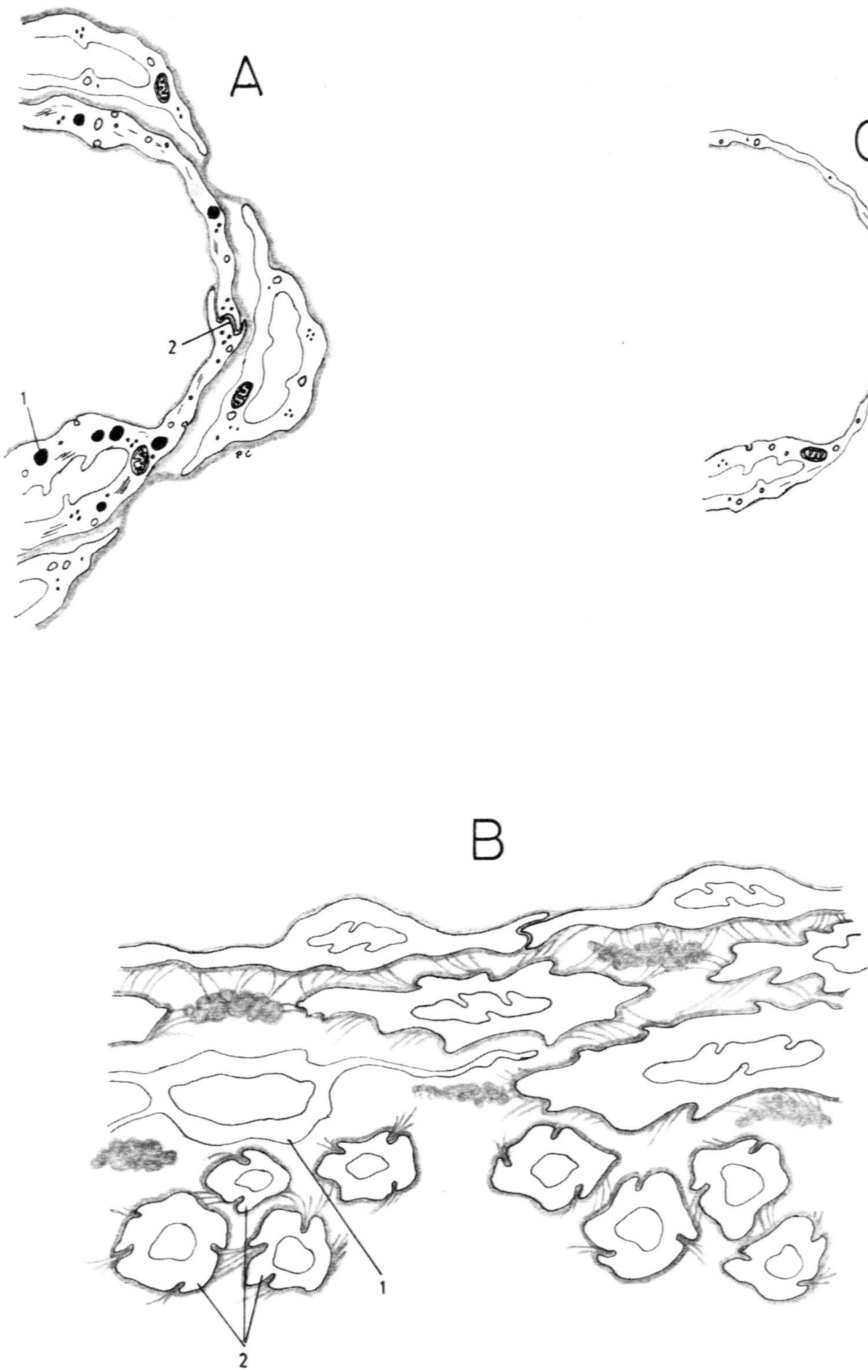

Plate 29

VI. HEART

The *endocardial lining* is identical to the endothelium of arteries, and the *myocardium* and *impulse-conducting* tissue have been described in the chapter on muscle. The mesothelial lining of the *pericardial sac* is similar to the peritoneal lining of the intestine (see chapter on alimentary system). Its endothelial-type cells are joined to one another partly by tight junctions and partly by very small, easily missed, desmosomes; they are rich in lysosomes and transport particles introduced into the pericardial sac (*e.g.* thorotrast) through pinocytosis.

Chapter 8

Respiratory System

I. GENERAL (Plate 30)

The respiratory system ensures a continuous delivery of oxygen into the blood and a continuous removal of CO_2 from it. It consists of a large tube, the trachea, which carries air from outside into the body interior where it branches repeatedly first into several generations of bronchi, and finally (Fig. A) into respiratory bronchioles[1] that expand into alveolar ducts[2], whose walls form small blind sacs, the alveoli[3]; each alveolus is surrounded by a basket of capillaries[4] through which blood exchanges gases with air. Since the crowded alveoli abut on one another, the spaces in any two adjacent alveoli[5] are separated by a partition (alveolar septum) consisting of a capillary network[6] which is lined on each side by flat alveolar epithelium[7]. Each lung represents a branching tree of air tubes and accompanying vessels, wrapped up by the simple squamous mesothelium of the visceral pleura which reflects at the lung roots to become the parietal pleura.

The trachea and the extrapulmonary bronchi have stiff walls of hyaline cartilage crescents that keep them permanently patent; they are lined by what appears under the L/M as pseudostratified columnar ciliated epithelium with goblet cells ("respiratory" epithelium) underneath which lie numerous sero-mucous glands whose secretion adds to that of the goblet cells. The wall of the air tubes undergoes the following main changes as one moves towards the alveoli: (a) in the intrapulmonary bronchi the cartilage breaks up into multiple plates, (b) in the terminal bronchioles the cartilage, the goblet cells and the sero-mucous glands disappear and smooth muscle gains prominence, and (c) in the short respiratory bronchioles, just before the alveolar ducts, the epithelium becomes simple cuboidal and smooth muscle largely disappears.

II. TRACHEA AND BRONCHUS EPITHELIUM ("RESPIRATORY" EPITHELIUM)

(1) Structure (Plate 30)

The epithelium is stratified and consists of basal, intermediate and three kinds of superficial cells: ciliated, brush and goblet cells (Figs. B, C, D), which are joined to one another by means of tight junctions. There are wide intercellular spaces in its middle and basal layers, and it is supported by a basement membrane (BM) which in turn is sitting on a thick layer of collagen fibrils. The BM and underlying collagen layer together constitute what looks like an unusually thick "BM" under the light microscope.

The *ciliated cells* (Fig. B) are characterised by more cilia[1] than microvilli[2], apical coils of very thin microfilaments (filosomes)[3] and numerous mitochondria[4], some of them branched and in contact with the basal corpuscles of the cilia. Ciliary structure is of the 9 + 2 type already described in general cytology. Both the cilia and the microvilli exhibit ATPase activity.

The *brush cells* (Fig. C) are very similar to the ciliated cells but they have more microvilli than cilia on their free surface and they occur much less frequently than the latter. Some of them are apparently enveloped by dendritic nerve fibers and are believed to be chemoreceptors.

The *goblet cells* (Fig. D) which are described in detail in the section on the alimentary system, are distinguished by a mass of confluent mucous droplets[1], an extensive Golgi system[2] and a prominent rough endoplasmic reticulum[3].

The *basal cells* (Fig. E) are characterised by small processes, numerous microfilaments[1] and ribosomes[2] and occasional lysosomes[3].

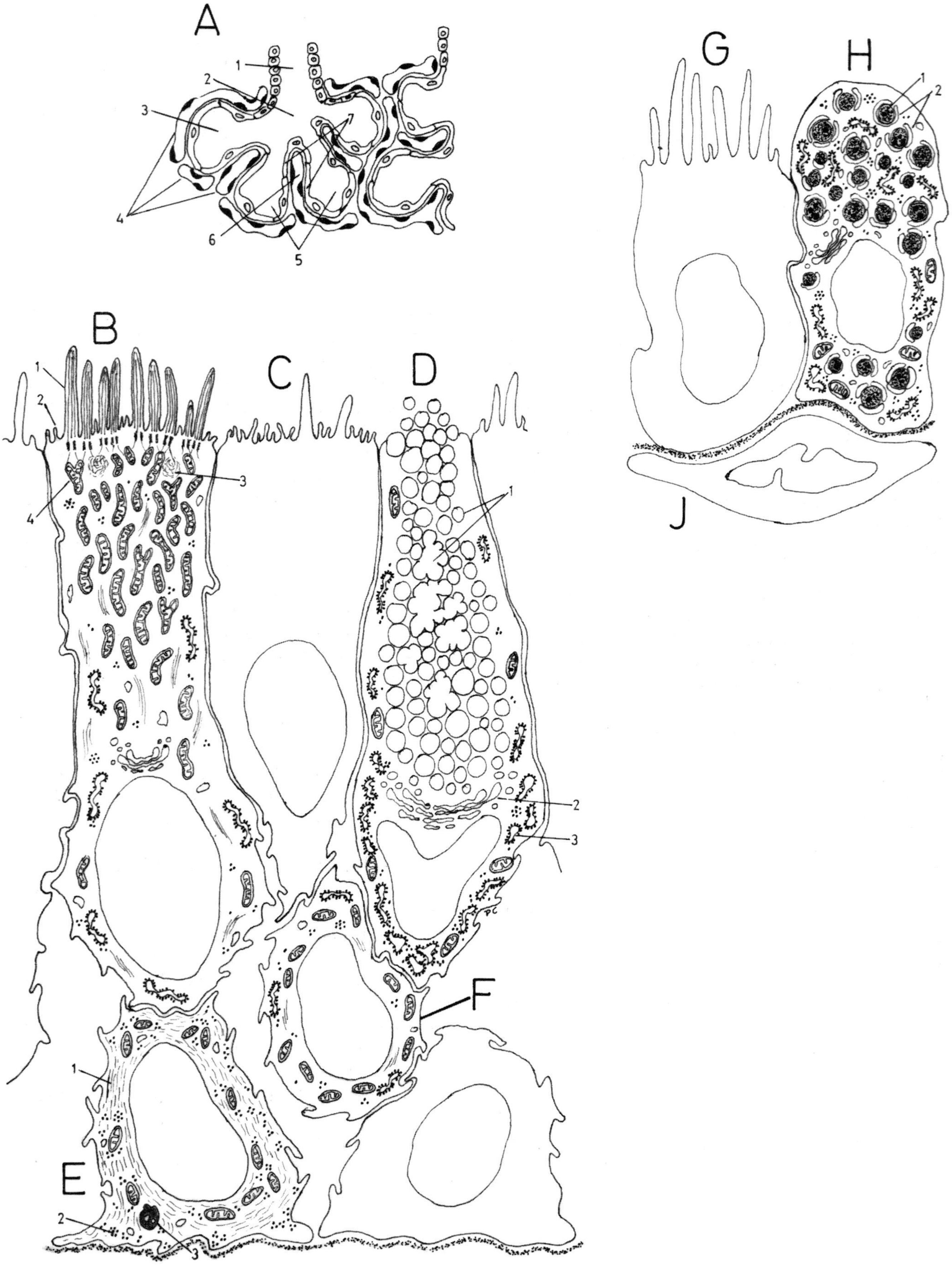

Plate 30

The *intermediate cells* (Fig. F) have no special features.

(2) Function

Besides providing a physical lining for the main air ducts, this epithelium is also concerned with (a) keeping its free surface constantly wet to prevent dehydration and shrivelling of its cytoplasm and to wet the instreaming air before it reaches the alveoli, (b) trapping and expelling some of the foreign particles (*e.g.* dusts, bacteria) that are carried into the bronchial tree by the inrushing air, and (c) offering some preliminary immunological resistance to airborne microorganisms.

The *wetting* is realised by (a) the mucus production of the goblet cells and (b) by additional mucus and also a serous (watery) secretion that are produced by subepithelial glands and are discharged on to the epithelial surface. Some of the fluid pool that is secreted evaporates but much of it is probably reabsorbed, accounting most likely in part for the extracellular spaces in the middle and basal epithelial layers. By virtue of antibodies of the IgA type that it contains, the secreted fluid also imparts some *protection against infection* to the epithelium it covers.

The *trapping* of some airbone particles is probably expedited through their adhesion to the sticky mucous film that forms on the epithelial surface while their *expulsion* is thought to be helped by movements of the cilia in the direction of the larynx.

As in all stratified epithelial linings, it is thought that the superficial cells of the respiratory epithelium are *continuously worn and sloughed off* into the lumen, to be replaced by new cells that push up from the bottom. Thus, the basal cells are thought to move up and differentiate into the brush cells and the latter to turn into ciliated cells, whereby the role and fate of the basal cell microfilaments is still not clear; conversely, the intermediate cells might turn into goblet cells. Appreciable study has been recently devoted to the *replication of ciliary basal corpuscles and centrioles* during this process of epithelial renewal; it seems that both organelles contain DNA and that their replication and ciliary development evolve structurally through the following visible stages, at least in amphibia: Small dense bodies (the "procentriole precursors") materialise in the apical cytoplasm of new prospective ciliated cells and are transformed into *ca.* 1500 Å wide cylinders whose wall consists of 9 microtubules (the "procentrioles") under the organizing influence of certain amorphous dense masses (the "procentriole organizers"). "Procentrioles", in turn, are transformed into *ca.* 2000 Å wide cylinders with a wall of 9 microtubule triplets (the "definitive centrioles") which become "basal bodies" when they become aligned perpendicularly to the apical PM and grow ciliary shafts (9 + 2 sets of microtubules) out of small dense bodies that develop at their apical end. The composition of the above structures in terms of DNA, RNA and protein has yet to be established.

III. TERMINAL BRONCHIOLE EPITHELIUM

(1) Structure (Plate 30)

This epithelium consists of a single layer of ciliated cells (Fig. G) alternating with granule-filled "Clara" cells (Fig. H). There are no goblet cells within or glands underneath this epithelium, which is supported by a basement membrane and underlaid by smooth muscle cells (Fig. J) that encircle the bronchiolar lumen.

The *ciliated cells* have the same structure as those of the trachea and bronchi. The *Clara cells* (Fig. H) are distinguished by numerous membrane-limited dense round bodies[1] which contain granular inclusions in their matrix, and are "wrapped" in concentric outlays of smooth endoplasmic reticulum (SER) cisternae[2] in the mouse but are free in the rat. Recently, some *argentaffine cells* have also been identified in this epithelium, squeezed in between its base and its basement membrane (See argentaffine cells in Chapter 9, Alimentary System, Section IV, 5, p. 109.

(2) Function

There are no goblet cells or glands in this mucous membrane because (a) the secretion of fluid at such a short distance from the alveoli would be dangerous, and (b) by the time it reaches the terminal bronchioles, the air is wetted by the secretions in the preceding bronchi.

The function of the *Clara cells* is at the moment obscure. Their numerous SER-wrapped bodies may represent phospholipoproteins secreted by exocytosis. Perhaps these cells will prove to bear a certain relationship to the phospholipid-producing great alveolar cells in the alveolar septa.

The contraction of the *smooth muscle cells* in the bronchiolar wall evidently reduces the diameter of the bronchiolar lumen. It is thus possible that these myocytes help to regulate air flow and adjust it in response to chemical feedbacks from the blood signalling the oxygenation degree of the latter; they are already known to respond to the rise of blood histamine and other substances by going into a spasm.

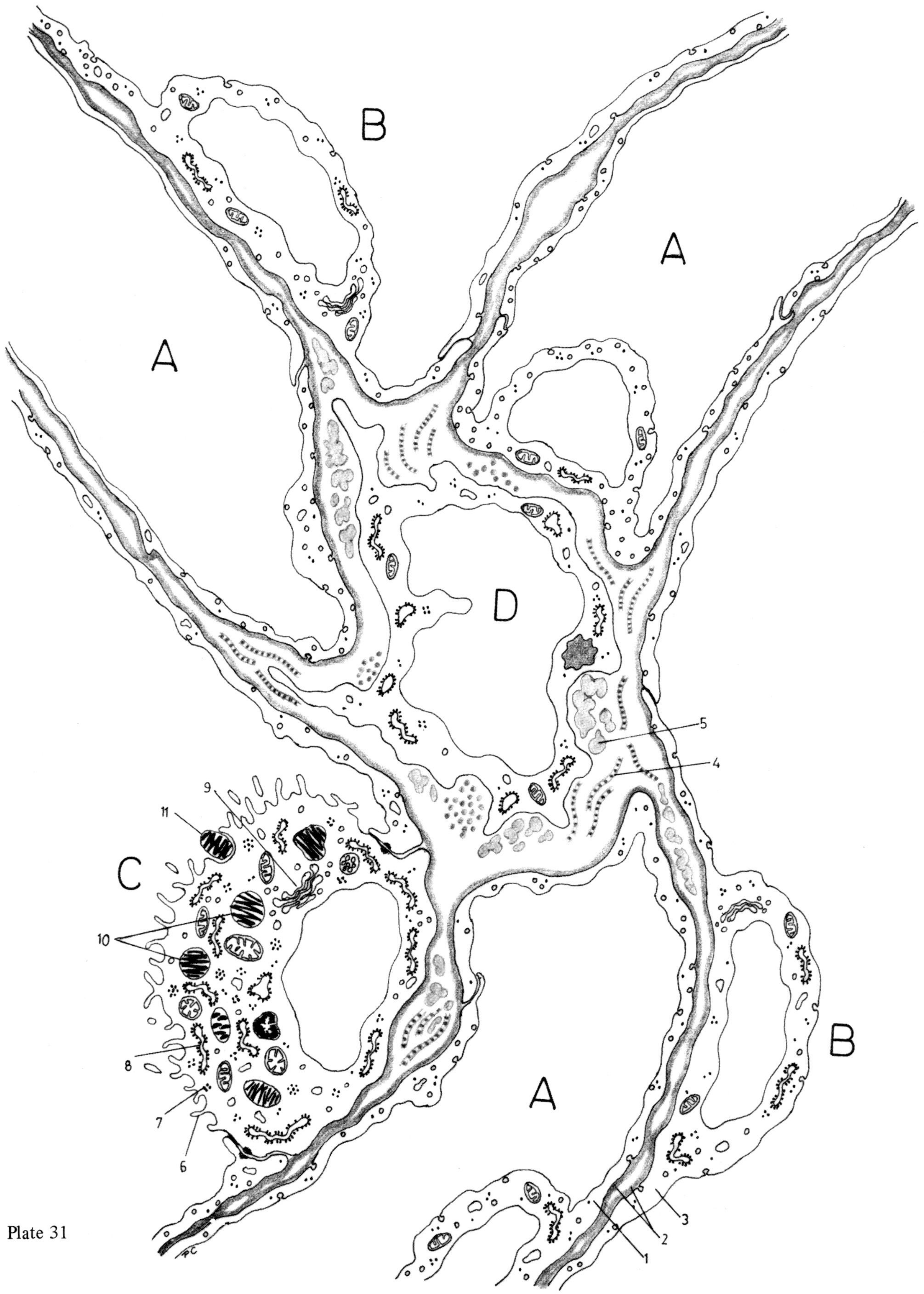

Plate 31

IV. ALVEOLAR SEPTUM

(1) Structure (Plate 31)

The alveolar septum is a partition between two neighbouring alveolar spaces that consists of a capillary loop (Fig. A) clothed by a continuous lining of alveolar epithelial cells of mainly two types: (a) flat small epithelial cells (Fig.B), the type I pneumocytes (the majority), interconnected by zonulae occludentes, and (b) round large epithelial cells (Fig. C), the type II or "granular" pneumocytes (the minority), connected to their neighbours by junctional complexes. Occasionally, "brush cells" with microvilli but no cilia, similar to those described in respiratory epithelium, are seen adjacent to type I pneumocytes. As a result of their direct juxtaposition, the basement membranes of the capillary and its epithelial lining often fuse. Thus the blood inside the capillary is separated from air by the following three layers which together form the "blood–air barrier": (a) a thin endothelial cytoplasm[1], (b) a double basement membrane[2], and (c) a thin epithelial cytoplasm[3]. In the small interstitial spaces between or in the center of capillary loops reside "interstitial" cells (Fig. D) which are surrounded by collagen fibrils[4] and some elastin flakes[5]; in corresponding positions at the free edges of alveolar septa smooth muscle cells have been described. Phagocytic cells that have picked up airborne foreign particles (*e.g.* various dusts, bacteria) or the debris of dead erythrocytes are often found in the alveolar spaces.

The capillary *endothelium* is of the type found in muscle with zonulae adherentes through which peroxidase molecules can pass. The *small epithelial cells* or type I pneumocytes (Fig. B) are very similar to the endothelial cells, possessing, like the latter, numerous pinocytotic vesicles in addition to small numbers of basic organelles. The *large epithelial cells* or type II pneumocytes (Fig. C) are characterised by microvilli[6], prominent ribosomes[7], rough endoplasmic reticulum[8] and a Golgi system[9] and numerous membrane-bound lamellated dense bodies[10] that contain phospholipids, are much denser in rats, mice, dogs, fetal rabbits and fetal sheep than in hamsters and guinea pigs, and are apparently secreted into the alveolar space by emiocytosis[11] Thus, lamellated or crystalloid phospholipid materials are often found in the alveolar spaces of some species (*e.g.* man, rat) and a continuous dense film that apparently contains phospholipids (*e.g.* dipalmitoyl lecithin) is seen to line the alveolar epithelium in others (*e.g.* chicks, lambs and guinea pigs) if very special techniques such as "tricomplex flocculation" are used to preserve it. Apart from the phospholipid lining, a thin acid polysaccharide coat (sialic acid) can be demonstrated to be closely attached to the outer leaflet of the alveolar epithelial plasma membrane in several species. The *interstitial cells* (Fig. D) are probably fibroblasts that produce the sparse amounts of septal collagen and elastin and that send processes into all recesses of the interstitial space but they might also have some endocrine function; the alveolar phagocytes are distinguished, like all macrophages, by processes, lysosomes and phagosomes.

(2) Function

The main function of the alveolar septa is to promote *gas exchanges* between blood and air across the triple-layered blood–air barrier which is very thin in order to accelerate such exchanges (the total thickness of the barrier is about 2000–4000 Å); both O_2 and CO_2 apparently diffuse passively across the plasma membranes, thin cytoplasmic sheets and basement membranes of the barrier.

Accessory functions of the alveolar septum include (a) the *dissipation of heat* from the blood by convection and by evaporation of water, and (b) the removal from the blood of appreciable amounts of *water* and of occasional volatile solutes such as *alcohols*, whereby liquid movements across both the endothelial and epithelial layers of the barrier may be expedited by pinocytotic transfer.

The secretion of a *phospholipid* material ("surfactin") on to the alveolar epithelial surfaces by the type II pneumocytes diminishes the surface tension of the latter and thus counteracts the collapse of the alveolar spaces. Since the numbers of lamellated dense bodies in the granular pneumocytes correlate well with the surfactant activity of lung extracts, these inclusions seem to represent the "surfactin" that lung physiologists discovered in recent years; they apparently develop from the interaction of Golgi-associated vesicles with multivesicular bodies.

Finally, the *alveolar phagocytes* play an important role in defense since they engulf invading foreign particles and remove them from the alveolar spaces (a) by being ejected out of the lungs (through coughing) or (b) by crawling into the interstitial space of septa and migrating from there into the pulmonary lymph nodes. While in the past these phagocytes had been thought to represent detached ("exfoliated") epithelial cells, there is now growing evidence that they represent blood monocytes which emigrate from the septal capillaries into the alveolar spaces where they turn into typical macrophages. This evidence is based on the ultrastructural and certain histochemical differences between alveolar phagocytes and alveolar epithelial cells, as well as on the finding that soon after introduction of foreign particles (*e.g.* thorium, pneumococci) into the lungs, phagocytes appear in the alveolar spaces and pick up the particles whereas the epithelial cells neither detach nor engage in phagocytosis. Smoking, like other particulate irritants, increases the number of phagocytes that can be retrieved from human lungs by bronchial lavage.

V. PLEURAL MESOTHELIUM

See peritoneal mesothelium (in Ch. 9, Alimentary System, Sect. V, 2, p. 111) which has the same ultrastructure.

Chapter 9

Alimentary System

I. GENERAL

The alimentary system consists of a long tube in which food is broken down chemically (digested) and absorbed into the blood stream. Its anterior end, the mouth, is specialised in the prehension and rough homogenisation of food through the cutting and grinding action of teeth, aided by the wetting and preliminary digestive effect of the salivary gland secretions and the voluntary movements of the tongue; the entire mouth-cavity is lined by squamous stratified epithelium which normally keratinises only at the tips of certain projections of the tongue surface, the filiform and fungiform papillae, and often contains primarily mucous small glands in its lamina propria. From the mouth, food passes through the pharynx and esophagus to the stomach, whose glands initiate the main protein digestion and whose powerful wall muscle completes the homogenisation process. Finally, food is transmitted from the stomach to the long intestinal tube, whose glands (including the liver and the exocrine pancreas) complete the digestive process and whose extensive epithelial surface absorbs the products of that process.

II. TOOTH

(1) General (Figs. A–C)

The development of a lower jaw tooth from its embryonic primordium to its definitive structure is summarised and simplified in the following three stages.

(A) Embryonic primordium (Plate 32, Fig. A)

From the floor of the mouth cavity between the lips[1] and the tongue[2] an ectodermal tissue mass in the form of an inverted cup, the "enamel organ"[3], grows down into the underlying mesenchyme. The mesenchymal cells withing the cup[4] proliferate in preparation for their differentiation into dentin-forming cells (odontoblasts) and pulp.

(B) Beginning enamel and dentin formation (Plate 32, Fig. B)

A cavity splits the cup of the enamel into two cell layers, the outer enamel cells[1] and the inner enamel cells or "ameloblasts"[2]. The ameloblasts produce enamel[3] between their tips; the most peripheral mesenchymal cells in the cup, the odontoblasts[4], line up in a row facing the ameloblasts and produce dentin[5] while the central ones remain undifferentiated[6] and are invaded by vessels[7] to form the tooth pulp. Figs. D and E represent E/M magnifications of ameloblasts and odontoblasts, respectively, from this stage.

(C) Definitive structure (Plate 32, Fig. C)

The adult tooth exhibits the following parts from the center out: (a) a *pulp chamber*[1] with mesenchymal pulp cells, vessels and nerves that reach it through the *root canal*[2], (b) a thick shell of *dentin*[3] which is penetrated radially by processes of numerous *odontoblasts*[4] (the cells that manufactured and maintain the dentin and still line its inner surface), (c) a thick cap of enamel[5] which has lost both the outer enamel cells and the ameloblasts that produced it (except at the lower sides where some of the latter persist), (d) a thin shell of bone-like tissue, the *cement*[6], around the lower dentin, (e) short collagen fibers, the *periodontal membrane*[7], attaching the tooth to its *bony socket*[8], and (f) the squamous stratified epithelium of the *gums*[9] pressing against the lower enamel sides and sealing off the periodontal space from the mouth cavity.

(2) Ameloblasts and enamel formation (Plate 32, Fig. D)

Ameloblasts are long prismatic epithelial cells that taper basally to a process[1] ("Tome's process") fringed with microvilli around which enamel[2] is laid down. They are characterised by (a) numerous RER cisternae[3] and a fair number of ribosomes, (b) an extensive and long Golgi system[4] at the enamelforming end, (c) numerous membrane-enclosed dense secretion granules[5] that originate

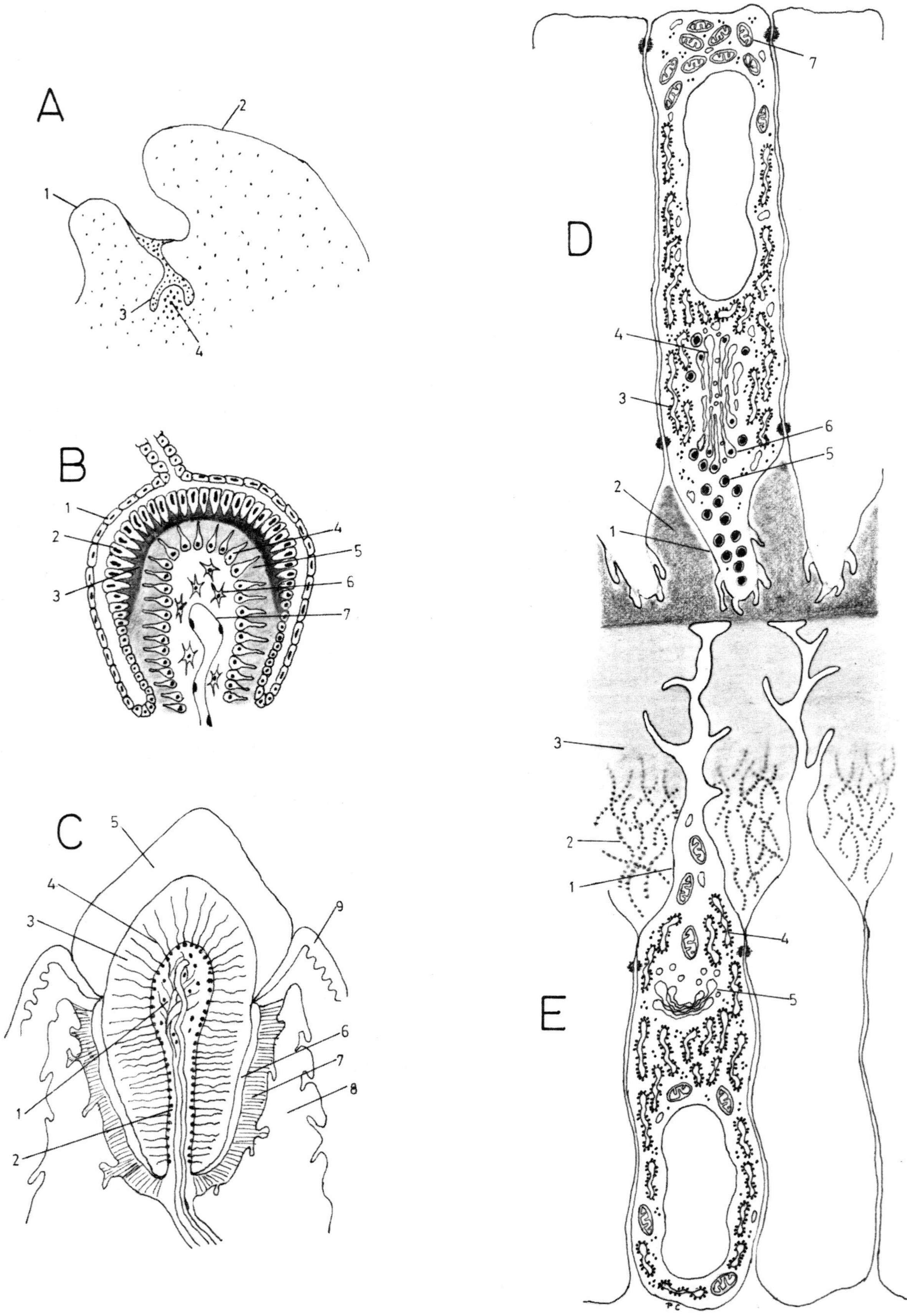

Plate 32

in the Golgi[6] and represent organic enamel precursors, (d) recently formed enamel around Tome's process with a crystalloid rodlet structure, (e) numerous apical mitochondria[7], and (f) zonulae adherentes that attach both ends of the ameloblast to its neighbours.

The ameloblasts secrete a protein component of enamel in the form of the membrane-enclosed granules that arise in their prominent Golgi; these granules are apparently released through emiocytosis and produce protein threads outside the cells that become mineralised (extracellularly) through the precipitation of a calcium phosphate–calcium carbonate–fluoride complex around them. Adult enamel constitutes the hardest substance in the body and consists of about 3% protein and 97% mineral. As the enamel grows in thickness by apposition, the ameloblasts always stay on top of it until the tooth erupts through the floor of the mouth, when they are rubbed off and further enamel formation ceases – except laterally at a very slow rate.

(3) Odontoblasts and dentin formation (Plate 32, Fig. E)

Odontoblasts face the ameloblasts; they taper apically into branching processes[1] around which first collagen fibrils[2] (predentin) and then dentin[3] (a bone-like material) is laid down. As the dentin layer thickens, the odontoblast processes elongate and – unlike the ameloblast processes – they stay buried in it for life (occupying narrow "canalicular" spaces molded to their shape). These cells are distinguished by (a) numerous RER cisternae[4] and several ribosomes, (b) a distinct apical Golgi[5], (c) a few SER vesicles and mitochondria, and (d) junctional complexes joining their "shoulders" with those of adjacent cells.

Dentin consists of about 28% collagen and 72% complex calcium phosphate–calcium carbonate salt. It is the same material as that found in bone and it seems to be produced in the same manner as bone is produced by osteoblasts, *i.e.* extracellularly, by the precipitation of mineral into a previously formed collagen framework (through extracellular enzyme activity). Odontoblasts not only function like fibroblasts and osteoblasts, but it seems possible that they also respond to heat, cold and chemical stimuli by generating and transmitting impulses to sensory pulp nerves.

III. SALIVARY GLANDS

(1) General (Plate 33, Fig. A)

Depending on the nature of their secretory portions, there are three types of salivary glands: serous, mucous and mixed. The mixed salivary glands possess (a) both serous[1] and mucous[2] secretory portions, and (b) mucous secretory portions surrounded by caps of serous cells[3] ("serous demilunes") all of which release their secretions into short intercalated[4] and then striated[5] ducts.

(2) Serous salivary glands

(A) Secretory portion cells (Plate 33, Fig. B)

Structure. These cells are distinguished by a prominent rough endoplasmic reticulum (RER)[1] at the base and sides, a large Golgi[2] and numerous membrane-bound secretory granules apically[3], some of them appearing to have broken envelopes (possibly due to artefact) or a dense periphery[4]; the contents of the secretory granules are discharged into the glands lumen (at the apical cell surface) through emiocytosis; the apical surfaces of the cells develop microvilli[5]; the lateral surfaces of adjoining cells (a) are joined through tight junctions apically, (b) interlock frequently, (c) often recede at a given site to form microvilli-lined tiny canals or canaliculi[6] that eventually reach the lumen, and (d) sometimes enclose what appear to be axon terminals[7] contacting the secretory cells; the basal surfaces are (a) often indented by tentacle-like smooth muscle "myoepithelial" cell processes[8], (b) underlaid by a basement membrane (BM), and (c) are sometimes approached by axons[9] which evidently penetrate the BM to move into the narrow intercellular cleft.

In addition to the above main secretory cell type, the acini (and ducts) of human salivary glands contain occasionally cells that are extraordinarily rich in mitochondria and have no known function, the so-called "oncocytes".

Function. The material in the secretory granules contributes to the thin "serous" component of saliva that consists of H_2O, electrolytes (to maintain a certain pH in the month) and the enzyme protein amylase (to initiate digestion of carbohydrates) and alkaline phosphatase; it is for the production of this enzyme protein that the serous cells have developed their prominent RER–Golgi systems. The function of the canaliculi in serous glands has not yet been adequately studied, nor is the significance of the occasionally ruptured envelope or heterogeneous content of secretory granules known. The contacts between axons and secretory cells represent the physical foundation of the long known nervous control of serous cell secretion while the tentacles of the myoepithelial cells (which envelop basket-like the whole secretory portion) presumably squeeze secretion out of the acinus lumen into the ducts.

Isoproterenol stimulates markedly the release and synthesis of secretory granules by these cells, and upon prolonged administration causes their mitosis and hyperplasia. By contrast, actinomycin inhibits the synthesis of

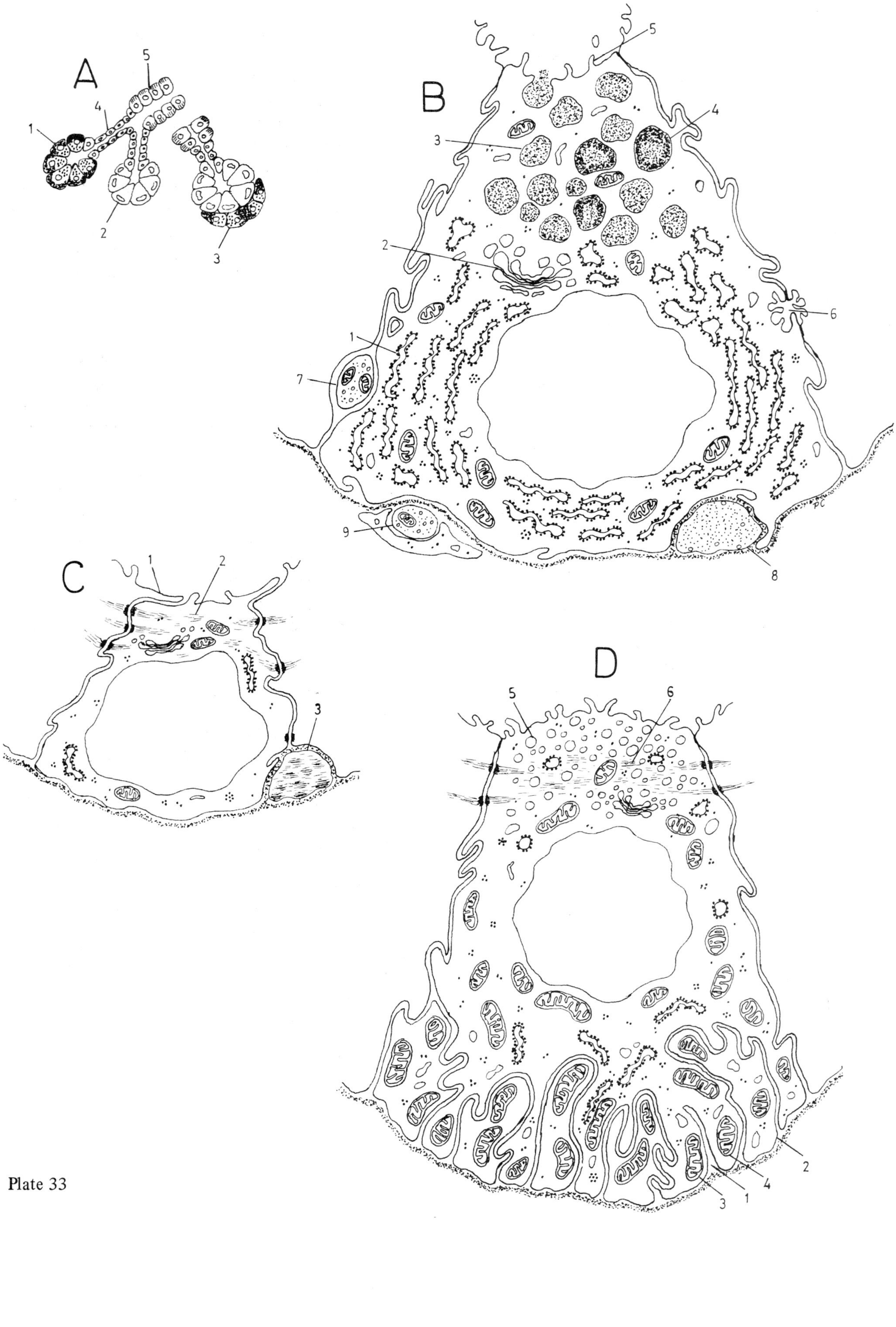

Plate 33

secretory granules by inhibiting RNA and therefore protein synthesis.

Mastication of solid food seems to be a powerful physiological stimulus for the function of serous salivary glands; when it is withdrawn (as after prolonged exclusively liquid diets), the parotid acini atrophy.

(B) Intercalated duct cells (Plate 33, Fig. C)

Apart from sparse basic organelles, a few apical microvilli and a basement membrane, these cells are characterised by (a) overlapping apical processes[1], (b) multiple desmosomes that join adjacent lateral surfaces, and (c) bundles of tonofilaments[2] that criss-cross their cytoplasm which is "taken up" during duct expansion. The myoepithelial cell tentacles[3] occasionally run under their basal surfaces.

The structure of the intercalated duct indicates that it is designed to merely conduct its fluid contents and to withstand some caliber expansion without leakage – hence the multiple desmosomes and the overlapping apical processes that probably represent "reserve" cytoplasm which is "taken up" during duct expansion. The myoepithelial processes around the duct possibly help to regulate the flow of secretion by varying their state of contraction and, therefore, the duct diameter.

(C) Striated duct cells (Plate 33, Fig. D)

These cells are distinguished by (a) a basement membrane, (b) numerous basal infoldings[1] and interdigitations with basal processes of neighbouring cells[2], (c) numerous mitochondria closely associated with the basal infoldings[3] and interdigitations[4], and (d) numerous microvesicles[5] in the apical cytoplasm; their apical surface forms microvilli and lateral surfaces are joined through tight junctions and multiple desmosomes from which bundles of tonofilaments[6] radiate into the apical cytoplasm. A sex difference has been reported in certain animals, the female apparently possessing a much more prominent striated tubule than the male.

The structure of the striated duct cells is in many ways similar to that of kidney tubule and apocrine sweat gland cells and indicates extensive fluid transport across the cell cytoplasm, either from the lumen to the base or the reverse. Unfortunately, there is no evidence at present as to whether fluid is being absorbed here from the lumen through the microvesicles into the blood or whether it moves in the opposite direction. Whether this duct segment proves to be a site of concentration or dilution of the primary secretion, it is certainly a modulator of the concentration of its solutes.

(3) Mucous and mixed salivary glands

(A) Secretory portion – mucous acinar cell (Plate 34, Fig. A)

This is very similar to the goblet cells (see section on intestine for further description). Most of its cytoplasm is occupied by a mass of translucent mucus[1] which is loculated by several thin cytoplasmic partitions[2] and results from the confluence of many membrane-bound mucus droplets[3]; the mucus mass probably flows into the lumen through an opening of the apical cell surface that represents a modified emiocytosis process, although the details of its exit mechanism are not quite certain yet. The sparse remaining cytoplasm of this cell is situated at the sides where it forms a "theca" (sheath) for the mucous mass and at the base, around the nucleus, where it exhibits a prominent rough endoplasmic reticulum[4] (RER) and Golgi system[5]. The lateral surfaces of adjacent cells are joined by tight junctions apically, interlock, and form canaliculi[6] that lead to the lumen, while the basal surfaces are underlaid by a basement membrane or serous demilune cells.

There is evidence that the protein component of mucus (a glycoprotein) is produced in the RER and passed on to the Golgi where it is packed together with carbohydrate into membrane-bound mucous granules.

Recently, axon terminals containing more empty than cored synaptic vesicles have been found to get very close to mucous acinar and myoepithelial cells (to within 200 Å of their PM) so that they are thought to innervate them.

(B) Secretory portion – serous demilune cells (Plate 34, Fig. B)

These are practically identical with the cell of the serous secretory portions already described but they seem to possess two types of secretory granules: some with a granular content[1], similar to that found in the RER cisternae[2], and some with an amorphous content[3]. The granule contents are discharged by emiocytosis into tiny microvilli-fringed canaliculi[4] between the demilune cells that connect with the upper canaliculi between the mucous cells and hence reach the gland lumen.

It is not known why serous is mixed with mucous secretion within the lumen of the mucous glands that possess demilunes, but it is possible that the demilune cells may produce carbohydrate-depolymerising enzymes that control the viscosity of the mucus.

(C) Intercalated and striated ducts

These are similar to the corresponding structures of

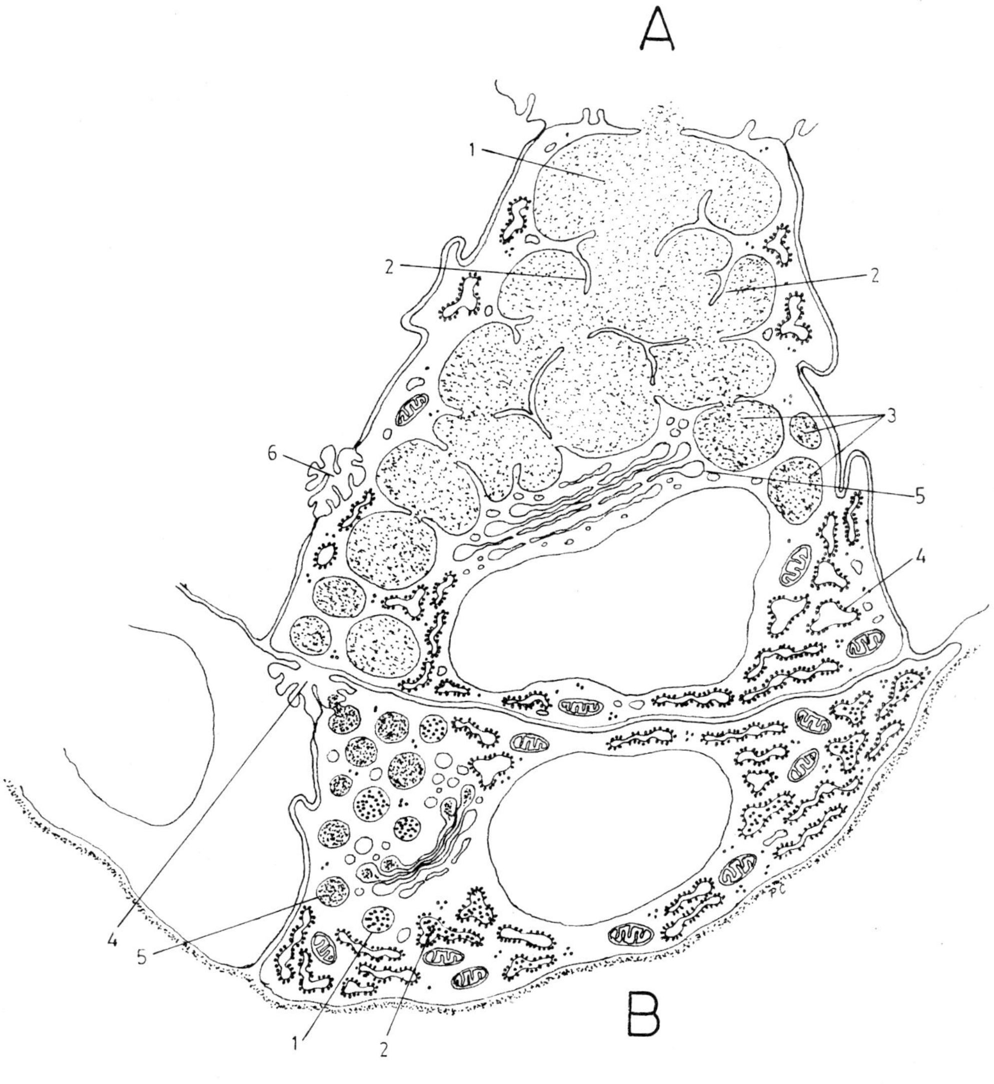

Plate 34

the serous glands, but the former possess *no* microvilli and the latter exhibit only a rudimentary system of basal infoldings and interdigitations, reflecting probably much less active fluid reabsorption from the viscous mucus than is the case with the watery serous secretion.

When a good part of the submandibular gland is extirpated, regeneration proceeds from the ductal cells, which differentiate into new secretory cells.

IV. STOMACH

(1) General (Plate 35)

The stomach is lined by a simple columnar surface epithelium that forms long tubular "gastric" glands (with a short neck) (Fig. A) in the main body of this organ and shorter branching "pyloric" glands in its pyloric segment; the cells of the surface epithelium [1], the pyloric glands and the necks [2] of the gastric glands are mucus-secreting, while those of the secretory portions of the gastric glands are of three types: (a) oxyntic (parietal) [3] cells, (b) zymogenic (chief) cells [4], and (c) argentaffine [5] cells. There are several smooth muscle layers in the wall of the stomach and its outer surface is lined by peritoneal mesothelium (a simple squamous epithelium).

(2) Mucous surface epithelium and mucous neck cells of gastric glands (Plate 35, Fig. B)

Like mucous salivary and goblet cells, these cells produce mucus, but at a slower rate (hence there is usually no confluence of mucus droplets to a huge mass) and of a different variety (hence its greater density). They are thus distinguished by (a) an only moderate development of rough endoplasmic reticulum, (b) a prominent, often multiple Golgi [1], (c) numerous membrane-bound mucus ("mucigen") granules [2] that tend to remain discrete, probably discharge their contents through emiocytosis (although this is not yet quite settled), and are much denser in the mucous cells of the surface than those of the gastric glands, (d) apical microvilli [3] that tend to have a fuzzy coat [4], and (e) lateral surfaces that interlock and are joined by tight junctions and multiple desmosomes.

Their function is to deliver into the stomach interior a glucoprotein material that (a) forms a protective film over the stomach lining, preventing its destruction by its own enzymes and acidity, and (b) helps to lubricate the stomach contents; recently gastric mucopolysaccharides have also been shown to possess antilipemic activity, but the significance of this is still unknown. Mucin secretion is inhibited by cortisone treatment.

(3) Oxyntic (parietal) cells (Plate 35, Fig. C)

These cells are characterised by (a) deep invaginations [1] lined by numerous long microvilli [2] that represent a huge increment of their surface area, (b) an extraordinary number of mitochondria [3], (c) several lysosomomes, (d) tight junctions and multiple desmosomes at their lateral surfaces, and (e) some basal microvilli [4].

They produce the hydrochloric acid of the stomach, most probably in the form of a HCl–protein complex that splits off free HCl after it has emerged from the gastric gland into the stomach cavity. The unusual number of mitochondria indicates that either some phase of the HCl production process requires much energy or that the ions of this acid are assembled with the direct physical participation of these organelles. When parietal cells are stimulated by the stomach hormone *gastrin* to secrete hydrochloric acid, they greatly increase their microvillous surface, apparently by feeding PM into it from intracytoplasmic tubulovesicles.

(4) Zymogenic (chief) cells (Plate 35, Fig. D)

The zymogenic cells have, like the serous salivary cells, a structure typical of protein secretion. They display (a) a very prominent rough endoplasmic reticulum [1] (RER) whose cisternae are packed along the base and sides, (b) a Golgi, (c) numerous dense secretory ("zymogen") membrane-bound granules [2] that reach a large size and discharge their contents through emiocytosis [3], and (d) microvilli [4] at their apical and tight junctions and desmosomes at their lateral surfaces.

The content of the secretory granules is a precursor of the proteolytic enzyme pepsin (pepsinogen) that is activated by HCl after it emerges from the gastric glands.

Hypophysectomy causes a marked atrophy of these cells and a shrinkage of their RER, Golgi and pepsinogen granule population.

(5) Argentaffine cells (Plate 35, Fig. E)

These cells are small and located at the periphery of the gastric gland so that they do not reach its lumen, but face a capillary instead. They exhibit (a) an appreciable (for their size) rough endoplasmic reticulum [1], (b) a Golgi, (c) numerous membrane-bound secretory granules [2] most of them with very dense nucleoids [3] and (d) numerous microvesicles [4]. They are separated by a basement membrane (BM) from the capillary.

There is strong evidence that the dense granules contain serotonine (5-hydroxy-tryptamine) which is probably secreted through an as yet unknown mechanism

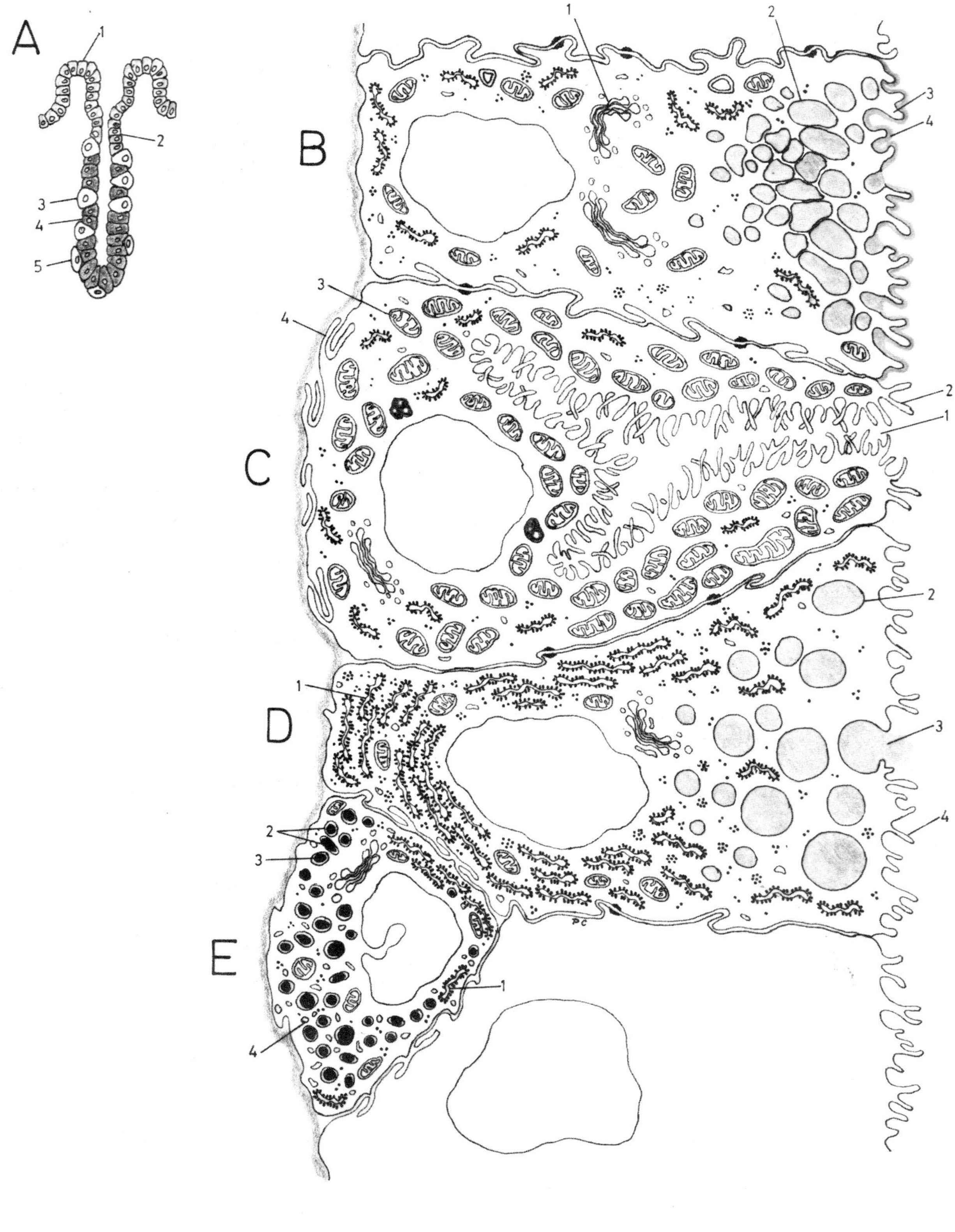

Plate 35

(perhaps diffusion) across the BM into the connective tissue space outside the gland and the facing capillary. The nucleated granules of the argentaffine cells resemble the nucleated serotonin granules of the platelets and the cored catecholamine vesicles of the adrenal medulla and adrenergic axon terminals; they become depleted by known catecholamine dischargers such as reserpine. The function of the serotonine from these cells is still uncertain; it may participate in the regulation of peristalsis by reaching smooth muscle cells via direct diffusion or via the bloodstream. It is now known that, in addition to their main product serotonin, argentaffine cells also produce other amines, polypeptides and the enzyme *kallikrein;* the latter releases bradykinin from α_2-globulin and is thus responsible for the vasodilator effect (flush) in patients with argentaffine cell tumors (*carcinoid syndrome*).

(6) Pyloric gland cells

Most cells of the pyloric glands are of one type and their ultrastructure seems identical to that of the mucous neck cells of the gastric glands, although the mucus they produce appears to be of a different variety in view of its different staining characteristics; like the mucous salivary glands they contain intercellular canaliculi; functionally, they seem to represent an additional source of glucoprotein.

Apart from mucous cells, the bottoms of pyloric glands are also inhabited by certain endocrine cells that look like argentaffine cells but contain the hormone *gastrin* in the dense homogeneous material of their capillary-oriented, 1500–2000 Å secretory vesicles. Gastrin, α-17-amino acid polypeptide, reaches the parietal cells of the stomach via the blood stream and stimulates them to secrete HCl; its own secretion is stimulated by acetylcholin.

V. INTESTINE

(1) General (Plate 36, Fig. A)

The lining of the intestinal canal consists of a simple columnar epithelium[1] that clothes the finger-like intraluminal projections (villi)[2] of the small intestine and forms the crypts of Lieberkuhn[3] in the lamina propria of the small and large intestine wall, as well as the mucoid Brunner's glands[4] in the submucosa of the initial part of the small intestine (the duodenum). The prevailing cell types of the villous and crypt epithelium are the absorptive[5] and mucoid[6] (goblet) cells, the percentage of the latter increasing progressively in caudal direction; in addition, there are some argentaffine cells and the bottoms of the crypts contain an appreciable number of enzyme-producing Paneth's cells[7]. The smooth muscle of the intestinal wall consists of an inner circular[8] and an outer longitudinal layer[9], while its free outer surface (like that of all abdominal viscera) is lined by peritoneal mesothelium[10].

The muscle of the intestinal wall is innervated by axons with the structural characteristics of both cholinergic and adrenergic nerves, their boutons (both terminal and "en passant") approaching myocytes to within about 800–900 Å from their PM in man; primarily cholinergic-type axons approach the epithelium but have not yet been seen to cross its BM.

(2) Absorptive cell (Plate 36, Fig. B)

These cells are characterised by (a) numerous densely packed microvilli[1] with a fuzzy, particle-containing coat[2] attached to the external leaflet of their apparently asymmetric plasma membrane (thicker inner leaflet) and an inner core of straight microfilaments[3] that extends deep into the underlying cytoplasm (see also insert B_1), (b) a prominent rough endoplasmic reticulum ranging over the entire cytoplasm with cisternae that tend to "hug"[4] the numerous mitochondria[5], and numerous ribosomes scattered between them, (c) a conspicuous Golgi[6] and (d) numerous smooth vesicles[7]. Their lateral surfaces are joined by "junctional complexes" (consisting of sequences of tight junctions[8], zonulae adherentes[9] and desmosomes[10]) and by interdigitations, and a band of filaments[11] runs horizontally through the apical cytoplasm apparently related to the zonulae adherentes (the "terminal web"). A basement membrane exists at the bottom.

The main known function of these cells is to *absorb* the products of enzymatic food digestion as well as small molecules (H_2O, electrolytes, etc.) from the lumen of the alimentary tube and to convey them to the blood or lymphatic (lacteal) capillaries of the intestinal villi. This involves absorption of hydrolysis products of proteins (amino acids), carbohydrates (monosaccharides) and various lipids (free fatty acids, monoglycerides, diglycerides, glycerin, etc.). While little is known about the ultrastructural modalities of the absorption of carbohydrates, some progress has been made in the study of protein and lipid (particularly triglyceride) absorption. As far as *protein* is concerned, it appears that, in addition to absorbing its hydrolysis products, the absorptive cells of the newborn of some species are also capable of absorbing certain whole maternal protein molecules. Thus in suckling pigs, these cells take up casein or labelled immunoglobulin IgG into their apical vesicles and are thought to transmit those protein-containing vacuoles directly to the cell base and the lamina propria; in suckling rabbits, on the other hand, while the same proteins are taken up into apical vesicles, they seem to trigger a lysosomal re-

A

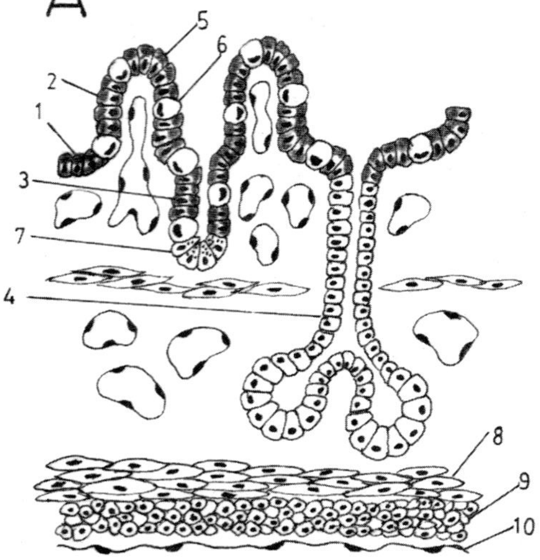

B₁

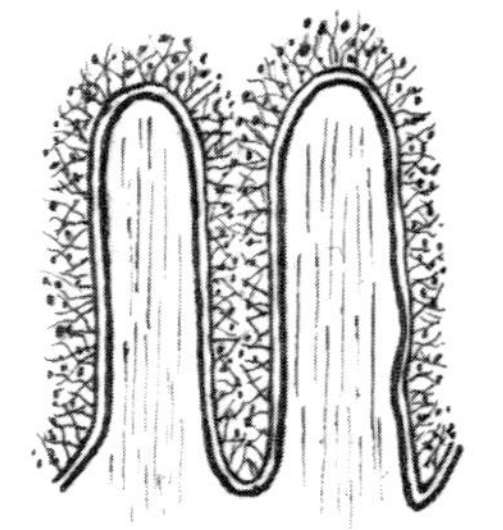

B

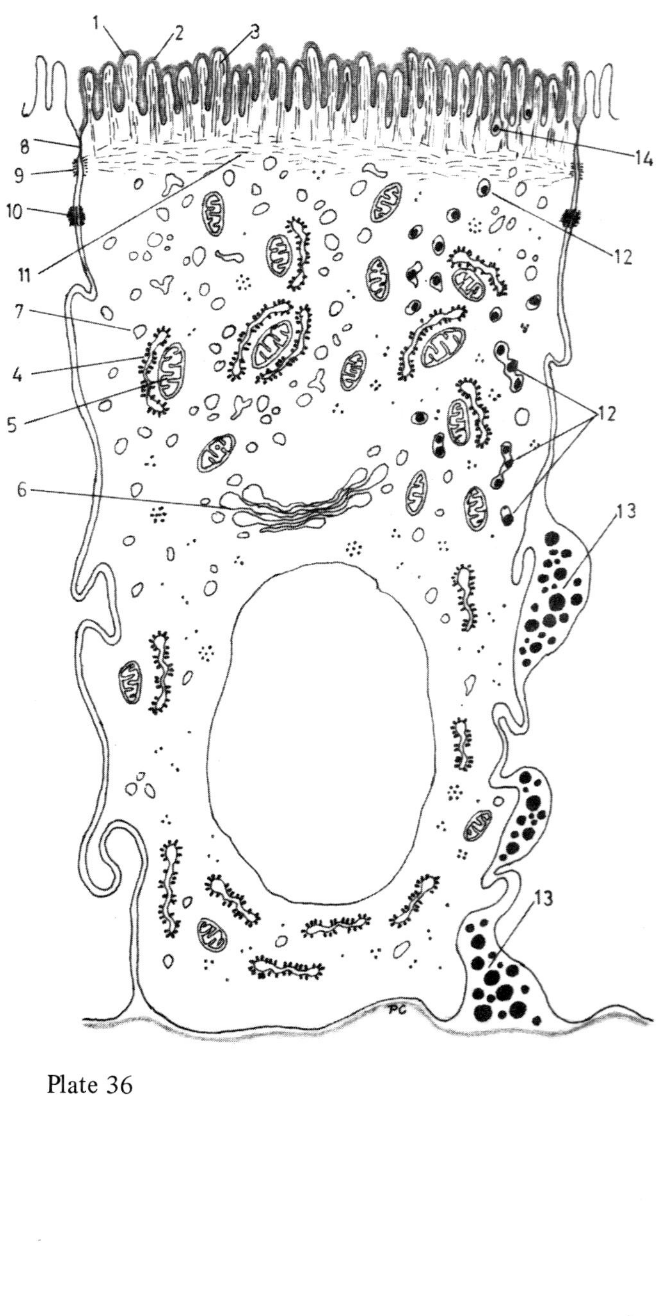

Plate 36

sponse and fuse with lysosomes to form phago-lysosomal sacs in which the protein molecules are apparently hydrolysed. As far as *lipid* absorption is concerned, it now seems that the free fatty acids and mono- and diglycerides which result from lipase action in the lumen form micelles with bile acids and "diffuse" invisibly across the plasma membrane of the microvilli into the apical cytoplasm and into its numerous smooth vesicles; there they become re-esterified into triglycerides (through the action of fatty acid CoA ligase and acyl-CoA monoglyceride acyltransferase) and are packed with some protein into chylomicrons, *i.e.* into visible particulate lipid[12], which somehow moves into the lower intercellular space[13] and somehow crosses the basement membrane and the lacteal lymphatic endothelium to enter the lymph, that will eventually carry it into the blood stream. While in the early intensive phase of lipid absorption the lipid particles generated in the cell are membrane-bound, later some large lipid particles also materialise free in the matrix (*i.e.* without an envelope) through an as yet obscure mechanism. According to recent views, an additional but definitely minor pathway of lipid absorption operates through the direct pinocytotic uptake[14] of some of the undigested lipid particles from the lumen. Like lipid, certain other substances, such as methoxychlor, seem to be absorbed by entering the apical cytoplasm and crossing from there to the lateral intercellular space. It is not certain whether these cells have any secretory besides their absorptive function.

The *fuzzy coat* seems to protect the apical cell surface from digestion by intestinal enzymes and the particles it contains may show some disaccharase and peptidase activity; it consists of acid mucopolysaccharides that apparently resist lysis by the ordinary enzymes of the alimentary canal and it adsorbs or binds several materials introduced into the gut such as vitamin B_{12} or ferritin. Its origin was uncertain and it was thought to represent mucus secreted by goblet cells and mucous glands and attached secondarily to the plasma membrane of the absorptive cells, but there is recent histochemical and autoradiographic evidence (with [^{3}H] fucose) that it may be produced in the Golgi of the absorptive cells.

The zonulae adherentes and the desmosomes of the *junctional complexes* seem to contain Ca^{++} and Mg^{++} as a structural component in their intercellular "glue" since they can be opened by chelating agents (with a resultant considerable increase in epithelial permeability). The same structures (but not the tight junctions) seem permeable to molecules of the size of peroxidase (about 40,000 MW); when the latter is injected intravenously it will move from capillaries into the lateral intercellular spaces of the intestinal epithelium and cross the desmosomes and zonulae adherentes but stop at the tight junctions.

(3) Mucoid and goblet cells (Plate 37, Fig. A)

These cells are distinguishable by (a) a prominent rough endoplasmic reticulum[1] (RER) basally, with cisternae that often "hug" the numerous mitochondria[2], (b) a large Golgi system, concave upwards, consisting of small "transfer" vesicles[3], flat cisternae[4] with dilated end-bulbs[5] and apical secretion-containing vesicles[6], (c) numerous membrane-bound mucus ("mucigen") droplets[7] that coalesce into a huge apical mass[8], (d) a few apical microvilli[9], (e) lateral surfaces that interdigitate and are joined by tight junctions and zonulae adherentes, and (f) underlying basement membranes.

Labelled hexose and amino-acid studies showed that the formation of mucus occurs in the Golgi as follows: Protein elaborated in the RER is moved into the Golgi cisternae through the transfer vesicles where it is coupled to locally synthesized carbohydrate to yield glycoprotein; the latter is concentrated in the dilated end-bulbs which detach and become first small secretory vesicles, then regular mucus droplets, growing in size by dilution and (or) coalescence. Support for the above view is found in the autoradiographic finding that when labelled glucose is made available to goblet cells it finds its way into the Golgi system within minutes and moves up from there into the lower and upper mucous droplets and the luminal mucus, in that sequence. The release mechanism of mucus is still uncertain although it is likely to take place through emiocytosis; the alternative hypotheses of secretion through a ruptured plasma membrane or of discharge of intact membrane-bound mucus droplets followed by rupture of their envelope in the lumen have not yet been proven.

(4) Paneth cells (Plate 37, Fig. B)

These exhibit (a) a prominent rough endoplasmic reticulum[1] with often dense or even crystalline inclusions[2] in its cisternae, (b) a conspicuous Golgi[3], (c) numerous secretory granules[4] with envelopes and very dense contents, (d) several lysosomes[5], (e) a few apical microvilli[6], (f) tight junctions laterally and (g) an underlying basement membrane.

The secretion granules represent enzyme protein, *i.e.* peptidases and lysozyme that originate in the Golgi and are released through an as yet unstudied mechanism into the intestinal lumen where they add to the activity of the pancreatic enzymes; they rapidly pick up and concentrate labeled zinc (an activator or a component of the active peptidase system), when it is made available to Paneth cells.

(5) Peritoneal mesothelium (Plate 37, Fig. C)

Peritoneal mesothelial cells are generally similar to capil-

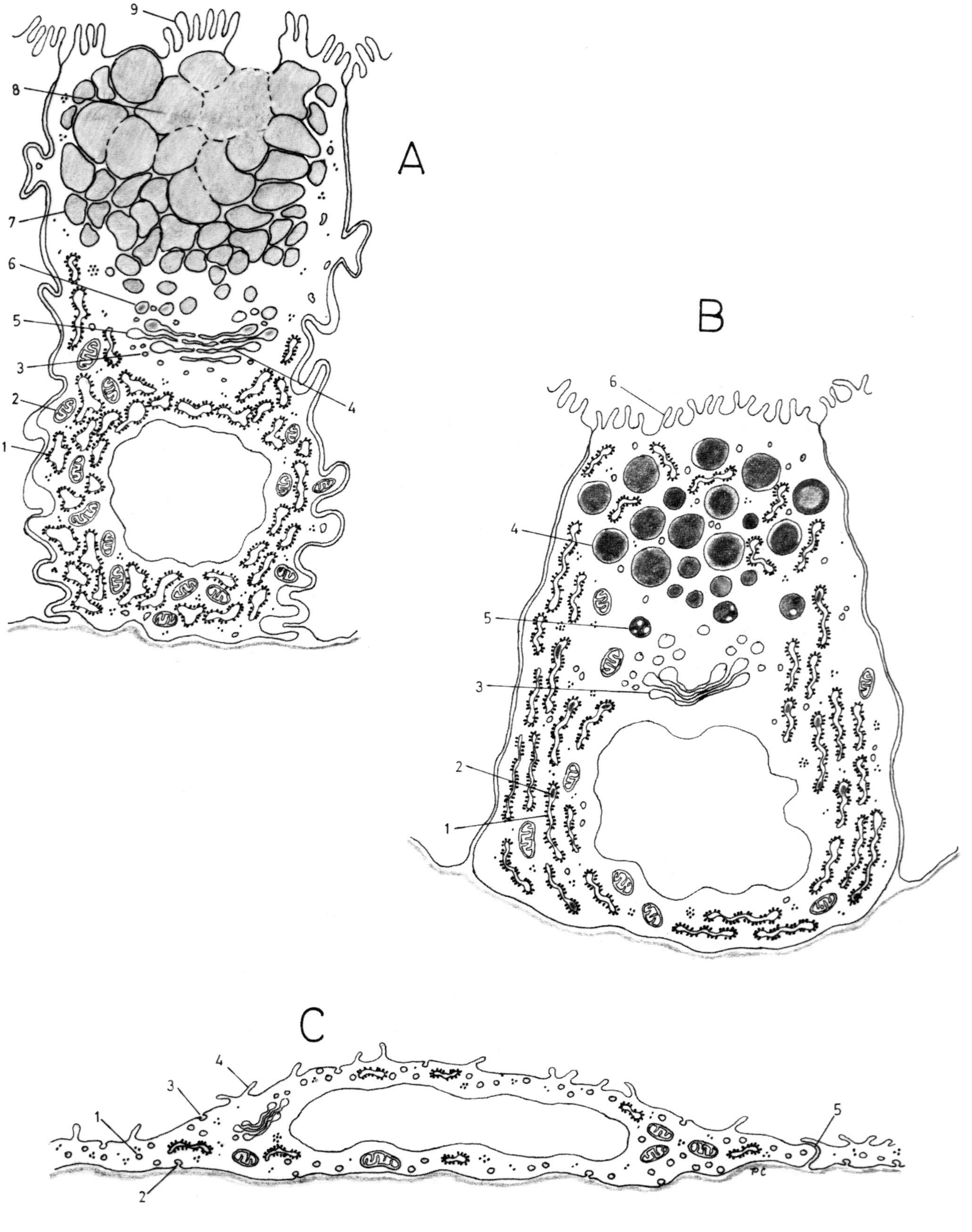

Plate 37

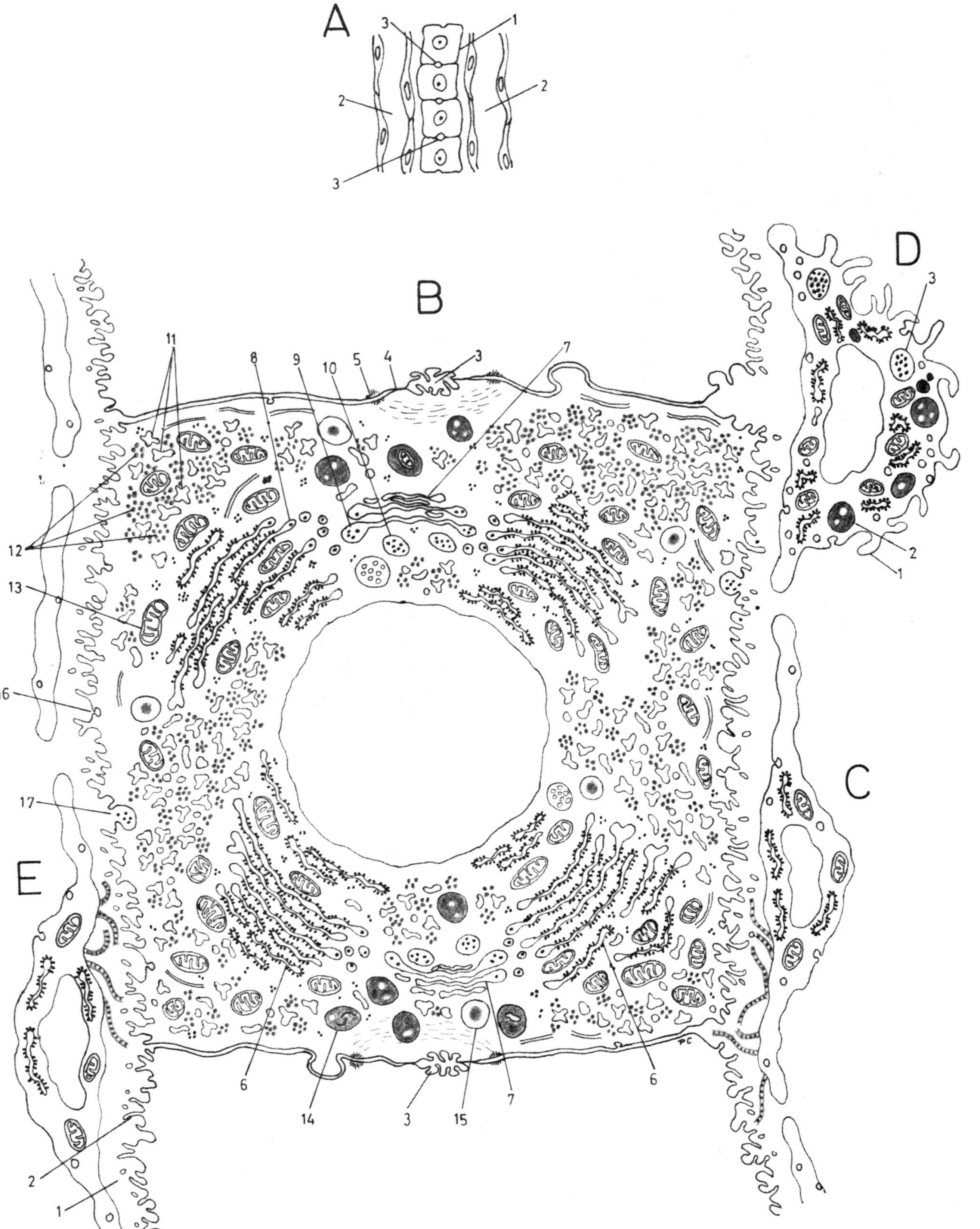

Plate 38

lary endothelial cells, but their structure indicates somewhat greater metabolic activity. They are distinguished by (a) numerous pinocytotic vesicles[1] that open on to both the free[2] and the attached surface[3], (b) appreciable numbers of basic organelles (ribosomes, RER and mitochondria), (c) a few superficial microvilli[4], (d) connections with adjacent cells through zonulae adherentes[5] and (e) a basement membrane, sometimes, demarcating them from the underlying connective tissue.

These cells are apparently capable of considerable fluid transport in both directions: from the underlying capillaries into the peritoneal cavity (generation of peritoneal fluid) and *vice versa* (absorption). The transport of fluid with small molecular solutes seems to be expedited through pinocytotic vesicle ferrying, but the transport of molecules of the size of peroxidase seems to take place by passive diffusion through the intercellular junctions. It is thought that the microvilli and the glycocalyx of mesothelial cells hold a film of fluid that lubricates serous surfaces and protects them from friction.

VI. LIVER

(1) General (Plate 38)

The liver has two major functions: (a) as the largest chemical factory of the body, it picks up countless millions of molecules from the blood, processes them and delivers the products back into the bloodstream, and (b) as an exocrine gland, it secretes bile acids, cholesterol and hemoglobin breakdown products into the gut.

At a certain stage of its development, the liver can be visualised as a large glandular bile duct tree that grows out of an outpouching of the gut wall, the rich sinusoid networks between its secretory portions receiving blood from both the portal vein and the hepatic artery and draining through central veins and hepatic veins into the inferior vena cava; at a later stage, its secretory portions fuse widely to form wall-like sheets (laminae) of hepatocytes within which the narrow secretory lumina (the bile canaliculi) establish a communicating network that drains through the bile duct tree into the gut. Whether the structural unit of its internal architecture (the lobule) is defined as centered around a vascular (central vein) or a glandular (bile duct) axis, the basic functional unit of this organ (Fig. A) is simply a wall of hepatocytes[1] which is flanked on both sides by sinusoid networks[2] and is crisscrossed internally by a network of communicating intercellular bile canaliculi[3], all of them eventually flowing together to drain into the gut.

(2) Hepatocytes (Plate 38, Fig. B)

Structure. These are cells with much cytoplasm, arranged in rows flanked on both sides by wide perforated capillaries (Figs. C, D, E) from which they are separated by the space of Dissé[1]. Their surfaces that face the capillaries are greatly increased by the formation of numerous microvilli[2]; they seem to be lined by a very thin carbohydrate (sialic acid) coat and no basement membrane separates them from the capillaries. By contrast, the lateral intercellular spaces are very narrow clefts (approx. 220 Å wide) and they form tiny canaliculi[3] which are lined by microvilli, sealed by tight junctions[4] and zonulae adherentes[5] and lead into the bile duct system. The hepatocyte cytoplasm is characterised by the following features: (a) an appreciable ribosome population and a prominent rough endoplasmic reticulum (RER) arranged in several stacks of cisternae[6], (b) multiple Golgi systems[7] that tend to lie between the RER stacks and face the bile canaliculi, (c) single or multiple lipoprotein particles 500–3000 Å or more wide (of a density that apparently depends on the unsaturated fatty acid content of the diet) contained within the dilated ends of RER cisternae[8], Golgi[9] and other vesicles[10], (d) extensive smooth endoplasmic reticulum (SER) systems that form 3-dimensional lattices (spongeworks) of communicating vesicles and tubes[11], with groups (rosettes) of glycogen granules[12] scattered among them, (e) mitochondria with relatively few cristae and dense matrix granules[13] associated with both the RER and SER systems, (f) lysosomes[14] that sometimes enclose organelles (mitochondria, SER vesicles) in various stages of degradation and are located close to the bile canaliculi, (g) microbodies[15] usually containing crystalline nucleoids, (h) small clear vesicles[16] and large lipoprotein-containing vesicles[17] that open on the capillary-facing surface, (i) long microtubules about 230 Å wide, and (j) a web of fine filaments close to the canaliculi.

Function. Hepatocytes (a) take in an enormous variety of molecules from the plasma, (b) transform most of them in their organelles, (c) secrete many of the products they elaborate back into the plasma, and (d) secrete some of their products into the bile canaliculi and thus into the intestine. The *uptake* of small molecules probably occurs through passive or active crossing of the PM, but the uptake of larger molecules and aggregates apparently takes place through vesicular transport (pinocytosis). Thus, injected protein peroxidase molecules (MW about 40,000) and alimentation-induced small chylomicrons (200–1000 Å) have been documented to enter the hepatocyte through pinocytosis which often generates large intracellular vesicles by confluence of smaller ones; heavy metals such as iron or copper are taken up into phagosomes which then turn into phagolysosomes or they enter lysosomes directly. Correspondingly, *secretion of materials into the plasma* probably takes place through both PM crossing and emiocytosis and, in the absence of specially designed kinetic studies, it is impossible to tell whether a vesicle that communicates with the cell surface represents uptake or release of its contents. While it is documented that the hepatocyte *secretes into the bile canaliculi* not only chemicals needed for intestinal function (*e.g.* bile acids) but also many materials that it wishes to eliminate (*e.g.* phagosomes, hemoglobin breakdown products, phagolysosomes, autophagic vacuoles, and lysosomes), the mechanism of the release of these chemicals and particles has not yet been thoroughly studied. Furthermore, it appears that while under normal conditions the contents of the bile canaliculi are sealed off (through the tight junctions) from the lateral intercellular clefts and, through them, from the space of Dissé, experimental infusion of fluids under pressure into either the bile ducts (common bile duct) or the space of Dissé (portal vein) can rupture the tight junction seals of the bile canaliculi.

The following specific functional information is associated with the various hepatocyte organelles and inclusions:

The *RER* manufactures (a) most plasma proteins (the albumins and α- and β-globulins) and (b) the hydrophilic component of most plasma lipoproteins. Autoradiographic studies after perfusion of labeled precursors indicate that proteins and phospholipids are synthesised in the RER cisternae, then move to the contiguous SER sacs where they are coupled with triglycerides (synthesized locally from free fatty acids and glycerin) to form low-density lipoprotein particles of about 150–500 Å or more diameter (liposomes) and finally pinch off to enter the Golgi system; from there the newly assembled lipoproteins drift off (carried within vesicles) towards the space of Dissé, into which they are unloaded by emiocytosis. The topography of cholesterol synthesis is not yet certain but it seems likely that, like that of triglycerides, it takes place in the SER. According to current views, the completed spheroid lipoprotein molecules consist of a sialic acid-coated protein (apoprotein) shell that encloses a triglyceride-cholesterol inner mass; the outermost sialic acid coat is apparently added to these molecules in the Golgi.

Hepatocytes build lipoproteins from building blocks that they either synthesize locally or absorb from the bloodstream. The mechanism of entry of lipid molecules of any size into liver cells has only begun to be explored. In the case of cholesterol, some findings following the i.v. injection of labeled cholesterol in the form of chylomicrons suggest that this molecule enters hepatocytes by crossing their membrane either esterified with fatty acids or free (after hydrolysis by a cholesterol esterase in the PM), but that it enters Kupffer cells through phagocytosis of the particles that carry it. However, the possibility that whole lipoprotein particles can, under certain circumstances, also be incorporated by pinocytosis into hepatocytes cannot be excluded at present since these cells have been documented to take up other large particles such as thorotrast and hemoglobin in this manner.

The *SER* vesicles and tubules seem to represent enzyme-charged sacs that develop from RER cisternae after removal of the attached ribosomes; in fact, since their unit membranes seem to be enzymes, it appears that the ribosomes of the RER manufacture both the membranes and the enzymes of this system. One of the main functions of the SER sacs is to polymerise glucose into its storage form, glycogen, and conversely, to release glucose from the latter when necessary – a key enzyme in these processes being glucose-6-phosphatase (which is contained in its membranes): glycogen granules increase in numbers after meals and after cortisone-induced gluconeogenesis and they practically disappear after severe fasting, accompanied by a surge of SER vesicle proliferation in both instances; injected labelled glucose appears within minutes in the SER system and cortisone-induced gluconeogenesis is accompanied by a marked conversion of RER to SER through ribosome removal. Another main function of the SER vesicles is the inactivation of numerous drugs and toxic chemicals through hydroxylating and other enzymes which are built into their membranes often by adaptive response. Thus, both the number and the enzymatic activity of the SER vesicles greatly increases in adaptive response to the administration of phenobarbital, dimethyl-aminoazobenzene and other chemicals. Finally, as mentioned above, the SER system is currently considered to be the site of triglyceride (and possibly cholesterol) synthesis and incorporation into the lipoprotein molecules that are manufactured in the liver.

The *lysosomes*, which have been found to originate in the Golgi, (a) fuse with pinocytic vesicles containing exogenous materials such as hemoglobin or thorium, (b) can engage in autophagic activity, and (c) are known to be discharged into the bile canaliculi under certain conditions. The *microbodies* seem to develop from the Golgi in the embryo and from the RER postnatally; they ordinarily contain catalase, *d*-amino oxidase and uricase and are thought to fuse with autophagosomes contributing to the oxidative degradation of their contents; their crystalline nucleoid seem to be the site of uricase activity and is absent from those species in which this enzyme has been lost; their catalase normally exhibits both catalase and peroxidase activity, but there is an "acatalasemic" strain of mice (the Csb strain) whose microbodies display very low or no catalase together with appreciable peroxidase activity. Recently, certain drugs have been found to have remarkable effects on these organelles; thus, chlorophenoxyisobutyrate (CPIB) stimulates an enormous proliferation of microbody numbers (aimed perhaps at oxidising CPIB), while aminotriazole practically abolishes their catalase and peroxidase activity. The *mitochondria* (already discussed in the first chapter) have a distinctly smaller number of cristae than those of muscle, but when hypermetabolism is induced through thyroid hormone treatment this number greatly increases (to 3–7 times normal) to provide the enzyme surface needed for the increased metabolic activity; the numerous dense granules in their matrix appear to be lipids since they have been found to disappear after lipid solvent treatment. The *nucleolar structure* and size can be manipulated dramatically by metabolic inhibitors in hepatocytes; actinomycin, which inhibits RNA synthesis by DNA, causes a shrinkage of the nucleolus (because the latter consists primarily of RNA) and it also induces a striking segregation of the latter into a granular and a fibrillar-amorphous component through an as yet obscure mechanism; by contrast, thioacetamide, which inhibits protein synthesis by RNA, causes a marked enlargement of the nucleolus to gigantic size (presumably because the lack of protein synthesis stimulates RNA synthesis by negative feedback and because ribosome transport out of the nucleolus is inhibited). Possibly for similar reasons, a marked increment of nucleolar size can likewise be induced by dietary deficiency in the amino acid threonine.

Nutritional conditions are known to influence hepatocytic structure profoundly. Thus, fasting and protein or choline deficiency all cause marked accumulation of lipids, but for different reasons: fasting mobilises lipids from the adipose tissue to the liver, protein deficiency interferes with the coupling of lipid to protein (and therefore with the movement of lipids out of hepatocytes) and choline deficiency presumably interferes with the synthesis of phospholipids that contribute to the solubilisation of triglycerides. Among other influences, dietary deficiency of essential fatty acids or riboflavin causes mitochondrial enlargement (to giant size, in the latter case) apparently as a compensation for the defects in respiratory processes induced by these deficiencies.

Finally, during the first few hours after partial hepatectomy, the surviving hepatocytes undergo significant changes in the direction of "dedifferentiation" as a preparation for mitosis and regeneration: their nucleolus enlarges, ribosomes proliferate, numerous autophagosomes develop, and most microvilli facing the space of Dissé disappear.

(3) Capillary (sinusoid) endothelium
(Plate 38, Figs. C, D, E)

The walls of the capillaries that flank the hepatocytes are like sieves due to the existence of large gaps between the endothelial cells throughout most of their length. There is no basement membrane around them but small groups of collagen fibrils are occasionally seen in the space of Dissé. The endothelial cells are of two types: (a) "regular" endothelial cells (Figs. C, E) with low pinocytotic activity, and (b) phagocytic, "macrophage-like" endothelial cells (Kupffer cells) (Fig. D) with tentacles[1], lysosomes[2], phagosomes[3] and occasionally ferritin.

The frequent, large endothelial gaps and the absence of basement membranes remove all barriers between hepatocytes and blood; the hepatocytes are literally bathed in plasma and this ensures the most rapid possible interaction between the two. The phagocytic Kupffer cells clear the blood of normal and pathological debris and of intravenously injected particles, acting like macrophages. The "regular" endothelial cells can apparently turn into phagocytic Kupffer cells whenever the need for phagocytic functions increases; thus, after repeated intravenous injections of particular matter (*e.g.* carbon) almost all endothelial cells of the liver sinusoids assume the structure and function of Kupffer cells. The attachment of particles to the surface of Kupffer cells and thus their phagocytosis can be inhibited by cortisone.

(4) Bile duct system

(A) General

This system of canals that convey the bile from the hepatocytes to the gut forms a tree whose tiniest twigs are the canaliculi that run between hepatocytes, and whose trunk is the common bile duct, with the gall bladder representing a sac-like dilation of the terminal trunk. It is probable that most of these canals not only conduct but also modify the bile that passes through them. The successive segments of the bile duct system, starting at the site of bile production, are as follows: (a) bile canaliculi, (b) the very short canals of Hering, (c) bile preductules, (d) bile ductules, (e) bile ducts, intrahepatic, and (f) bile ducts, extrahepatic and gallbladder. The walls of the bile canaliculi are formed by two hepatocytes, as already described; those of the canals of Hering are formed by one hepatocyte and one "duct type" epithelial cell. As the bile canals increase in diameter, the duct epithelium that lines them grows taller, the intrahepatic ducts acquire a connective tissue sheath of increasing thickness and the extrahepatic ducts and the gall bladder acquire a muscular coat in addition; the muscular coat of the extrahepatic ducts serves to control the flow of the bile in the latter while that of the gall bladder reservoir serves to eject (detrusor) or retain (sphincter) the stored bile. What follows is a brief discussion of the epithelial lining of the different segments of the duct system.

(B) Bile canaliculi

These have been described with the hepatocytes.

(C) Hering canals (Plate 39, Figs. A and B)

The walls of these very short transitional conduits between canaliculi and pre-ductules are formed by one hepatocyte (Fig. A) and one "duct" type epithelial cell (Fig. B). They are lined by microvilli and sealed by tight junctions. The hepatocytes are as already described, while the duct cells are undifferentiated cells that possess a high nucleus/cytoplasm ratio, a fair amount of the basic organelles (ribosomes, RER, Golgi, SER and mitochondria) and a basement membrane on their surface.

While duct cells have been traditionally thought to represent reserve elements that can proliferate and differentiate into hepatocytes whenever this becomes necessary, some recent evidence has challenged this concept; it has been reported that after liver injury both duct cells and hepatocytes proliferate but that each cell species seems to reproduce only its own kind.

(D) Bile pre-ductules

These are short shunt channels between the canals of Hering and the ductules. In cross-sections their walls are made of 2–3 duct type epithelial cells.

(E) Bile ductules (Plate 39, Fig. C)

In cross-sections, their walls consist of rings of more than three duct type epithelial cells which are as already described, with luminal microvilli[1] plus occasional dense lipid inclusions[2] which increase in frequency as one follows the ducts towards the gut.

It is probable that starting at about this level, the duct epithelium begins to play some active role in modifying the bile that flows past it through either absorption or secretion of some materials.

(F) Bile ducts, intra- and extrahepatic

The point at which ductules begin to be called "ducts" is vague. It seems that channels with more than about six duct cells in cross-section, and an appreciable amount of surrounding connective tissue are called by most workers "ducts". The lining duct cells here are qualitatively similar to those of the ductules but they grow increasingly taller.

(G) Gall bladder epithelium (Plate 39, Fig. D)

This consists of tall cells with much cytoplasm and the following specific features: (a) a prominent RER[1], particularly at the base and sides, (b) a fair amount of smooth vesicles[2] and a conspicuous Golgi[3], (c) numerous mitochondria[4] mainly apically, (d) numerous membrane-limited granules[5] that contain a homogeneous dense material apically, (e) several lysosomes[6], (f) a microvillous free border (partly covered by a fuzzy coat)[7], and (g) tight junctions and desmosomes and extensively interdigitating lateral surfaces. The intercellular clefts are narrow (about 200 Å wide) when little or no fluid absorption from the bile occurs[8], but extremely wide when the bile in the gall bladder is being dehydrated[9]. A basement membrane (BM) underlies the epithelium.

Fluid apparently crosses this epithelium by entering into the apical cytoplasm of these cells somehow (by pinocytosis and/or transmembranous passage) and moving from there to the lateral (intercellular) spaces. The presence of Na^+ or Cl^- ions in the lumen has been found to be indispensable for this fluid transport.

The structure of most of these cells indicates that they are very active. Of their probable several functions only one is at present established: They absorb great amounts of water (and probably certain solutes) from the bile and pass it through the intercellular clefts and the BM to the underlying capillaries; they thus concentrate the bile. It now appears that the apical granules represent a glycoprotein material (mucus) which is secreted on and protects the apical PM from the effects of concentrated bile. The function of the apical lysosomes remains to be elucidated.

VII. EXOCRINE PANCREAS

(1) General

The exocrine pancreas is a gland that, like the liver, develops from an outpouching of the intestine, its secretory portions (acini) draining through short intralobular and interlobular channels into its main central duct; it secretes a whole battery of powerful digestive enzymes into the gut. The endocrine islets of Langerhans represent certain secretory portions that become pinched off from their ductules at an early development stage.

(2) Acinar cell (Plate 40, Fig. A)

This cell is distinguished by (a) an extraordinarily luxuriant rough endoplasmic reticulum (RER) which forms parallel stacks of cisternae[1] at the base and sides, (b) a conspicuous Golgi[2], (c) numerous dense secretion granules apically[3] that are contained in not always easily discernible and occasionally fractured envelopes and are secreted by emiocytosis into the lumen[4], filling it with a dense material[5], and (d) microvilli at the free surface, tight junctions laterally, and a basement membrane at the base. Axon terminals[6] of both the cholinergic and adrenergic type approach several acinar cells closely.

As the unusual development of the RER indicates, this is a cell of intensive protein synthesis; it manufactures three enzyme proteins (trypsin, diastase, lipase) which are identical with the dense apical granules and

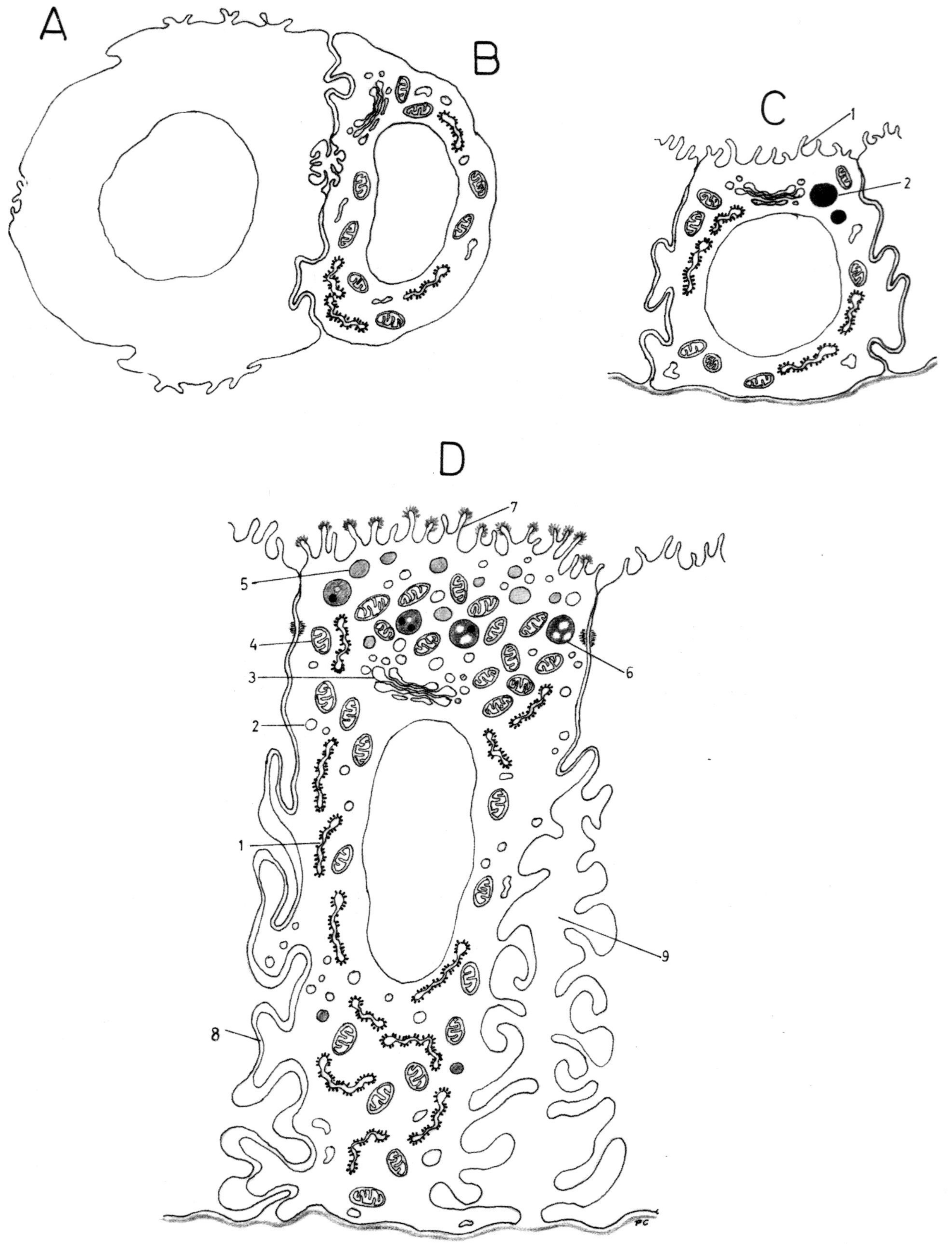

Plate 39

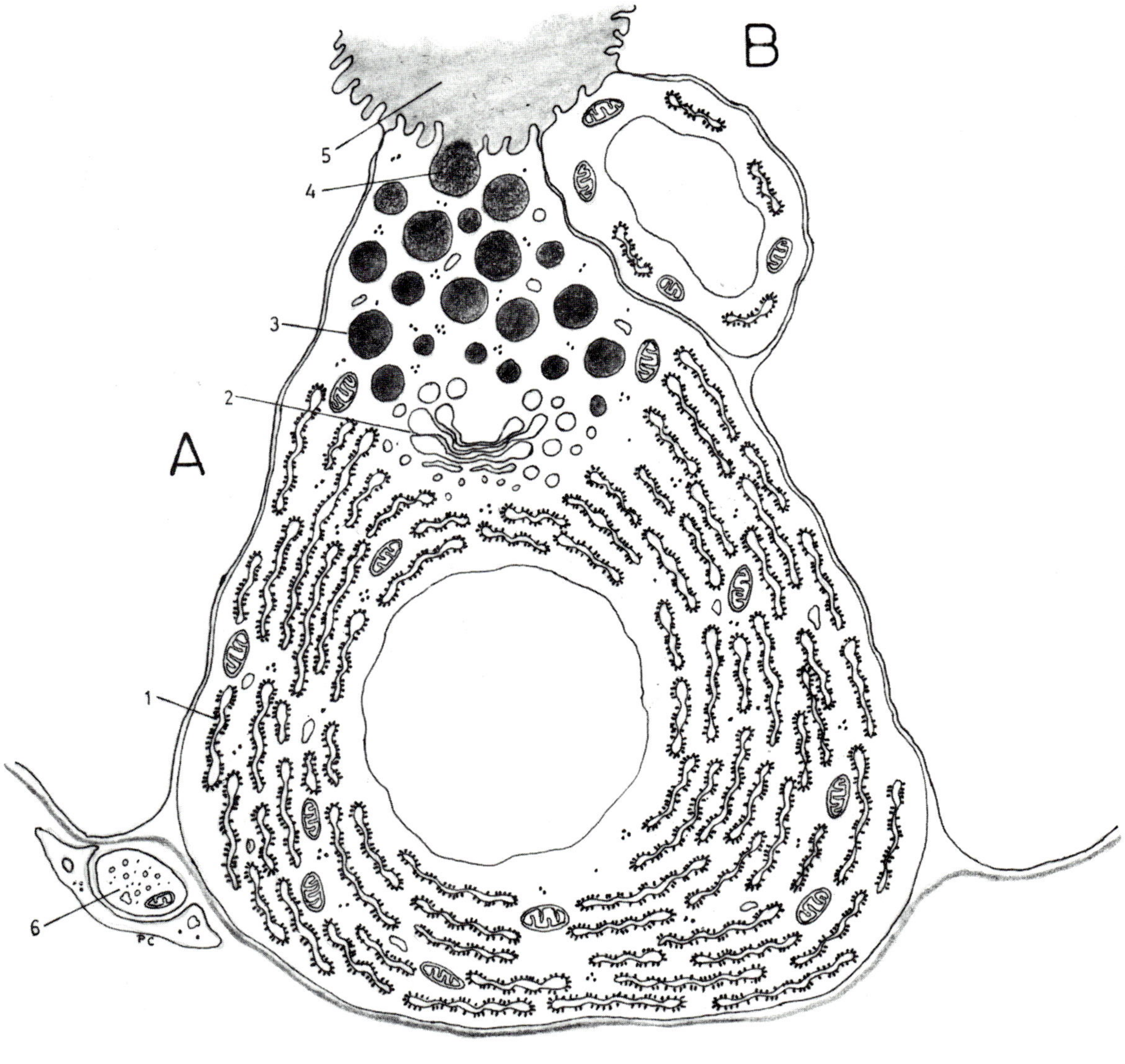

Plate 40

the dense material in the lumen; the enzymes are probably activated only after they reach the alkaline pH environment in the intestine. The topology of the various phases of the *enzyme secretion* process has been much studied with the administration of labelled protein precursors (*e.g.* [^{14}C] or [^{3}H] leucine) and subsequent autoradiography or radioactivity studies of cell fractions; as a result, it is now accepted that enzyme precursors are manufactured in the RER and move from there to the Golgi, the lower granules, upper granules and lumen, in that sequence. The secretion process is under both nervous and hormonal control; thus, secretion is stimulated by parasympathetic (vagal) impulses or vagomimetic drugs and by secretin and pancreozymin (substances elaborated in the stomach wall). The release of enzyme granules from the cell apex into the lumen can be observed within minutes of the injection of vagomimetic drugs such as pilocarpine.

Within 2–3 weeks of its extensive destruction by ethionine, the exocrine pancreas is *regenerated* completely, apparently through extensive mitosis of the surviving and some reversibly injured acinar cells as well as some ductal cells.

(3) Centro-acinar cells (Plate 40, Fig. B)

These are small undifferentiated cells with a high nucleus/cytoplasm ratio that are occasionally seen wedged between the tips of acinar cells. They possess basic organelles and a few rudimentary microvilli and they are joined to their neighbours through tight junctions. They probably represent the first cells of the duct epithelium and thus a reserve population that may differentiate into acinar cells when the latter are destroyed by various insults.

(4) Pancreatic duct system

This is similar in most respects to the duct system of the serous salivary glands.

Chapter 10

Urinary System

I. GENERAL (Plate 41, Figs. A and B)

The principal known functions of this system are (a) the elimination of metabolic wastes through the filtration of blood and the excretion of the modified filtrate (urine) from the body, (b) the maintenance of a steady water and electrolyte concentration in the blood through the variation of the excretion of these materials, (c) the hormonal regulation of blood pressure, and (d) the hormonal regulation of erythropoesis in the bone marrow. Its main parts are the kidneys, the ureters, the urinary bladder and the urethra.

In the kidney, the renal artery divides repeatedly until it forms hundreds of thousands of afferent arterioles (Fig. A). Each afferent arteriole[1], in turn, breaks up into a small knot of anastomosing capillary loops[2] (the glomerulus) which is invaginated into the blind sac-like end of a renal tubule[3]; the blind tubule end forms Bowman's capsule around the glomerulus, with a parietal layer[4], a visceral or podocytic[5] layer that hugs the glomerular loops and a space between the two; blood is collected from each glomerulus into an efferent arteriole[6] which breaks up into capillaries[7] that surround and supply the rest of the tubule before draining into a renal venule.

Every renal tubule together with its glomerulus constitutes a nephron (Fig. B) and exhibits the following successive segments, starting with its glomerular end: the proximal segment[1], the thin part[2] of the loop of Henle (with a long descending and a short ascending limb), the thick part[3] of the loop of Henle, and the distal segment[4]; several distal segments drain into a collecting tubule[5] and several collecting tubules join repeatedly to form ever larger collecting channels[6] until a few dozen large terminal ducts[7] (of Bellini) are created which drain the urine into the expanded beginning of the ureter (the renal pelvis). The ureter finally transmits the urine into a large contractile storage vesicle, the urinary bladder, which expels its contents periodically through the urethra. Blood is filtered through the glomerular loops of each nephron into its tubule and, as filtrate passes down the various segments of the latter, it is modified by the removal or addition of various components, until it becomes the definitive urine at the level of the collecting tubules.

The distal tubule of each nephron returns briefly to its own glomerulus (Fig. A) where it approximates[8] the afferent arteriole and the mesangial cells[9] (a midglomerular group of intercapillary myocyte-like cells); the whole "juxtaglomerular" complex of afferent and efferent arteriole and approximated distal tubule is functionally interrelated and concerned with blood pressure regulation.

II. GLOMERULUS

(1) Capillary loops and podocytes (Plate 41, Figs. C–E)

Structure. The *endothelial tubes* (Fig. C) are extremely thin and of the completely perforated type[1], with endothelial cell bodies[2] that are distinguished by the absence of pinocytotic vesicles, the presence of appreciable numbers of polyribosomes and a thin coat of acid mucopolysaccharide. They are surrounded by a substantial basement membrane[3] which is about 3300 Å wide in adult humans (increasing in thickness with age) and which in turn is surrounded by numerous small processes, the "foot processes"[4] of the podocytes or visceral epithelial cells; on close-up (Fig. D) it is seen to consist of three layers: a lucent external and internal layer (the lamina rara externa[1] and interna[2], respectively) and a dense middle layer, the lamina densa[3]. The lamina densa appears to represent a tight mat of 30–40 Å thick filaments and to contain much glycoprotein. The foot processes of the podocytes[4] seem to be attached to the lamina densa with fine filaments[5] and to one another with extremely thin diaphragms[6]; the distance between them varies from 200–500 Å depending on species.

The *podocytes* (Fig. E) are characterised by (a) moderate numbers of ribosomes, RER cisternae, mitochondria and a distinct Golgi, (b) numerous smooth vesicles, some large but most of them small[1], (c) several multivesicular bodies[2], (d) several 50–70 Å thick fine fila-

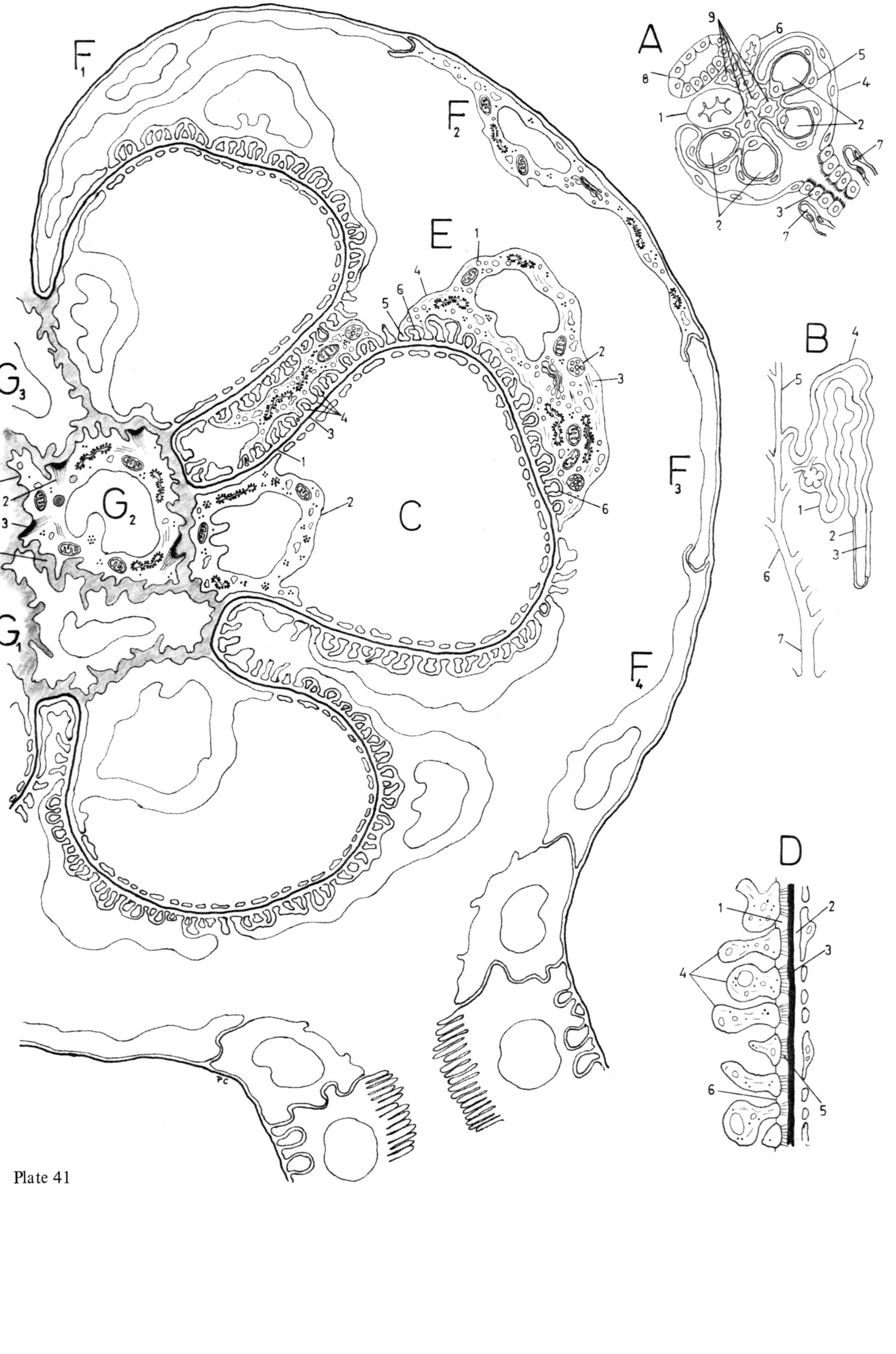
A
B
C
D
E
F1
F2
F3
F4
G1
G2
G3

ments[3] scattered randomly throughout the cytoplasm, and (e) a relatively low matrix density in the cytoplasm but a higher one in the foot processes. They give off major processes, the trabeculae[4], which in turn branch into the many small foot processes[5]; the foot processes of neighbouring trabeculae interdigitate extensively[6]. A thick coat of acid mucopolysaccharide can be demonstrated with colloidal iron to cover the podocyte surface, fill the slits between the foot processes and line the internal surface of the large vesicles within the podocytic cytoplasm.

Function. The hydrostatic pressure of blood in the capillaries filters out of plasma water and molecules with a molecular weight of less than 45,000 through the walls of the capillary loops into Bowman's space to form the "primary" urine; the barrier across which this filtration process occurs consists of the capillary basement membrane (BM) and the thin diaphragms between the podocytic foot processes. From Bowman's space the primary urine enters the nephronic tubule and runs through its various segments where it is modified by the removal and the addition of several materials, until it leaves the kidney as the "definitive" urine at the open end of the terminal collecting tubules.

The function of the podocytes is not quite settled yet, but it is likely that they perform at least two tasks: First, they probably *maintain the BM* of the capillary loops as indicated (a) by the finding that after the latter is marked by heavy silver deposits (through the addition of $AgNO_3$ to the drinking water for a given period), new BM material is visibly added to the old BM on the podocytic rather than the endothelial side, and (b) by the finding of secretory bodies within their RER cisternae. Secondly, they probably remove certain molecules from the primary urine through a process that perhaps involves their multivesicular bodies; this is supported (a) by the finding that podocytes incorporate certain large molecules such as ferritin that reach them by intratubular or intravenous injection – the latter under conditions of pathologically increased BM permeability – and (b) by the extensive interdigitation of their processes, which is a structural pattern that is always associated with intensive transcellular transport processes in the other parts of the nephron, *e.g.* the proximal tubule cells, and in other parts of the body (*e.g.* sweat glands, stria vascularis, ciliary epithelium). In addition to the above two functions, the recent finding of myosin-like coarse filaments in podocytes with the freeze substitution procedure suggests that these cells may also be contractile.

(2) Parietal Bowman's epithelium (Plate 41, Figs. F_1–F_4)

These flattened cells are continuous with the podocytes on the one hand (Fig. F_1) and with the beginning of the proximal tubule on the other (Fig. F_4). They form a spherical shell around the cluster of glomerular capillaries, from which they are separated by Bowman's space. They are relatively undifferentiated cells with (a) few ribosomes, RER cisternae and mitochondria, (b) a small Golgi, and (c) simple interlocking junctions; their BM is continuous with that of the glomerular capillaries and the proximal tubule.

Their function is unsettled but it is known that (a) they can absorb unusually large molecules such as ferritin when the latter get into the primary urine, and (b) they can proliferate vigorously under pathological stimulation; it is also possible that they represent an undifferentiated cell "reservoir" that can differentiate into either podocytes or proximal tubule cells.

(3) Mesangial cells (Plate 41, Figs. G_1–G_3)

This term describes a few cells in the glomerular center that are probably undifferentiated smooth muscle cells and very similar to the renin-producing (juxtaglomerular) myocytes in the wall of the afferent arteriole. They probably develop from the media of the afferent arterioles, with which they are anatomically continuous; those mesangial cells that are closest to the arteriolar pole of the glomerulus are called the "Polkissen" or "lacis" cells (Fig. G_3).

Mesangial cells (*e.g.* Fig. G_2) are characterised by (a) many processes[1], (b) moderate numbers of ribosomes, RER cisternae and mitochondria, (c) bundles of thin filaments[2], some of them attached to densities of the PM[3] (as in smooth muscle), (d) occasional dense bodies, and (e) surrounding pools of dense "BM-like" material[4] which seems continuous with the BM of the capillary loops and may also contain a few collagen fibrils.

The function of mesangial cells is not settled yet but there is evidence that (a) they produce the intercellular materials that surround them, (b) they have phagocytic properties, and (c) they react to certain stimuli like the renin-producing cells in the wall of the afferent arterioles, *e.g.* they enlarge and develop many dense granules in response to mineralocorticoid deficiency.

III. THE JUXTAGLOMERULAR COMPLEX

(1) Afferent arteriole (Plate 42, Fig. A)

The media of this vessel is very unusual since it consists of modified myocytes with a secretory function. These cells exhibit (a) appreciable numbers of ribosomes and RER cisternae[1], and a prominent Golgi system[2], (b) numerous membrane-bound secretory granules[3] of moderate density, (c) moderate numbers of mitochondria, (d) several myofilament bundles in the cell periphery[4], and (e) a fair number of pinocytotic vesicles[5], mostly on

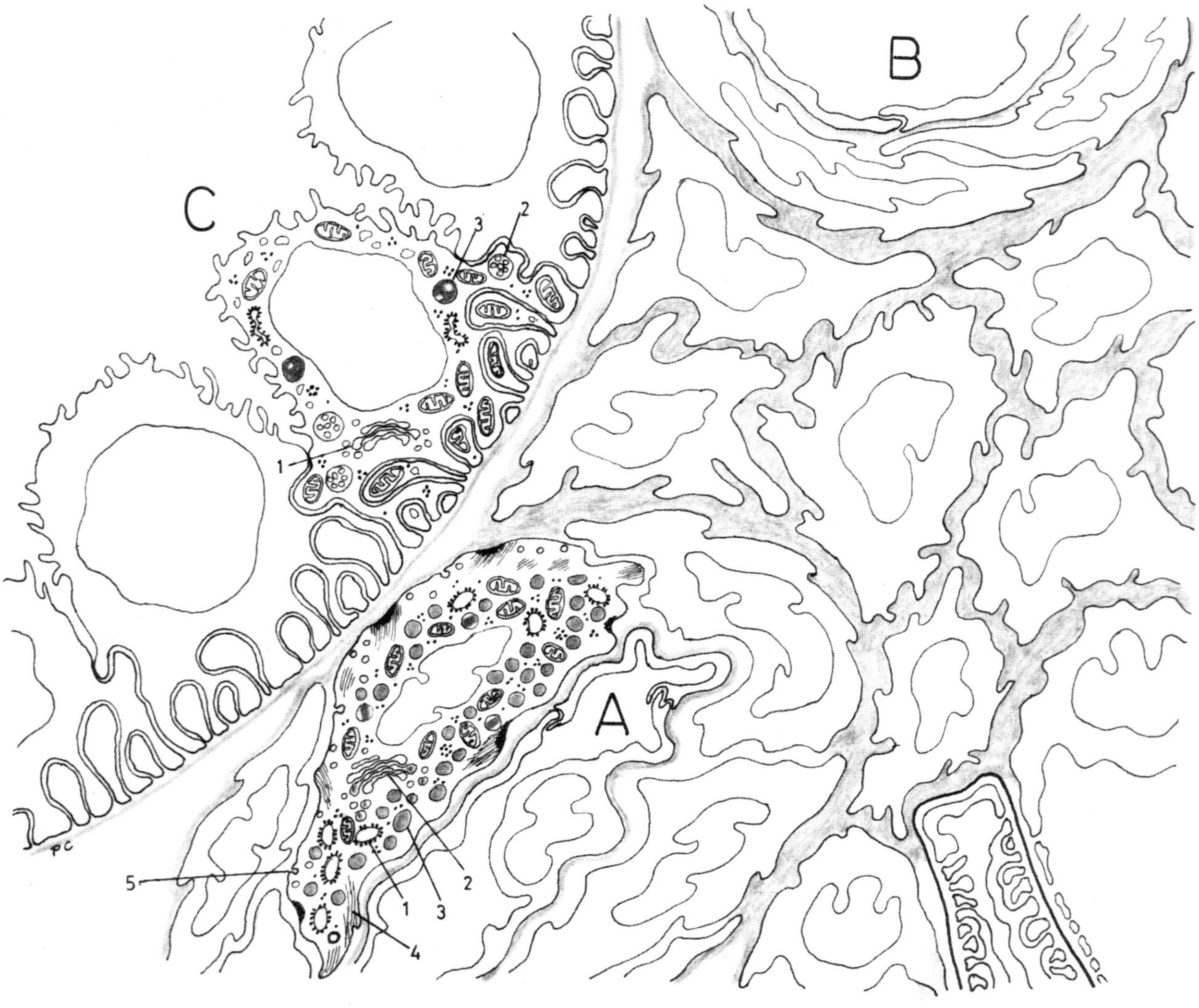

Plate 42

their basal side; they are surrounded by a BM except at sites at which they are closely approached by unmyelinated axon terminals of an apparently adrenergic type.

The secretory granules represent renin, an enzyme that turns angiotensinogen into angiotensin in the blood and through the latter stimulates (a) contraction of arteriolar smooth muscle, (b) adrenal production of mineralocorticoids, and (c) the sympathetic nervous system – its ultimate physiological effects thus being the raising of blood pressure and blood sodium levels. The presence of renin in the granules has been established with immunofluorescent anti-renin and through the correlation of kidney renin assays with its content of such granules. Renin is produced in the RER cisternae of the afferent arteriole myocytes in the form of crystalloid subunits (the "protogranules") which then travel to the Golgi vesicles where they are conglomerated into the definitive granules. It is not yet certain how renin is released into the bloodstream; since emiocytosis has not yet been documented, perhaps it diffuses out of the secretory granules and through the myocyte PM in molecular quanta.

Renin secretion by the modified myocytes of the afferent arteriole contributes substantially to the regulation of blood pressure in the body by responding to appropriate humoral feedback mechanisms and nervous stimuli. Thus, renin synthesis and release is stimulated (a) by a drop of the blood pressure, apparently "sensed" through the corresponding change in arteriolar myocyte stretch, (b) by a drop of the sodium ion concentration in the blood and urine (such as caused by a low sodium diet or adrenalectomy) which may be "sensed" through the diffusion of some chemical signal from the distal tubule to the basal surface of the arteriolar myocytes, (c) by a drop of angiotensin levels in the blood, and (d) by sympathetic nerve stimulation. Conversely, renin release is inhibited by the reverse of the above conditions, *i.e.* by high blood pressure, high blood sodium concentrations (as *e.g.* after high sodium diet or mineralocorticoid treatment) and high blood angiotensin levels. The number of visible renin granules in the arteriolar myocytes at any given time depends on the balance between renin synthesis and release at that time. For this reason, granules will be numerous when synthesis outpaces release but scarce or even absent when synthesis lags behind release – as in all endocrine secretions.

Recently, the possibility has been raised that some of the secretory granules with crystalline substructure may represent not renin but the renal erythropoietic factor.

(2) Efferent arterioles (Plate 42, Fig. B)

These have a thinner wall than the afferent arterioles; their contraction increases filtration pressure in the capillary loops of the glomerulus; their myocytes are mostly of the ordinary smooth muscle type although granular myocytes of the renin-secreting type are occasionally observed in their wall.

(3) Macula densa of distal tubule (Plate 42, Fig. C)

The segment of the distal tubule (see Sect. VII) that establishes very close contact with the vascular pole of the glomerulus exhibits the following special features that distinguish it from the rest of the distal tubule: (a) the epithelial cells on the side that faces the glomerulus are narrower and therefore their nuclei are distinctly more crowded than on the other side – hence the term "macula densa" for that part of the tubule wall, (b) the Golgi is located basally[1], (c) unusually numerous multivesicular bodies[2] and several dense cytosomes[3] are located in the basal portions of the tubule cells. The above structural features indicate a functional orientation of the macula densa cells towards the afferent and efferent arterioles and the mesangial system, although the nature of this relationship is not yet clear; it probably involves the emission of a humoral feedback signal concerning urinary sodium concentration from the macula densa to the arteriolar and mesangial cells.

IV. PROXIMAL TUBULE (Plate 43, Fig. A)

The cells of this part of the renal tubule are distinguished by (a) numerous long slender microvilli[1] with a glycocalyx (not shown) on their luminal surface, (b) numerous smooth tubules[2] and vesicles[3] apically, many of them opening on to the surface[4] between the bases of the microvilli, (c) appreciable numbers of ribosomes, RER cisternae and mitochondria and a distinct Golgi, (d) numerous basal invaginations[5] into which protrude mitochondria-rich basal processes[6] of neighbouring cells (*i.e.* extensive interdigitation between adjacent epithelia), (e) several cytosomes[7] (lysosomes), cytosegresomes[8] (the "hyaline droplets" of the L/M), microbodies[9] (with crystalloid and non-crystalloid nucleoids) and multivesicular bodies[10], (f) apical junctional complexes with terminal bars and zonulae adherentes, (g) a "cell web" of tonofilaments running below the cell surfaces, most bundles apparently originating from the lateral junctions, and (h) a BM.

The main function of these cells is to absorb from the plasma filtrate various materials including sodium, sugar and any large molecules that find their way into it (small protein molecules at normal and large protein molecules at abnormal permeability of the glomerular BM), and to return these materials to the blood that flows in the peritubular capillaries (Fig. E); since this transport takes place against osmotic gradients it requires energy, hence the numerous mitochondria in the interdigitating processes. Thus sodium can be demonstrated in the apical

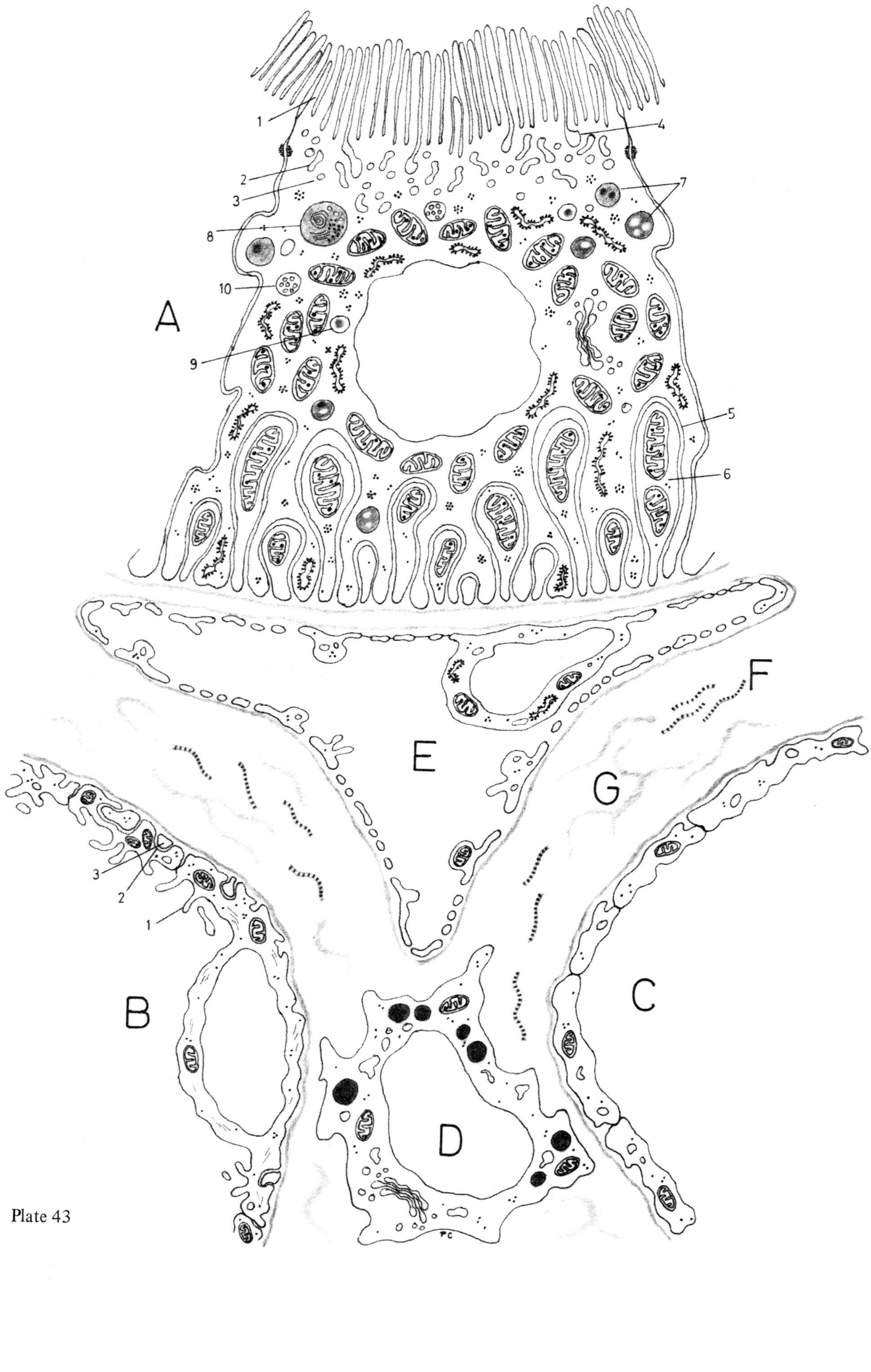

Plate 43

cytoplasm at all times; parenterally administered sucrose (^{14}C-labeled) is absorbed into large vacuoles; parenteral hemoglobin, albumin (^{125}I-labeled), iron and intratubularly administered ferritin are picked up through an as yet uncertain mechanism (perhaps by pinocytosis between the microvilli) and land in large apical vacuoles (phagosome equivalents) which fuse with lysosomes to form phagolysosomes and residual bodies, the latter being eliminated into the intercellular space. Finally, parenteral gold has been found to enter mitochondria causing their destruction and expulsion into the tubular lumen. It should be noted that in addition to entering from the luminar surface, large molecules could also reach the basal surface of these cells from the peritubular capillaries, but this possibility has not yet been adequately explored.

Although it is certain that the extensive basal interdigitations of the proximal tubule cells are associated with the intensive re-absorption that occurs in these cells, the specific role of the interdigitations in these processes remains to be elucidated; microdensitometric studies indicate that the basal folds are filled with a material that has the same density as the cytoplasmic matrix of the proximal tubule cells and is perhaps involved in the expedition of molecular traffic between cells and capillaries.

Among external influences that have been studied is that of drugs such as phenacetin which cause an expansion of the SER and lysosome system and the appearance of large cytosegresomes that are apparently eliminated into the lumen after withdrawal of the drug. This reaction is homologous to that which occurs in the liver after high dosage drug treatment and probably represents the synthesis of drug-metabolizing enzymes bound to the SER membranes. Another influence is that of hibernation which causes proteinuria, dilatation and fluid-filling of the SER vesicles (presumably due to retardation of the energy-consuming transport processes within the cells) as well as the appearance of nuclear inclusions.

When one kidney is removed, the cells of the other proliferate in compensation; during this process many proximal tubule cells "dedifferentiate" as evident by the loss of microvilli and basal infoldings, the rise in ribosome numbers and the appearance of many microtubules.

V. LOOP OF HENLE (Plate 43)

(1) The *descending thin limb* (Fig. B) consists of very thin, relatively undifferentiated cells that exhibit (a) a few ribosomes, smooth vesicles and mitochondria, (b) no RER or Golgi (c) several luminal microvilli[1] and basal invaginations[2] into which protrude basal processes of neighbouring cells[3] (basal interdigitation of adjacent cells), and (d) mostly narrow zonulae adherentes and a BM. The main function of this segment of the renal tubule is to promote the diffusion of fluid and certain ions from the lumen through the thin epithelium and stroma into the adjacent capillaries (Fig. E). This molecular movement is thought to be powered by physical forces inherent in the close proximity of two liquid streams (the primary urine in Henle's loop and the blood in the adjacent capillary) that run in opposite directions and possess different temperatures (a "counter-current ion exchange" situation). It is not certain yet whether the diffusion of fluid across Henle's epithelium is mainly intracellular or intercellular.

(2) The *ascending thin limb* (Fig. C) differs from the descending thin limb in that its cells (a) have no microvilli, and (b) have no basal interdigitations between adjacent cells.

(3) The *ascending thick limb* is very similar in structure to the distal tubule (see next section) but has a thinner wall than the latter, and its cells are held together mostly by tight junctions; it possesses apical vesicles exhibiting marked glumatic oxalacetic transaminase activity and, therefore, may excrete ammonia.

VI. STROMA OF KIDNEY

(1) Interstitial cells (Plate 43, Fig. D)

The structure of the interstitial cells resembles that of fibroblasts but (a) they are distinguished by a conspicuous number of dense osmiophilic (lipid) granules that contain arachidonic acid and prostaglandins A and E, and (b) they send out several processes that attach to the neighboring tubules and capillaries, often with expanded end-feet. It is currently thought that these are endocrine cells, manufacturing prostaglandins from the precursor material arachidonic acid and secreting it somehow into the bloodstream of adjacent capillaries. The prostaglandins relax constricted arterioles (and thus lower the blood pressure) in nanogram quantities but cause smooth muscle contraction in microgram quantities. It is, therefore, probable that the interstitial cells of the kidney participate in the regulation of blood pressure.

(2) Intertubular (peritubular) capillaries (Plate 43, Fig. E)

These have a thin wall, with numerous perforations that are sealed by very thin diaphragms. Their structure permits a very rapid and extensive exchange of materials with the renal tubules.

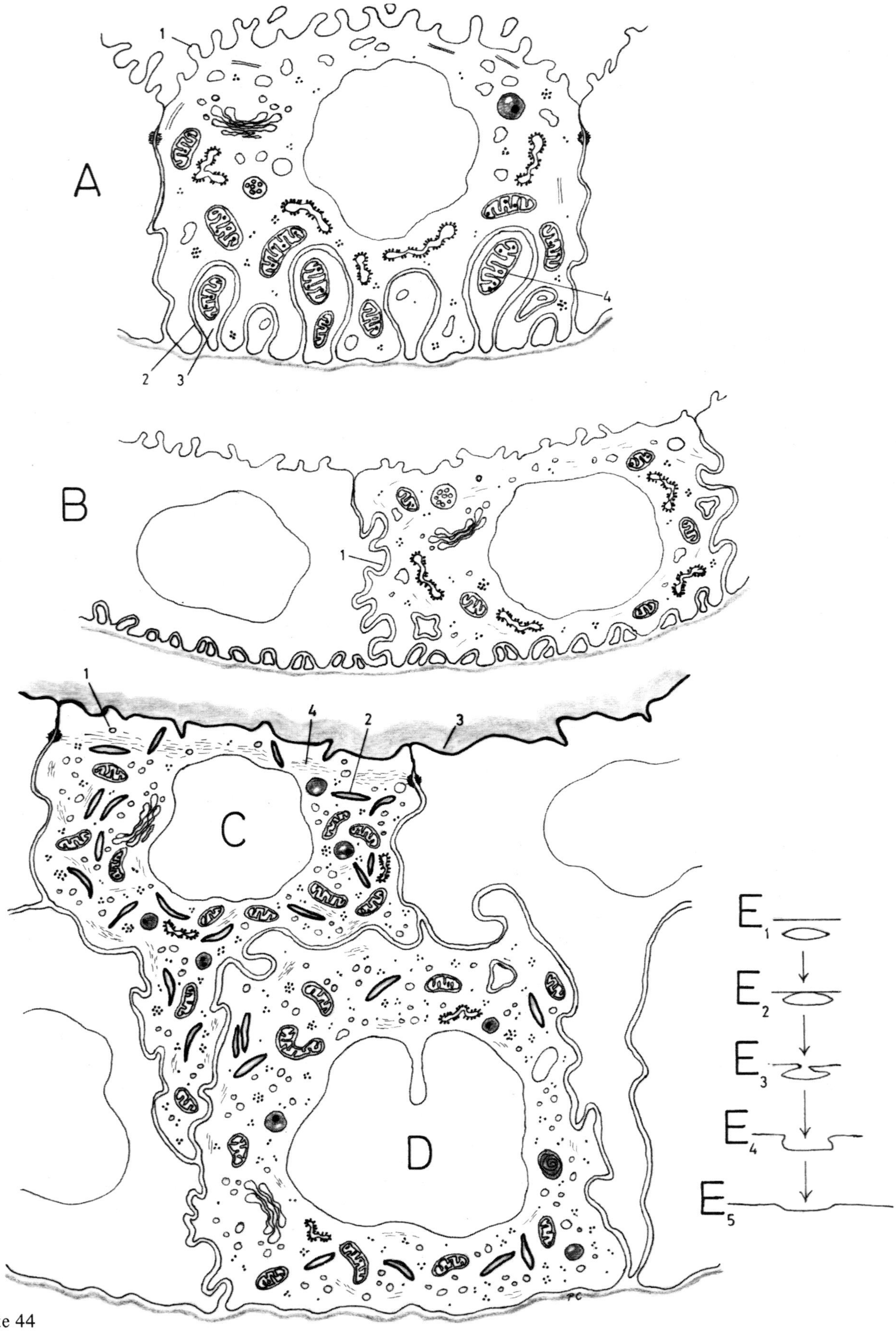

Plate 44

(3) Extracellular materials

These consist of (a) a few scattered collagen fibrils (Fig. F), (b) a few wisps of protein-like material (Fig. G), and (c) a variable amount of low density interstitial fluid (presumably plasma filtrate) that fills the narrow stromal space between tubules and capillaries and probably represents a carrier for the molecular traffic between them.

VII. DISTAL EPITHELIAL TUBULE (Plate 44, Fig. A)

Its cells are characterised by (a) moderate numbers of ribosomes, RER cisternae, large smooth vesicles, mitochondria and a Golgi, (b) several short stubby microvilli[1] at the apical surface, which is covered by a thin acid mucopolysaccharide coat, (c) a few cytosomes and multivesicular bodies but no microbodies (in man), (d) several basal invaginations[2] occupied by basal processes[3] of adjacent cells which usually contain large mitochondria[4], (e) tight junctions and a BM. The special features of the part of the distal tubule known as "macula densa" have been already described in the section on the juxtaglomerular complex.

The function of this segment of the renal tubule is absorptive as well as secretory.

VIII. COLLECTING TUBULE (Plate 44, Fig. B)

The majority of the cells (the so called "light cells") have the same structure as those of the distal tubule, with the following differences: (a) their apical microvilli are rudimentary, (b) their basal invaginations and the interdigitating neighbouring processes are very small and (c) there is appreciable interlocking[1] between the lateral cell surfaces. A few cells in the beginning of the tubule have an appreciably denser cytoplasm than the rest (the so called "dark cells") because of more ribosomes, more mitochondria and a denser cytoplasmic matrix. Both light and dark cells are joined by tight junctions and are lined by an acid mucopolysaccharide coat on their luminal surface.

The epithelium of the collecting tubule seems to be capable of much water absorption under proper stimulation. Vasopressin, the posterior pituitary water-conserving hormone causes an appreciable proliferation of the smooth vesicles and a marked dilatation of the lateral intercellular spaces; these structural changes express the stimulation of an increased uptake of water from the lumen into vesicles and of its release into the intercellular spaces (and hence into the capillaries) by the action of this hormone.

IX. URETER AND URINARY BLADDER EPITHELIUM (Plate 44, Figs. C–E)

Although for reasons of space economy this epithelium has been drawn to show two layers, it usually consists of three layers in man. It is a "pseudostratified" epithelium, *i.e.* all of its cells reach the BM (the upper ones through processes). The cells of all three layers are characterised by (a) many ribosomes, very few RER cisternae and a conspicuous Golgi, (b) numerous small smooth vesicles[1], (c) many large smooth flattened sacs[2] (the "discoid" or "fusiform" vesicles) whose membrane is asymmetric and distinctly thicker than the ordinary unit membrane (with a total thickness of 115 Å due to a 65 Å thick inner dense leaflet) and whose inner surface is lined by a sialomucin-like coat, and (d) appreciable numbers of mitochondria and lysosomes. The cells of the superficial layer exhibit (a) an unusually thick luminal plasma membrane that has a total thickness of 115 Å and is asymmetric, with a 65 Å thick outer dense leaflet, (b) an approximately 4000 Å thick sialomucin-like coat[3] over their luminal surface which can be visualised with ruthenium or lanthanum, (c) tight junctions and zonulae adherentes, and (d) bundles of tonofilaments[4] running through their apical cytoplasm. A small percentage (2–3%) of the epithelial cells, the so called "bundle cells" contain appreciable mucin-like granules. There is much interdigitation between all cells when the epithelium is in the contracted state.

The primary function of the urinary bladder epithelium is to be distensible so as to accommodate large volumes of urine. The epithelium can apparently stretch enormously (and at the same time become much thinner) through (a) the ironing out of the interdigitating folds between adjacent cells and, (b) the gliding of deeper cells into more superficial positions (which is feasible since junctions exist only between the apical portions of the superficial cells. An intriguing third process through which these cells may be stretched has been recently suggested by the elucidation of their fine structure: there are indications that the large "discoid" vesicles with the thick asymmetric membranes may fuse with the equally thick and asymmetric plasma membrane and add membrane material to it, *i.e.* lengthen it through an emiocytosis-like process (Figs. E_1–E_5). Since the discoid vesicles seem to be generated by the confluence of several small vesicles which are produced in the Golgi apparatus, it has been speculated that a "membrane flow" takes place from the Golgi towards the cell PM.

The function of the substantial sialomucin coat of the epithelial surface is presumably to protect the latter from maceration by the urine, but its origin is uncertain: it either represents a secretion of the "bundle cells" already mentioned, or it is carried to the surface by the emiocytosis-like movement of the discoid vesicles.

There is evidence that the bladder epithelium can absorb substantial amounts of fluid from the urine and pass them on to the underlying capillaries, at least under conditions of vasopressin stimulation (particularly in lower vertebrates). Thus administration of the latter hormone increases transepithelial water transport and widens the intercellular spaces in a manner reminiscent of its effects on collecting tubules.

One of the most intriguing observations has been the finding that deficiency of vitamin A produces keratinisation in urinary bladder epithelium, transforming it into epidermis-like tissue.

Chapter 11

Female Reproductive System

I. GENERAL

This system is concerned with (a) the production of ova, (b) their maintenance throughout the stages of fertilisation and embryonic development and (c) the production of female sex hormones that induce anatomical and behavioral changes favorable to fertilisation and embryonic development. It consists of the ovum-producing gonad (the ovary) and the ducts in which the ovum is fertilised and developed into a mature fetus before it is delivered (the oviducts, the uterus and the vagina). During its intra-uterine life, the embryo is nourished and oxygenated by the villi (branching processes) on the external surface of an enveloping trophoblastic shell; these villi absorb nutrients and oxygen from the surrounding uterine tissues and blood and transmit them to the embryo; they enlarge particularly within a circumscribed trophoblastic area to form the placenta.

II. OVARY

(1) General (Plate 45, Fig. A)

The ovary is a connective tissue (stroma) mass[1] that is lined by a simple cuboidal germinal epithelium[2]. Cell clusters[3] grow out of the germinal epithelium into the underlying stroma where they become ovarian follicles[4], one cell in the center of each follicle differentiating into an ovum[5] and the rest proliferating to form a granulosa[6] around it; in their mature (Graafian) stage[7], follicles secrete estrogen and develop a large cavity (the antrum)[8] filled with fluid (the liquor folliculi) but the ovum, enveloped by a thick membrane (the zona pellucida)[9], lies buried under a pile of granulosa cells (the cumulus oophorus)[10] at one end of the antrum. Upon appropriate hormonal stimulation, the mature follicle ruptures[11] through the germinal epithelium and the ovum with a few adhering granulosa cells is detached from the cumulus and ejected into the open end of the oviduct[12]. Soon after ovum ejection (ovulation), the cells of the ruptured follicle and of its stromal sheath (theca)[13] enlarge, acquire much cytoplasmic lipid (*i.e.* become "luteinised") and secrete progesterone in addition to estrogen – the follicle is transformed into a corpus luteum[14]. A corpus luteum turns into a scar, *i.e.* dense fibrous tissue ("corpus albicans"), upon reaching the end of its hormone-producing life span.

(2) Germinal epithelium (Plate 45, Fig. B)

This is an undifferentiated cell with a high nucleus/cytoplasm ratio and all basic organelles. It is characterised by (a) numerous ribosomes, including spiral polyribosome clusters[1] (cochleosomes), (b) a few lipid inclusions[2], and (c) microvilli[3] and a basement membrane. It is not joined to its neighbours by tight junctions.

The high ribosome and polyribosome content of this cell expresses its readiness for the high level of protein synthesis which it has to undertake since it is destined to proliferate and differentiate into a large ovum and its surrounding follicular epithelial cells. The absence of tight junctions with its neighbours probably facilitates the "drop-out" of this cell from epithelial formation and its descent into the underlying stroma where it proliferates and differentiates.

(3) Growing follicle with ovum

(A) Ovum (Plate 45, Fig. C)

This is a cell of huge size. It is distinguished by (a) some ribosomes[1] but practically no rough endoplasmic reticulum (RER), (b) perinuclear accumulations of mitochondria of very variable structure[2], several with a few or no cristae at all[3] ("oval bodies"), (c) cisternae of smooth endoplasmic reticulum[4] (SER) in very close association with the perinuclear mitochondria, (d) a fair number of smooth vesicles[5], some of them in pinocytosis-like communication with the cell surface[6], (e) several multivesicular bodies[7], (f) occasional annulate lamellae[8], (g) lysosomes, (h) a few lipid inclusions[9] in the mammalian ovum, but great numbers of yolk platelets[10] in ova of egg-laying animals (sacs with large cristalloid cores), and (j) a concentric Golgi[11] usually encircling the centrosome. The surface of the ovum (a) forms numerous

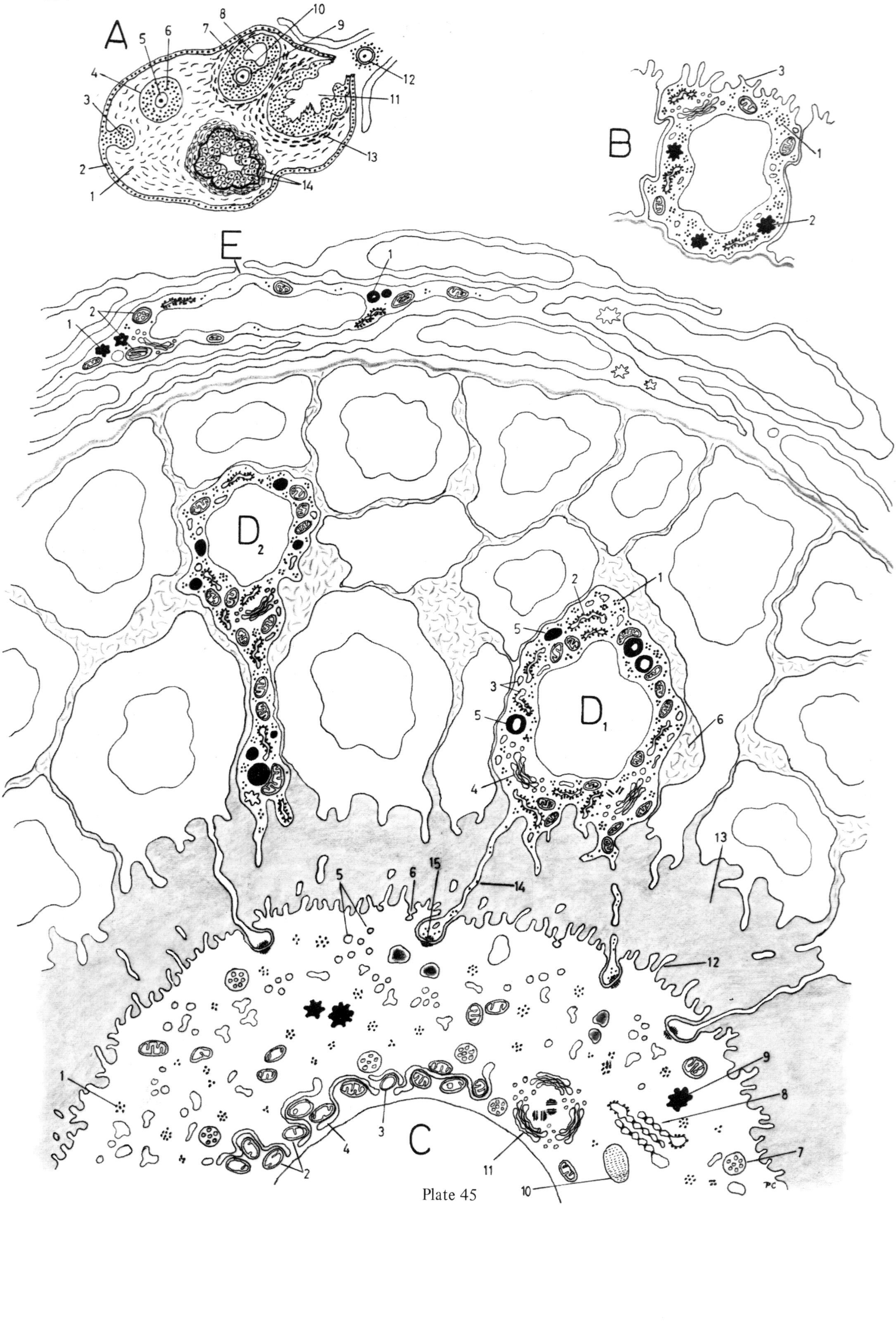

Plate 45

microvilli[12], (b) is surrounded by a thick glucoprotein layer of low density[13] (the "zona pellucida"), and (c) receives long thin processes[14] of the surrounding follicular epithelium cells with attach to the bottom of invaginations of the ovum plasma membrane through zonulae adherentes[15].

The *mechanism of nutrition* of the ovum is not certain yet; it is probable that certain nutrient materials (coming from the blood or manufactured by the follicular epithelium) diffuse across the zona pellucida and then enter the ovum by transmembrane diffusion and pinocytosis; it is also possible that some materials may be transmitted to the ovum by the processes of the follicular epithelium that anchor on its surface and that have as yet obscure functions. The *presence of ribosomes but no RER* is the structural expression of the fact that this cell does not synthesize its proteins for secretion but for growth and proliferation. The *loss of cristae* in many perinuclear mitochondria of the mammalian ovum and their transformation into "oval bodies" probably represents a mock-production of yolk platelets, ("pseudovitellogenesis") *i.e.* a phylogenetically vestigial process; it is a likely evolutionary remnant or homologue of the intense yolk-forming activity in the ova of some egg-laying animals in which perinuclear mitochondria are turned into yolk platelets by losing their cristae and accumulating cristalloid phospholipoproteins in their matrix. It is intriguing that yolk platelets are strikingly similar to certain other structures with phospholipoprotein contents, the premelanosomes (see chapters on skin and eye). The *multivesicular bodies* may represent aggregated pinocytotic vesicles (as is indicated by the appearance of intravenously injected dense particles within such bodies in certain kidney cells) or, like the mitochondrial decristation, they may be part of a vestigial yolk-formation process since they seem to participate in the manufacture of yolk platelets in certain egg-laying species. Finally, the function of *annulate lamellae* is unknown; these multiple constricted sacs are found in certain fast growing tumors besides ova and they seem to originate from the outer nuclear envelope – at least in some cell species. The close relationship of annulate lamellae and nuclear envelope is shown by the fact that the periodic fusions of the two membranes of the former represent structures that are practically identical with nuclear pore complexes with regard to both profile and "en face" details; thus annulate lamellae can be considered as multiple expansions of nuclear envelope into the cytoplasm.

During fertilisation, the head of a spermatozoon attaches to the zona pellucida (z.p.), penetrates it, and migrates 15–20 μ away from the entry site to perforate the ovum plasma membrane (PM), which breaks up into vesicular units at that point. Both the z.p. and the PM gap are re-sealed after the sperm head passes through them, and certain Golgi-derived vesicles migrate to the ovum surface to discharge their contents by emiocytosis as soon as the above events have occurred.

Soon after fertilisation, an appreciable RER system develops in the ovum and during the first divisions the number of polyribosomes rapidly increases in the daughter cells (blastomeres); perhaps as a result of incomplete cytoplasmic divisions, the blastomeres of early invertebrate embryos are interconnected by very thin cytoplasmic bridges.

(B) Follicular epithelium (granulosa cells) (Plate 45, Figs. D_1–D_2)

These small cells surround the ovum in several layers. Depending on the density of their cytoplasmic matrix, there are two kinds of them: the "light" (Fig. D_1) and the "dark" (Fig. D_2) granulosa cells. Both types have essentially the same structure and are characterized by: (a) a relatively high nucleus–cytoplasm ratio, (b) numerous ribosomes[1], (c) an appreciable rough endoplasmic reticulum (RER)[2], (d) increasing amounts of smooth endoplasmic reticulum (SER)[3] that develop from the RER as the follicle matures, (e) distinct and often multiple Golgi systems[4], (f) numerous mitochondria, and (g) a few lipid inclusions[5], often with extracted (translucent) centers. Small pools of intercellular fluid with reticular contents[6] ("the liquor folliculi") are scattered through the follicle epithelium and the cells of its innermost layer send off long, slender processes that cross the zona pellucida and attach to invaginations of the ovum surface, as already described in the preceding section.

The function of these cells is not entirely elucidated yet. It is probable that they help to *maintain the ovum, before it implants* into the uterine endometrium, by contributing to its nutrition either through secretion into the zona pellucida or through a more direct cytoplasm-to-cytoplasm transmission by means of their processes which dip into pockets of the ovum's surface; they certainly have the structural equipment to secrete since they possess a well developed RER and Golgi system. It is further established that they *produce hormones* (estrogens and later progestogens) which act at a distance to prepare and maintain a favourable environment for the development of the ovum after fertilization (within the uterine endometrium). The functional significance and the origin of the *liquor folliculi* are not yet entirely clear; this material may represent a transudate of blood, a secretion of the follicular cells, or both; it may serve as a vehicle for the storage or transport of follicular hormones from their production site to blood or for the transport of nutrients to the ovum; its reticular contents represent coagulated protein and it has been found to contain estrogen.

Steroid synthesis seems to be associated with the SER, since the latter expands in the last (Graafian) stage of follicle development, as well as after *FSH* injection.

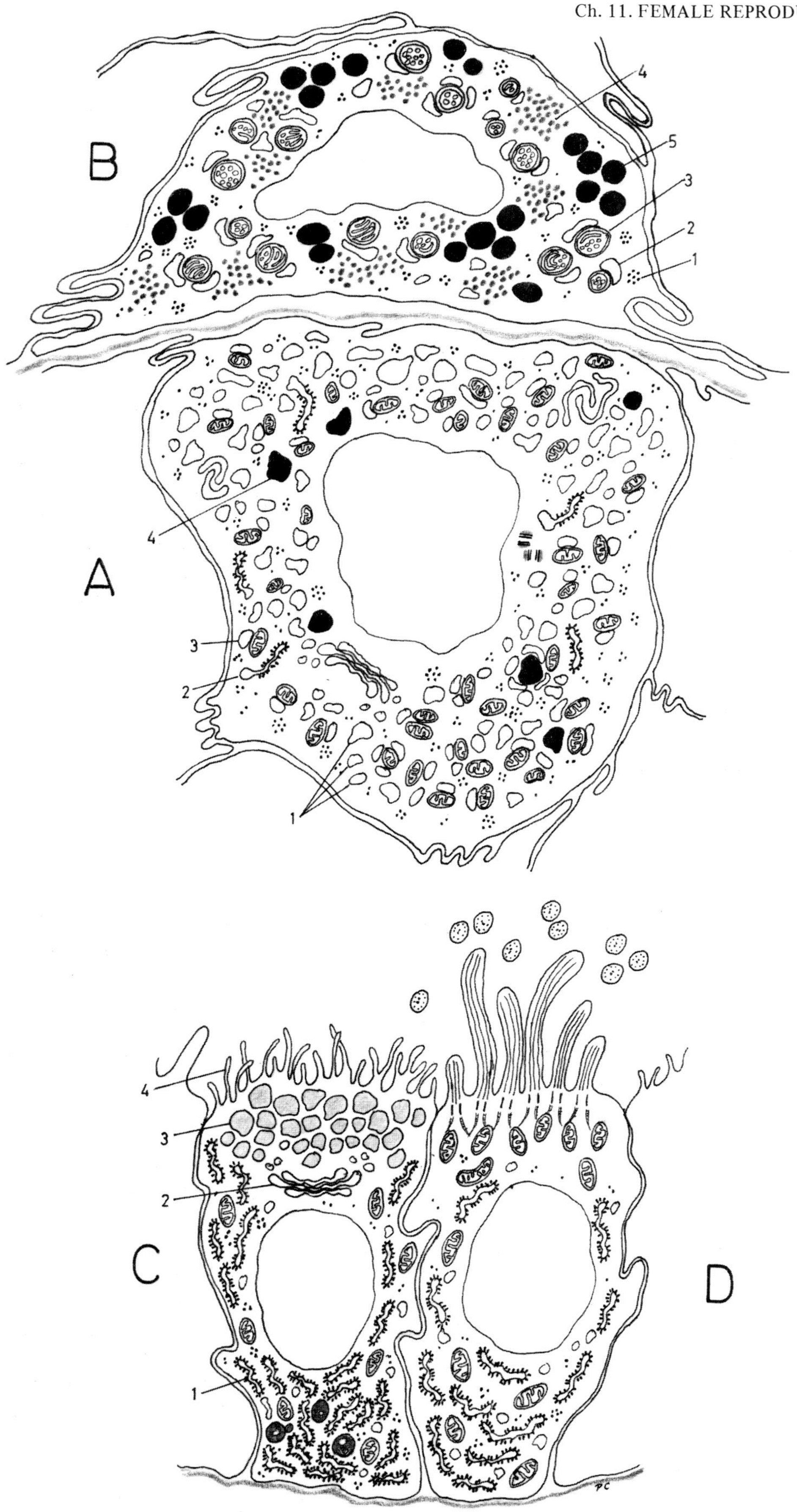

Plate 46

LH, given after FSH, stimulates the development of ribosomes and RER, apparently in preparation for the further great expansion of SER that occurs after ovulation. Both FSH and LH induce a marked rise of granulosa cell phospholipids, which probably reflects the increased synthesis of internal cell membranes (SER and RER).

(C) Theca (Plate 45, Fig. E)

Theca cells are like fibroblasts but they exhibit (a) greater than usual numbers of lipid inclusions[1], (b) mitochondria of the type found in the adrenal cortex and the Leydig cells, *i.e.* with tubular cristae[2], and (c) only sparse collagen fibrils in the intercellular spaces. They represent a ring of several concentrically packed stroma cells around the follicle, separated from the latter by a BM.

Their function at the stage of the growing follicle is uncertain; they seem to be undifferentiated mesenchymal cells which, however, undergo dramatic differentiation when they participate in the formation of the corpus luteum after ovulation (see next section).

(4) Corpus luteum

(A) Granulosa-lutein cells (Plate 46, Fig. A)

As the granulosa cells turn into lutein cells after fertilization, they retain all their previous basic organelles and, in addition, develop (a) much more cytoplasmic matrix, (b) an enormous smooth endoplasmic reticulum system (SER)[1] which develops from the rough endoplasmic reticulum (RER)[2], tends to form whorls and become closely associated with mitochondria[3], (c) a moderately greater number of lipid inclusions[4] which may become associated with SER sacs, (d) multivesicular bodies (originating from the nuclear membrane), and (e) at least in human corpora lutea during pregnancy, terminal web, desmosomes connecting the cells and long filament bundles streaming from the latter.

These cells produce much greater amounts of steroid hormones than before and they secrete them into the blood of the numerous capillaries that invade the follicle after ovulation. Their *luxuriant SER* is associated with marked 5-3-hydroxysteroid dehydrogenase activity and seems to be the site of the intensive estrogen and progestogen synthesis, since other cells that produce steroid hormones (*e.g.* those of the adrenal cortex or the Leydig cells) also possess extraordinarily extensive SER systems. It is not certain how the steroid hormones are released from the granulosa-lutein cells. Perhaps they diffuse out of the cells as lipoprotein molecules in a very low aggregation and fine dispersion state so that they never form large visible molecular packages; and perhaps the relatively few visible lipid inclusions represent stores of precursor materials for the manufacture of the steroids.

Luteotrophic hormone (prolactin) stimulates the manufacture and release of progesterone by corpus luteum cells, an effect that is expressed morphologically by an expansion of RER, SER and number of Golgi complexes and by a shrinkage of lipid globules.

During regression of a corpus luteum the lutein cells develop increased lysosome numbers and concentric "myelin-like" membrane systems, presumably as an expression of organelle degradation.

(B) Theca-lutein cells (Plate 46, Fig. B)

As the theca cells of the follicle turn into lutein cells they develop (a) a large amount of cytoplasm, (b) a fair number of ribosomes[1] but a very rudimentary rough endoplasmic reticulum (RER) and Golgi, (c) an appreciable number of smooth endoplasmic reticulum (SER) cisternae[2] which become closely associated with large mitochondria possessing tubular cristae[3], (d) many glycogen granules[4], and (e) many lipid globules[5]. The above changes can be induced, in theca and interstitial cells of immature animals by the combination of follicle-stimulating (FSH) and luteinising (LH) hormone.

The function of these cells is as described for the granulosa-lutein cells. It is not yet known whether theca-lutein and granulosa-lutein cells produce the same or different hormones.

III. OVIDUCT

(1) General

The oviduct is a moderately muscular tube lined by a folded columnar epithelium of ciliated and secretory cells. It picks up the ovum after ovulation, holds it during the period of its fertilisation and early cleavage and propels it to the uterus.

(2) Secretory cell (Plate 46, Fig. C)

This cell is characterised by (a) a prominent rough endoplasmic reticulum[1] (RER), (b) a conspicuous Golgi[2], (c) numerous mucous secretory granules of low density[3] apically, (d) a few lysosomes, and (e) apical microvilli[4], tight junctions with neighbors and a basement membrane.

The function of the secretory cells of the oviduct is to manufacture mucus (through the mechanism already discussed for the mucous-producing cells of the respiratory and alimentary systems) and to release it into the lumen of this tube in order to lubricate it and thus facilitate the propulsion of the ovum towards the uterus. This secretion is under cyclic hormonal control: in rodents, it is maximal during every metestrus – *i.e.* at the time of maximal need for it, since copulation in these animals occurs only during estrus.

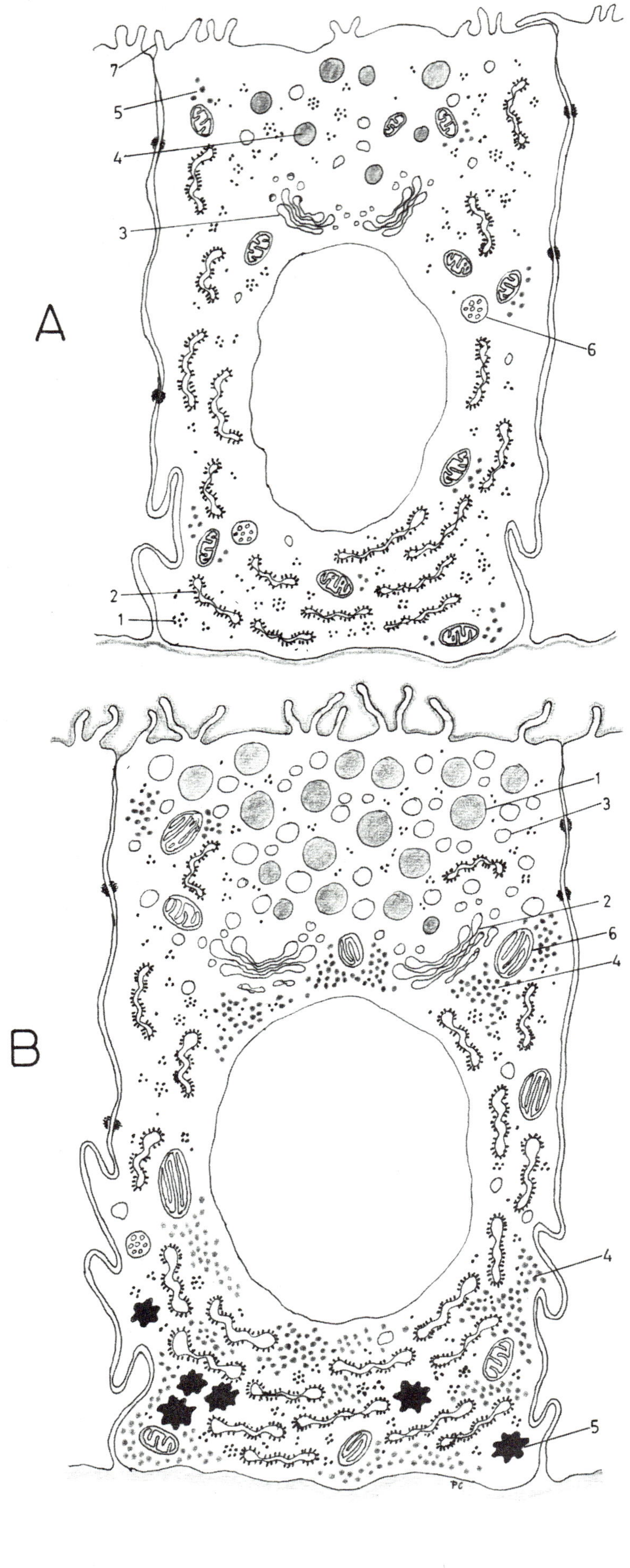

Plate 47

(3) Ciliated cell (Plate 46, Fig. D)

The structure of these cells is as described for the ciliated cells in the epithelial lining of the trachea and bronchi, but they usually have no apical microvilli between the cilia. Often "glycogen bodies" (SER whorls intermingled with glycogen granules) are seen in the apical cytoplasm of the ciliated cells, presumably representing fuel depots for the action of cilia.

Their role is to help propel the fertilized ovum towards the uterus through the beating of their cilia, in cooperation with the presumed peristaltic contractions of the oviduct's muscular coat.

IV. UTERUS – ENDOMETRIUM

(1) General

The uterus is a tube with a very thick wall whose main substance is smooth muscle (the myometrium) and whose inner surface is lined by a mucosa (the endometrium) with a simple columnar surface epithelium and numerous tubular glands embedded in a highly cellular stroma. When an ovum is fertilised by a spermatozoon, it is implanted into the endometrial lining of the uterus and stays embedded in it throughout its whole intrauterine growth period. Thus, in expectation of a possible implantation of a fertilised ovum, the endometrium undergoes periodic changes designed to prepare it for the above event; before each ovulation, the uterine gland cells are stimulated hormonally to proliferate and then to secrete. If fertilisation occurs, further "decidual" changes take place in the fibroblasts of the endometrial stroma; if no fertilisation occurs, the thickened secretory endometrium is peeled away and is discarded (menstruation) and a new one is built up in its place.

(2) Gland epithelium – Proliferative stage (Plate 47, Fig. A)

These cells are characterised by (a) the development of more cytoplasm than in the immediate postmenstrual stage, (b) many ribosomes[1], (c) a prominent rough endoplasmic reticulum[2] (RER), (d) a conspicuous Golgi system[3], (e) a few secretory glycoprotein (mucus) granules[4] of much greater density than those of the oviduct epithelium, (f) a fair number of mitochondria, (g) a few smooth vesicles, (h) a few clusters of glycogen granules[5], (j) occasional multivesicular bodies[6], and (k) sparse apical microvilli[7], tight junctions and multiple zonulae adherentes laterally and a thin basement membrane.

The function of these gland cells is (a) to proliferate so as to increase the thickness of the tissue that is destined to become the bed of the fertilised ovum, and (b) to start secreting glycoproteins into the gland lumen which are to serve as nutrients for the fertilised ovum. The glycoproteins seem to be produced and secreted through the same mechanisms as in the case of the mucoid cells of the alimentary tube.

Castration (hormone withdrawal) decreases the size of the cells and diminishes their populations of ribosomes and other organelles; by contrast, *estrogen* increases the cell size and ribosome population.

(3) Gland epithelium – Secretory stage (Plate 47, Fig. B)

The following changes occur in the uterine gland cells during the secretory stage of the cycle: (a) a further increment in cell size and length of microvilli, (b) a great increment in the number and size of the glycoprotein secretion granules[1], which appear first in the Golgi, (c) an increment of the size of the Golgi apparatus[2], the number of smooth vesicles[3] and the number of glycogen granules[4], (d) the appearance of lipid inclusions[5], (e) a great enlargment of mitochondria, some of which become giant organelles with longitudinal cristae[6] and allegedly visible DNA threads, (f) an enlargement of nuclei and nucleoli, and (g) swelling and loss of density of the basement membrane.

It is not known what the significance of the large numbers of *smooth vesicles* is; perhaps they represent a secretion of an unknown material. The other changes (development of large amounts of glycoprotein and glycogen and of some lipid) evidently greatly enrich the glands with nutrients to be utilised by the growing embryo – since the early embryo's trophoblast digests the endometrial glands. When the endometrium, however, is about to be sloughed off, these cells begin to develop serious anoxic damage as a result of the sustained spasm of the endometrial arteries: first they swell (presumably due to collapse of the sodium pump function of their PM), then their plasma membranes break and several cells disintegrate.

Combined *estrogen and progesterone* given to castrate animals causes marked RER development and nucleolar expansion and migration to the nuclear membrane which reportedly develops widened pores at the nucleolus attachment site; these changes express the accelerated nuclear synthesis and transport of RNA and the increased glycoprotein production induced by the combined hormone stimulation.

Recent studies on the *mechanism of action of steroid hormones* with labeled compounds showed that steroids are trapped within the cytoplasm of responsive target cells by receptors (possibly proteins); the resulting steroid–receptor complex then moves to the nucleus where it "turns on" specific DNA segments (genes) and thus sets in motion the sequence of events that lead to production of specific cell proteins or to cell growth. The

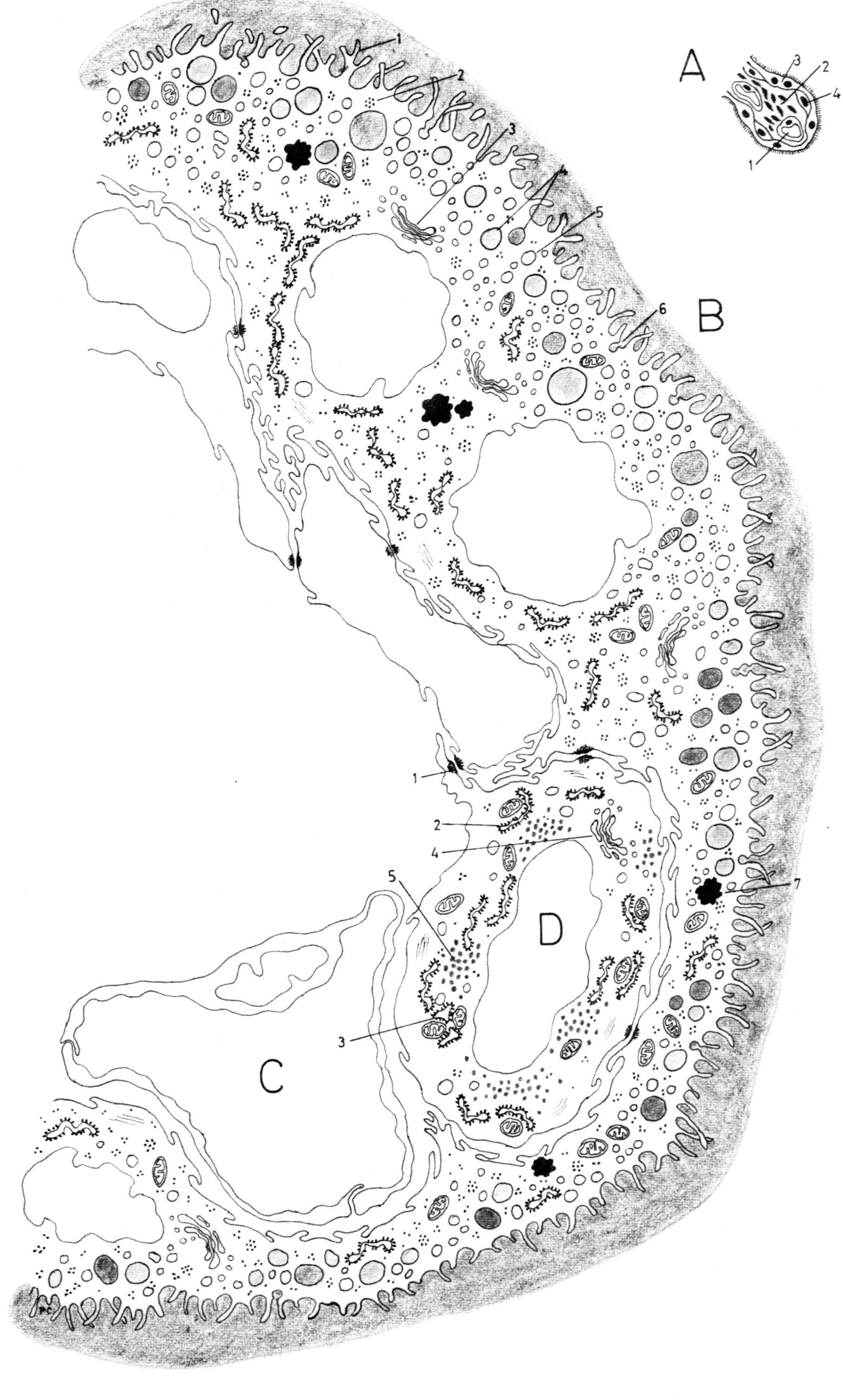

Plate 48

process through which the steroid–receptor complexes activate DNA is unknown; perhaps they "derepress" certain genes, *i.e.* they remove some proteins that are believed to attach to – and inactivate – all of the resting DNA (the DNA that is not active at a given moment).

(4) Decidual changes

When the blastocyst attaches to the endometrium, the epithelial cells develop great numbers of lysosomes (which are thought, but not proven, to cause their lysis) while the fibroblasts of the latter undergo certain rapid and dramatic changes: their cytoplasm, nucleus and nucleolus enlarge considerably, they develop glycogen and lipid inclusions, they become joined to one another by zonulae adherentes and occludentes and they proliferate. These "decidual changes" are designed to thicken the endometrial bed of the growing embryo and to increase its content of nutrients; they can be induced experimentally not only by the implantation of an ovum but also by a variety of mechanical and other stimuli in an endometrium that is sensitized by progesterone.

(5) Postpartum involution

A great increment of the number of lysosomes and autophagic vacuoles containing mitochondria, RER and other structures develops in endometrial cells during this period.

V. UTERUS – MYOMETRIUM

The myocytes of the myometrium are harnessed to one another by collagen and by unusually frequent *junctions* of three types, presumably because of the unusual need for mechanical cohesion of the uterus during the powerful contractions of delivery. *Estrogen* causes hypertrophy of the nucleus, organelles and cytoplasmic size of these cells as it builds up the size of the uterus to accommodate the growing fetus. During the first few days of the uterine *involution* that the follows delivery, the collagen content of this organ declines and histiocytes have been reported to phagocytize collagen fibrils.

VI. UTERUS – METRIAL GLAND

During pregnancy, clusters of fibroblast-like cells with extensive RER, large Golgi and numerous dense membrane-bound granules develop in the mesometrial triangle of rat uteri; they constitute the "metrial gland" and are thought to have an endocrine function, perhaps secreting relaxin, the hormone that loosens the pubic symphysis to increase the diameter of the birth canal. Similar cells have also been described as "granular cells" in the lamina propria of the endometrium of many vertebrates including man.

VII. VAGINA

The epithelial lining of the vagina consists of a stratified squamous epithelium similar to that which constitutes the epidermis of the skin. In the absence of estrogen (as *e.g.* after ovariectomy) the epithelium is thin (2–3 cell layers) infiltrated by polymorph leucocytes and its superficial layers are *not* keratinised – in ordinary laboratory rodents such as the mouse; estrogen injections will thicken and keratinise this epithelium by inducing mitotic proliferation in its basal layers and keratinisation in its superficial layers through a process which is similar to that operating in the epidermis at all times (see Ch. 14, Skin, p. 167). During the various phases of the *estrous cycle*, the structure of the vaginal epithelium varies continuously between extremes imposed by a minimum estrogen level at "diestrus" (appearance as after ovariectomy) and a maximum level at "estrus" (appearance as after estrogen injections). The maximal thickening and keratinisation of the vaginal lining during "estrus" (the ovulation time) is probably geared to the maximal likelihood of copulation during that period.

VIII. PLACENTAL VILLUS (LATE STAGE)

(1) General (Plate 48, Fig. A)

A placental villus is one of numerous branching processes which grow out of the external surface of the trophoblastic shell that envelops the embryo. At its mature stage it projects into a lake of uterine (maternal) blood and consists of a richly capillarised[1] areolar tissue core[2] which is lined by a single continuous layer of syncytial cells with a brush border, the syncytiotrophoblast[3]; immediately underneath the latter is located a discontinuous layer of single cells, the cytotrophoblast[4]. Various materials are absorbed from the maternal blood by the syncytiotrophoblast and transmitted to the villus capillaries through which they reach the embryonic circulation.

(2) Syncytiotrophoblast (Plate 48, Fig. B)

Ultrastructural study has confirmed that the cells of the syncytiotrophoblast form a pool of cytoplasm that contains several nuclei. This common cytoplasm pool is characterised by (a) numerous long and slender microvilli[1] coated by a glycocalyx on its free and a few short microvilli on its basal surface, (b) many ribosomes[2] but only a moderate number of rough endoplasmic reticulum (RER) cisternae, (c) multiple Golgi systems[3], (d) numerous membrane-bound granules of variable size and density[4], (e) many smooth vesicles[5] and occasionally large vacuoles, (f) plasma membrane invaginations of the pinocytotic type[6] at the free surface, (g) a moderate number of mitochondria, and (h) a few lipid inclusions[7], that are sometimes surrounded by SER whorls.

This syncytium functions as the lung, the intestine and the kidney of the embryo and as an independent endocrine system which produces hormones vital to its maintenance. Thus, (a) *oxygen* crosses the free villous surface from the maternal blood, traverses the cyncytiotrophoblast and the capillary endothelium (Fig. C) to enter the fetal blood, (b) *nutrients* are absorbed from maternal blood at the free microvillous surface (probably partly by pinocytosis) and transmitted to the fetal capillaries inside the villus, (c) embryo *waste products* (urea, etc.) move out of fetal capillaries, enter the syncytiotrophoblast at its basal surface and leave it at its free surface to plunge into the maternal blood, and (d) at first *protein hormones* (placental gonadotrophins) and later *steroid hormones* (placental estrogen and progestogen) are synthesized in the syncytiotrophoblast and released into the maternal blood. Of the above hormones, chorionic gonadotrophins have been demonstrated in the human syncytiotrophoblast with fluorescent anti-gonadotrophin antibodies. It is not known whether the numerous *dense granules* represent absorption, secretion or both; similarly, it is uncertain whether the *smooth vesicles* stream towards the maternal surface or away from it. It has been shown, however, that particles such as thorium and protein molecules such as peroxidase and ferritin are taken up by coated pinocytic vesicles at the microvillous surface and ferried across the entire thickness of the syncytiotrophoblast to be released by emiocytosis at its basal surface; from there, peroxidase has been found to enter the lumen of villus capillaries by crossing their endothelium through both pinocytosis and trans-junctional passage. The high ribosome content of this syncytium is explained by the need for the synthesis of many enzymes for its diverse transport functions and its hormone manufacture.

Occasionally, the surface of placental villi becomes coated by thick layers of *fibrin* that are reportedly initiated by the aggregation of maternal platelets on the syncytiotrophoblast. The cause of this aggregation and the possible role of direct fibrin precipitation in this phenomenon is unknown at the moment; the possibility of changes of the syncytial surface, of immunological rejection of maternal platelets by some embryos (or of placentae by some mothers), and of release of placental thromboplastin will have to be explored before this problem is resolved. When such fibrin thrombi develop, they become lined by a layer of syncytiotrophoblast (just as mural thrombi in blood vessels become lined by endothelium), but they are not usually organized into scar tissue.

During *early implantation*, the syncytiotrophoblast attaches itself firmly to endometrial epithelial cells and to the external surface of endometrial capillaries through the formation of junctional complexes, including desmosomes.

(3) Cytotrophoblast (Plate 48, Fig. D)

This consists of relatively undifferentiated cells that are equipped with a moderate number of basic organelles and are attached to each other and to the syncytiotrophoblast by zonulae adherentes[1]. They contain (a) ribosomes, (b) RER cisternae[2] which are often associated with mitochondria[3], (c) a Golgi[4], (d) smooth vesicles, and (e) glycogen[5].

Although their function is not definitively settled yet, the cells of the cytotrophoblast are currently considered as reserve (stem) cells that feed into the syncytiotrophoblast and contribute to its growth. The fusion of cytotrophoblastic cells to form syncytium is supported, among other things, by the frequent finding of PM-lined clefts (residues of intercellular spaces) and by the absence of mitoses in the growing syncytiotrophoblast.

(4) Stroma of placental villus

The stroma of a placental villus consists of fibroblasts swimming in a sea of amorphous and translucent glycoprotein, macrophages (Hofbauer cells) and capillaries. The endothelial cells of the latter have been described to develop large vacuoles through the curving and fusion of sizable PM folds with their luminal surface; such macrovacuoles could perhaps allow a faster removal of soluble wastes from the embryonic blood than ordinary micropinocytic vesicles.

Chapter 12

Male Reproductive System

I. GENERAL

The function of this system is to produce and deliver the spermatozoa (male gametes) as well as to manufacture hormones which control the structures and the activities associated with their delivery. It consists of the testis (in which the spermatozoa arise), a long duct that transports the gametes to the urethra (the epididymis and its continuation, the vas deferens) and several glands that add their secretion to the passing semen (the seminal vesicle, the prostate and the mucous glands of Cowper). Within the testis, the spermatazoa are born in numerous seminiferous tubules from which they are conveyed through the rete tubules and efferent ductules to the epididymis. Situated between the seminiferous tubules are groups of male hormone producing cells, the Leydig cells (interstitial cells).

II. SEMINIFEROUS TUBULES

(1) General (Plate 49)

Lodged in these tubules are several layers of cells comprising the "spermatogenic epithelium". The immature stem cells or spermatogonia (Figs. A, B) occupy the most peripheral position; they proliferate and differentiate through the stages of spermatocytes (Fig. C) and spermatids (Figs. D_1, D_2, D_3) to become spermatozoa (Fig. E) at the top of the pile. The whole sequence of stages from spermatogonium to spermatozoon is called "spermatogenesis" while its terminal segment (from spermatid to spermatozoon) is referred to as "spermiogenesis". Filling out the spaces between the spermatogenic cells and embracing them in their cup-shaped processes are the Sertoli cells (Fig. F). The seminiferous tubule is bound by a BM, which in turn is surrounded by a few collagen fibrils.

(2) Spermatogonium (Plate 49, Figs. A and B)

There are two types of spermatogonia: type A and type B. Type A (Fig. A) is an undifferentiated cell with a moderate number of ribosomes, smooth vesicles and mitochondria that has (a) no RER, (b) an inconspicuous or absent Golgi, (c) several microtubules[1], (d) a nucleus with two or more nucleoli which are attached to the nucleur membrane, and (e) often a "vacuole" in the nucleus (apparently an invagination of the latter).

Type A spermatogonia are stem cells that divide to yield more type A and some type B spermatogonia. Their prominent and marginally placed nucleoli express the high rate of RNA synthesis that is taking place in these continuously dividing cells.

Type B spermatogonia (Fig. B) are similar to those of type A but (a) they possess only one nucleolus which is not marginal and (b) they usually exhibit a prominent centriole; they differentiate into primary spermatocytes.

Recent studies indicate that proliferation of spermatogonia is regulated by a "chalone", *i.e.* by a substance which is produced by dividing spermatogonia and inhibits its mitosis in the remaining stem cells.

(3) Spermatocytes (Plate 49, Fig. C)

There are primary and secondary spermatocytes and they have similar structures. These cells are characterised by (a) larger size than that of spermatogonia, (b) the development of a conspicuous Golgi[1], (c) appreciable numbers of smooth vesicles[2], (d) a conspicuous centriole[3], and (e) conspicuous heterochromatin strands. They give rise to spermatids of various stages.

(4) Spermatid (Plate 49, Figs. D_1–D_3)

The *early spermatid* (Fig. D_1) exhibits (a) development of extraordinary Golgi[1] activity that leads to the elaboration of secretion in many vesicles[2] which then pinch off and coalesce to form a large "acrosomal vesicle"[3], (b) a condensation of secretion within the latter to form a large dense "acrosomal granule"[4] that contains hyaluronidase (a glycoprotein splitting enzyme), (c) mitochondria with sometimes dilated cristae, and (d) a dense cytoplasmic mass called the "chromatoid body"[5], which

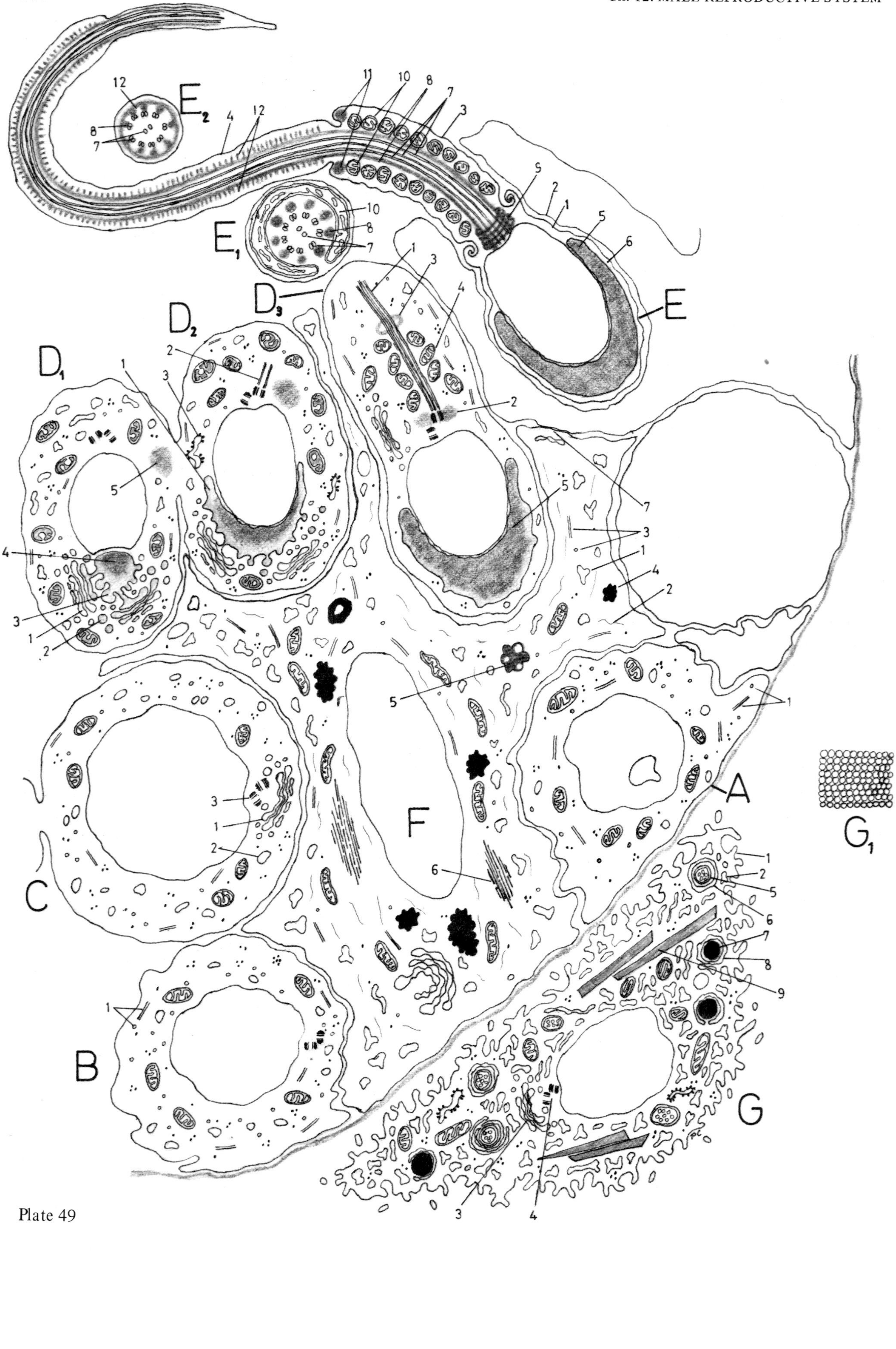

Plate 49

represents amorphous RNA and basic proteins and is destined to contribute to the synthesis of the microtubules of the spermatozoon tail that occurs later in the centriole region.

In the *intermediate spermatid* (Fig. D_2), (a) the acrosomal vesicle flattens and curves to form a "head cap"[1] that attaches to and embraces one half of the nucleus, (b) the Golgi begins to disengage from the acrosomal vesicle, (c) the distal centriole begins to generate the rudiments of an "axial filament"[2] (a cilium-like complex of 9 + 2 microtubule pairs), (d) a few RER cistenae may appear[3], (e) the nuclear chromatin begins to condense into predominantly fibrillar strands, and (f) the nucleus becomes elongated, perhaps as a result of the stretching of helical microtubules.

In the *late spermatid* (Fig. D_3), (a) the Golgi has detached completely from the acrosomal vesicle, (b) the axial filament grows longer[1], (c) the chromatoid body forms a sleeve[2] around the distal centriole as well as a ring ("annulus")[3] around the axial filament that glides towards it caudal end, (d) the mitochondria begin to crowd[4] around the axial filament, (e) the main cytoplasmic mass moves away from the nucleus to surround the axial filament, (f) the dense material[5] within the acrosomal vesicle expands to fill it up completely, and (g) the chromatin condenses even more vigorously.

Thus, the spermatid develops in several stages the principal organelles needed by the spermatozoon (the axial filament and the acrosomal cap) as well as the foundation of its definitive shape.

(5) Spermatozoon (Plate 49, Fig. E)

The spermatozoon, whose structure varies with the species, consists of a head[1] which is buried in an invagination of a Sertoli cell[2], and of a middlepiece[3] and a tail[4] that lie free in the lumen of the seminiferous tubule. The head consists of a nucleus with an extremely compact and uniform chromatin, an acrosome cap[5] and a very thin surrounding film of cytoplasm[6]. The middlepiece (see Fig. E_1 for a cross-section) consists of an axial filament[7] (a 9 + 2 microtubule pair complex), surrounded by 9 coarse fibers[8] ("columns"), which are in turn surrounded by (a) a ribbed sleeve proximally[9] (from the chromatoid body), (b) a spiral sheath of elongated mitochondria[10] along the entire length of the middlepiece, and (c) a ring structure[11] at the distal end of the middlepiece. The tail consists of the continuation of the axial filament of the middlepiece and its surrounding 9 columns as well as an outermost sheath of fibrous rings[12] (see Fig. E_2 for a cross-section). Most other organelles disappear, partly by sequestration into autosegresomes and extrusion from the cell. The function of the spermatozoon is to make an incredibly long and rapid trip up the uterus and the oviduct to reach the ovum (in proportion, the approximate equivalent of a 15 foot miniature submarine traversing 2000 miles at 150 miles per hour). This journey is accomplished by the propeller-like movements of the tail and it is powered by the mitochondria which surround the initial segment of the axial filament, using perhaps the glycogen of the uterine secretions as fuel. Once the spermatozoon reaches the ovum, its anterior PM and acrosomal membrane rupture, releasing hyaluronidase that enables it to "digest" its way through the corona radiata and the zona pellucida of the female gamete; a rod-like "perforatorium" then grows from the posterior membrane of the acrosomal vesicle and attaches to the PM of the ovum, which breaks at that point, allowing the nucleus of the spermatozoon to enter the ovum cytoplasm. After the spermatozoon nucleus enters, its own envelope as well as that of the ovum nucleus break up, permitting a pooling of the chromatins of the two gametes and launching the first division of the fertilized ovum.

(6) Sertoli cell (Plate 49, Fig. F)

Sertoli cells exhibit (a) relatively few ribosomes and RER cisternae, (b) a conspicuous SER[1], (c) long, slender mitochondria, (d) some fine filaments[2] and numerous microtubules[3], (e) a fair amount of lipid droplets[4] and lipofuscin granules[5], (f) spindle-shaped crystalloids of Charcot–Böttcher[6], found only in man (bundles of *ca.* 150 Å thick filaments), (g) a prominent nucleolus, and (h) peculiar *ca.* 80 Å wide broad junctions[7] with neighbouring Sertoli cells that are accompanied by flattened RER cisternae.

Their function is not completely elucidated. It is possible that they "nurse" the numerous spermatogenic cells embedded in their invaginations (*i.e.* transport nutrients and other metabolites to them). They have been also reported to phagocytise autosegresomes discarded from the mature spermatids during spermiogenesis or even whole parts of degenerating gametes. Finally, there is some evidence that they secrete estrogen, probably in their SER. Injections of FSH apparently stimulate steroidogenesis and expand the number of nuclear invaginations as well as the polyribosome and SER system of Sertoli cells. The role of the Charcot–Böttcher crystalloids is still obscure.

III. INTERSTITIAL (LEYDIG) CELLS (Plate 49, Fig. G)

These cells are characterised by (a) numerous microvilli[1] along their entire surface, (b) relatively few ribosomes and RER cisternae, (c) a very extensive SER[2], (d) distinct Golgi[3] and centriole[4] systems, (e) mitochondria with tubular cristae[5] that are often wrapped in several concentrically arranged SER cisternae[6], (f) a fair num-

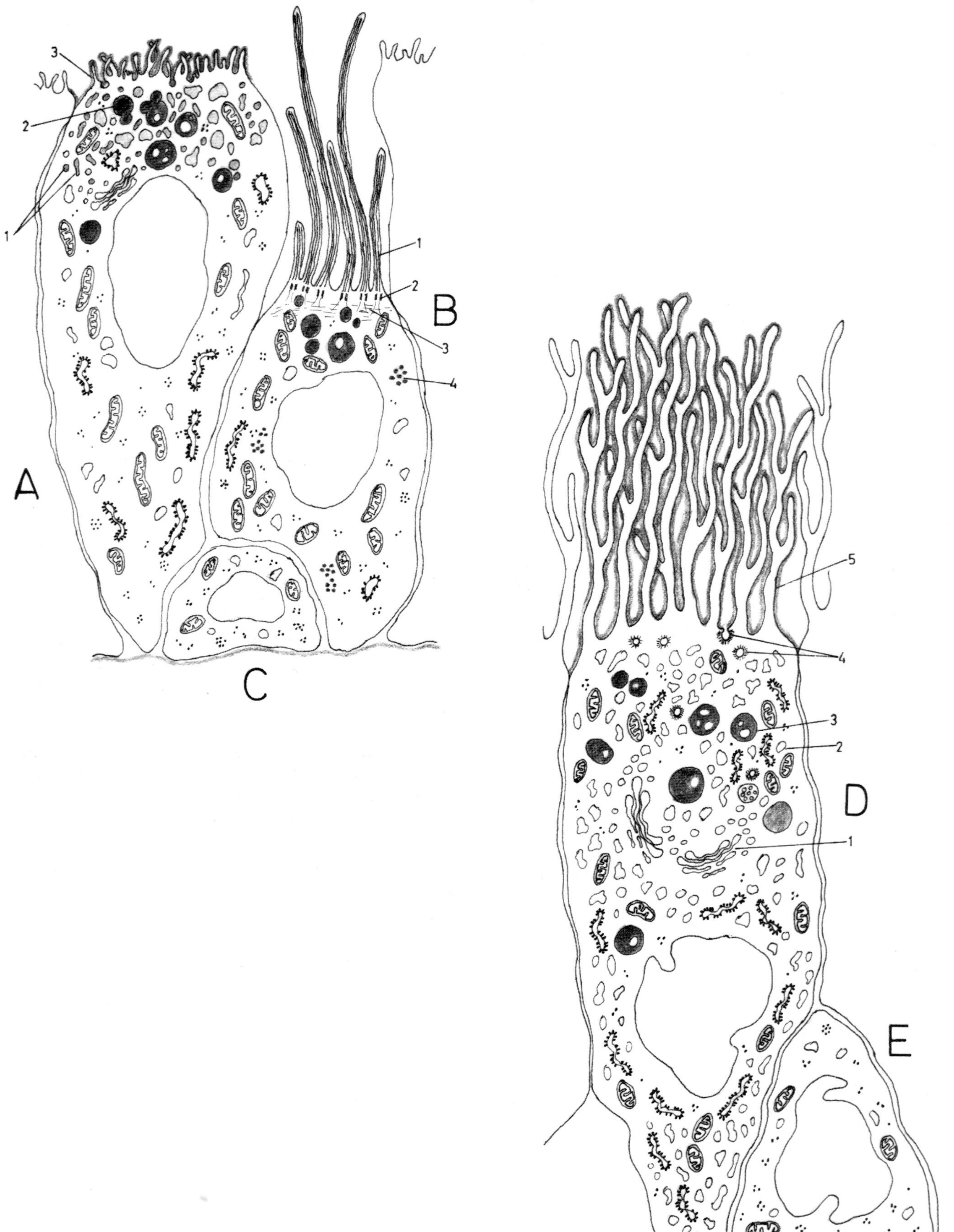
3
2
1
A
1
2
B
3
4
C
5
4
3
2
D
1
E
PC

ber of lipid globules[7] surrounded by SER sacs[8] (in man and some other species), and (g) several crystalloids[9] (of Reinke) with a substructure of tightly packed tubules (inset G_1).

Leydig cells produce androgens (testosterone and related steroids) and secrete them into the extracellular space, from where they find their way into the adjacent capillaries The biogenesis of androgen probably involves the transformation of cholesterol (absorbed from outside or synthesized in the SER) into pregnenolone within the mitochondria and the subsequent conversion of the latter to testosterone within the SER (whose membranes contain the necessary enzymes and perhaps also store the newly synthesized male hormone). The release mechanism of testosterone is unknown and probably similar to that discussed for the steroids of granulosa and corpus luteum cells. As expected, injections of interstitial cell stimulating hormone (LH) cause a marked expansion of the SER and an increment of the intramitochondrial lipid content.

IV. RETE TESTIS

The cells lining the canals of the rete testis are relatively undifferentiated cells with appreciable numbers of ribosomes, interlocking lateral margins and tight junctions. It is possible that they differentiate into the epithelium of the ductuli efferentes.

V. DUCTULI EFFERENTES EPITHELIUM

(1) General

This epithelium consists of brush border cells, ciliated cells and basal cells.

(2) Brush border cells (Plate 50, Fig. A)

They are characterised by (a) moderate numbers of ribosomes and RER cisternae, (b) several smooth vesicles and tubules containing a light, often reticular material[1], (c) numerous mitochondria, (d) several lysosomes[2] apically, (e) microvilli[3], junctional complexes and a BM. Their function is obscure. They perhaps absorb materials from and secrete materials into the semen; they may also remove debris from the latter since they have been observed to phagocytise HgS particles injected into the rete.

(3) Ciliated cells (Plate 50, Fig. B)

They have the same general structure as the brush border cells but (a) they possess cilia[1] instead of microvilli, along with basal bodies[2] and a terminal web[3] of filaments, (b) they have less RER then the brush border cells, and (c) they contain some glycogen granules[4]. They probably contribute to the forward propulsion of the semen through the movements of their cilia.

(4) Basal cells (Plate 50, Fig. C)

They are undifferentiated cells with a few basic organelles. They probably represent reserve elements that differentiate into either of the two overlying cell types.

VI. EPIDIDYMIS AND VAS DEFERENS EPITHELIUM

(1) General

This epithelium consists of stereocilium and basal cells.

(2) Stereocilium cells (Plate 50, Fig. D)

They exhibit (a) a few ribosomes and several RER cisternae, (b) a conspicuous Golgi[1] and SER system[2], (c) large, dense bodies which are probably lysosomes[3], (d) a fair number of mitochondria, (e) several coated apical pits and vesicles[4], (f) stereocilia[5], *i.e.* long branching processes of an unusual type that are coated by a fuzzy material, (g) tight junctions and a basement membrane.

Their structure suggests a secretory function (possibly the secretion of glycosidase and phospholipids) but they have also shown phagocytic ability since they can take up injected peroxidase from the duct lumen into phagosomes and form phagolysosomes. The presence of coated pits and multivesicular bodies furthermore suggests absorption of some solutes from the semen as it passes by. Castration causes the development of several stacks of annulate lamellae from the outer nuclear membrane of these cells and greatly depresses all structural evidence of synthetic activities while testosterone reverses these changes.

(3) Basal cells (Plate 50, Fig. E)

These are undifferentiated cells resembling those of the ductuli efferentes. They possibly mature into stereocilium cells.

VII. SEMINAL VESICLE EPITHELIUM

(1) General

The seminal vesicle epithelium consists of secretory and basal cells.

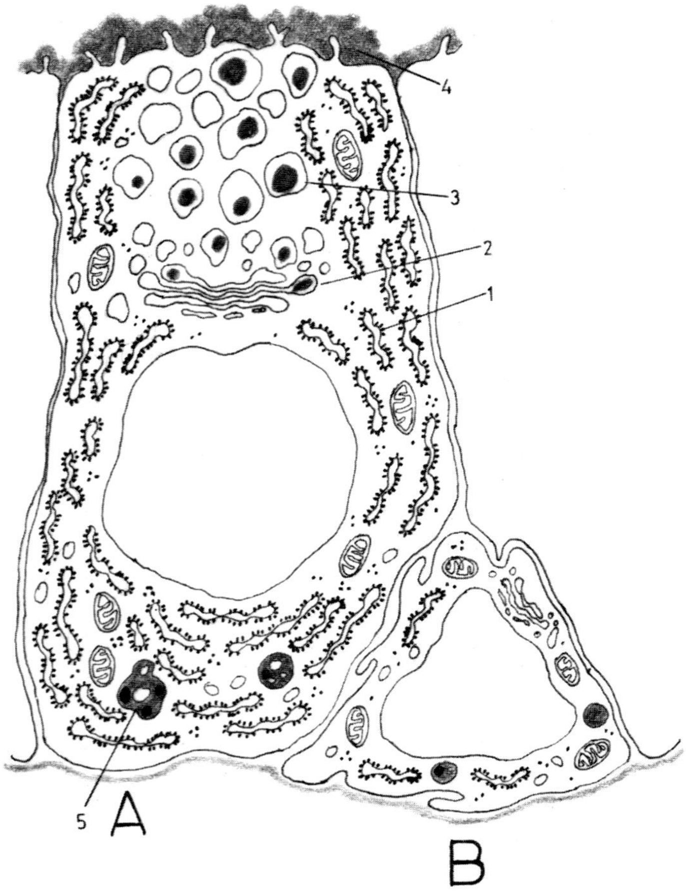

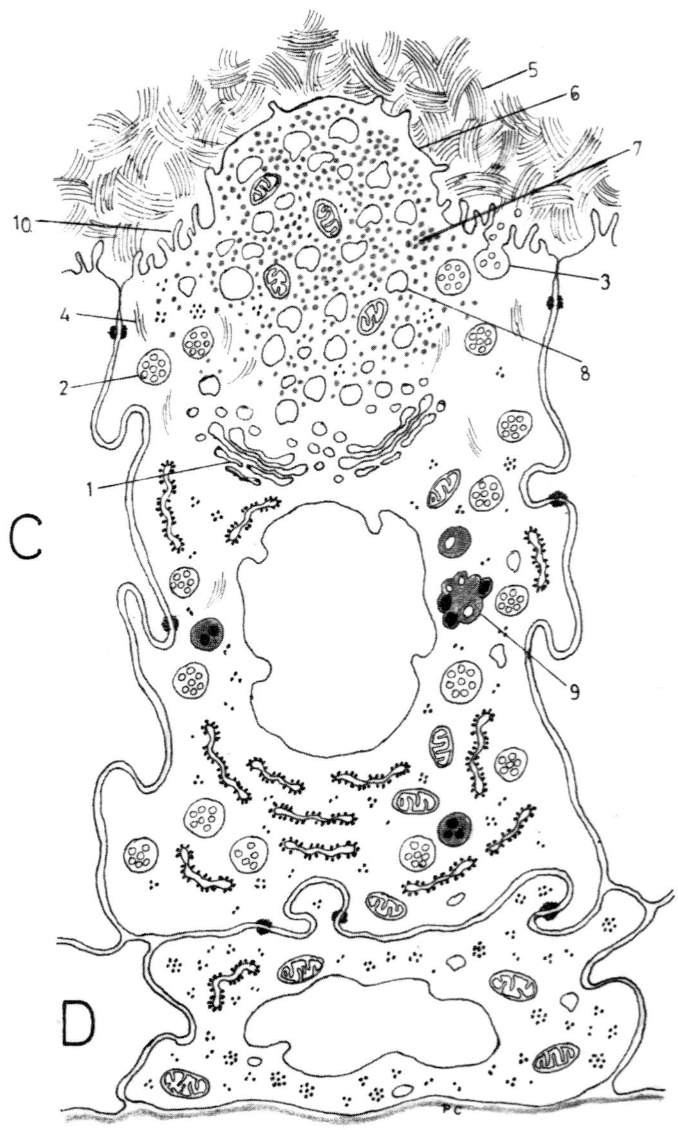

Plate 51

(2) Secretory cells (Plate 51, Fig. A)

They are characterised by (a) a fair number of ribosomes and an extensive RER[1], (b) a very prominent Golgi[2], (c) numerous dense membrane-bound secretion granules[3] that originate in the Golgi vesicles, (d) amorphous dense secretion in the lumen[4], (e) moderate numbers of mitochondria, (f) a few lysosomes[5], (g) microvilli, tight junctions and a BM, (h) frequent filamentous nuclear inclusions of unknown significance.

They secrete a material that includes fructose and citric acid and presumably contributes to the survival of the spermatozoa. Castration causes (a) an enormous shrinkage of these cells, (b) the disappearance of fructose and citric acid from their secretion, (c) a marked regression of RER, Golgi and an eventual disappearance of the secretory granules, and (d) an increment in the number of lysosomes.

(3) Basal cells (Plate 51, Fig. B)

These are undifferentiated cells resembling those of the basal cells of the vas deferens. They probably differentiate into secretory seminal vesicle cells.

VIII. PROSTATE EPITHELIUM

(1) General

This epithelium consists of secretory and basal cells.

(2) Secretory cells (Plate 51, Fig. C)

These cells are distinguished by (a) a fair number of ribosomes and RER cisternae, (b) a very large supranuclear Golgi[1], (c) numerous multivesicular bodies[2] that apparently represent a secretion and release their vesicles through emiocytosis[3] into the lumen, (d) several smooth vesicles and mitochondria, (e) a few bundles of filaments[4] within the cytoplasm, and masses of tightly packed filament bundles in the lumen[5] (the "corpora amylacea"), (f) an apical cytoplasmic lobe[6] rich in glycogen granules[7] and large smooth vesicles[8], (g) several lysosomes and lipofuscin granules[9], (h) microvilli[10] on either side of the apical lobe, and (i) multiple desmosomes and interlocking of plasma membranes with their lateral and basal neighbour cells.

The human prostatic epithelium cells secrete a material that contributes to the motility of spermatozoa and according to recent studies represent a mixture of stuff from the vesicles of the multivesicular bodies (merocrine component) and the detached, glycogen-rich apical lobe (apocrine component). Both the intracellular and extracellular filament bundles seem to consist of keratin-like protein masses with a very high sulfur content, but the production and release mechanism of the extracellular filament masses, their function and their relationship to the intracellular filaments are unknown. Castration causes a marked involution of the RER and an increment of the lysosome-segresome population while ageing increases the number of lipofuscin granules.

(3) Basal cells (Plate 51, Fig. D)

These are undifferentiated with numerous ribosomes but only moderate numbers of other basic organelles and no Golgi or myofilaments. They possibly turn into secretory cells.

Chapter 13

Endocrines

I. GENERAL

The endocrine gland cells secrete certain substances (hormones) into the blood stream which are carried to distant tissues to regulate their function. The main endocrine glands are the anterior, posterior and intermediate pituitary, the pineal, the thyroid, the calcitonin cells, the parathyroid, the adrenal cortex and medulla, the male and female gonads (already considered with the reproductive systems) and the pancreatic islets. In addition to the above, a number of other cells in the body have been discovered to secrete hormones into the blood stream and, therefore, to be "endocrine" by definition (*e.g.* the renin-secreting juxtaglomerular cells of the afferent renal arterioles, the hemopoietic hormone producing cells of the kidney, and the gastrin and secretin producing cells of the intestine).

II. ANTERIOR PITUITARY

(1) General (Plate 52).

While routine techniques revealed the presence of three cell types (acidophils, basophils and chromophobes) with the L/M, the following six types of cells can presently be distinguished by the E/M in this gland: luteotrophs and somatotrophs (corresponding to the "acidophils"), gonadotrophs, corticotrophs and thyrotrophs (corresponding to the "basophils"), and small granule-free cells that correspond to the "chromophobes". Luteotrophs produce luteotrophin (prolactin), somatotrophs growth hormone, gonadotrophs FSH and LH, corticotrophs ACTH, thyrotrophs thyrotrophic hormone and the small chromophobe cells secrete nothing. All above hormones are membrane-bound protein granules, secreted into the numerous capillaries around which the pituitary cells are clustered. In the adjacent drawing (Figs. A–F), the various cells of this gland are arranged clockwise in order of decreasing granule size around a capillary with diaphragm-sealed perforations (Fig. G).

(2) Luteotrophs (Plate 52, Fig. A)

The number of these cells is much greater in the female than in the male. They exhibit (a) moderate numbers of basic organelles, (b) moderate numbers of dense 6000–9000 Å thick luteotrophin (prolactin) granules[1], (c) smooth surfaces, no intercellular junctions and a BM on their side that faces the capillary, like all anterior pituitary cells.

Luteotrophin induces progesterone production in the corpora lutea, lactation in the mammary glands and maternal behavior. Studies with [^{3}H] leucine uptake have shown that a precursor form of this hormone is produced in the RER, then transferred to the Golgi and finally matured in the large membrane-bound secretion granules from which it is possibly (but not certainly) released through emiocytosis. The function of these cells can apparently be stimulated through nervous (sensory) impulses arising in the mammary nipples during suckling. During lactation, the amount of the RER, the size of the Golgi and the number of secretion granules increase while the interruption of lactation has the opposite effects and also induces autosegresome formation.

(3) Somatotrophs (Plate 52, Fig. B)

These cells exist in equal numbers in the male and female pituitary and they are the most numerous of all granulated ("chromophil") cells. They exhibit (a) approximately the same basic organelles as the luteotrophs, but a much more prominent Golgi[1] and (b) numerous membrane-bound dense 3000–6000 Å thick growth hormone (somatotrophin) granules[2].

Like the hormones of all the other anterior pituitary glands, somatotrophin seems to be produced in the RER in an immature form, transferred to the Golgi and matured in the secretory sacs from which it is released into the adjacent capillary through an uncertain mechanism (emiocytosis is possible, but not yet proven). Somatotrophin has been identified with the granules of these cells because (a) it can be localised in this granule fraction upon fractional centrifugation of anterior pituitary

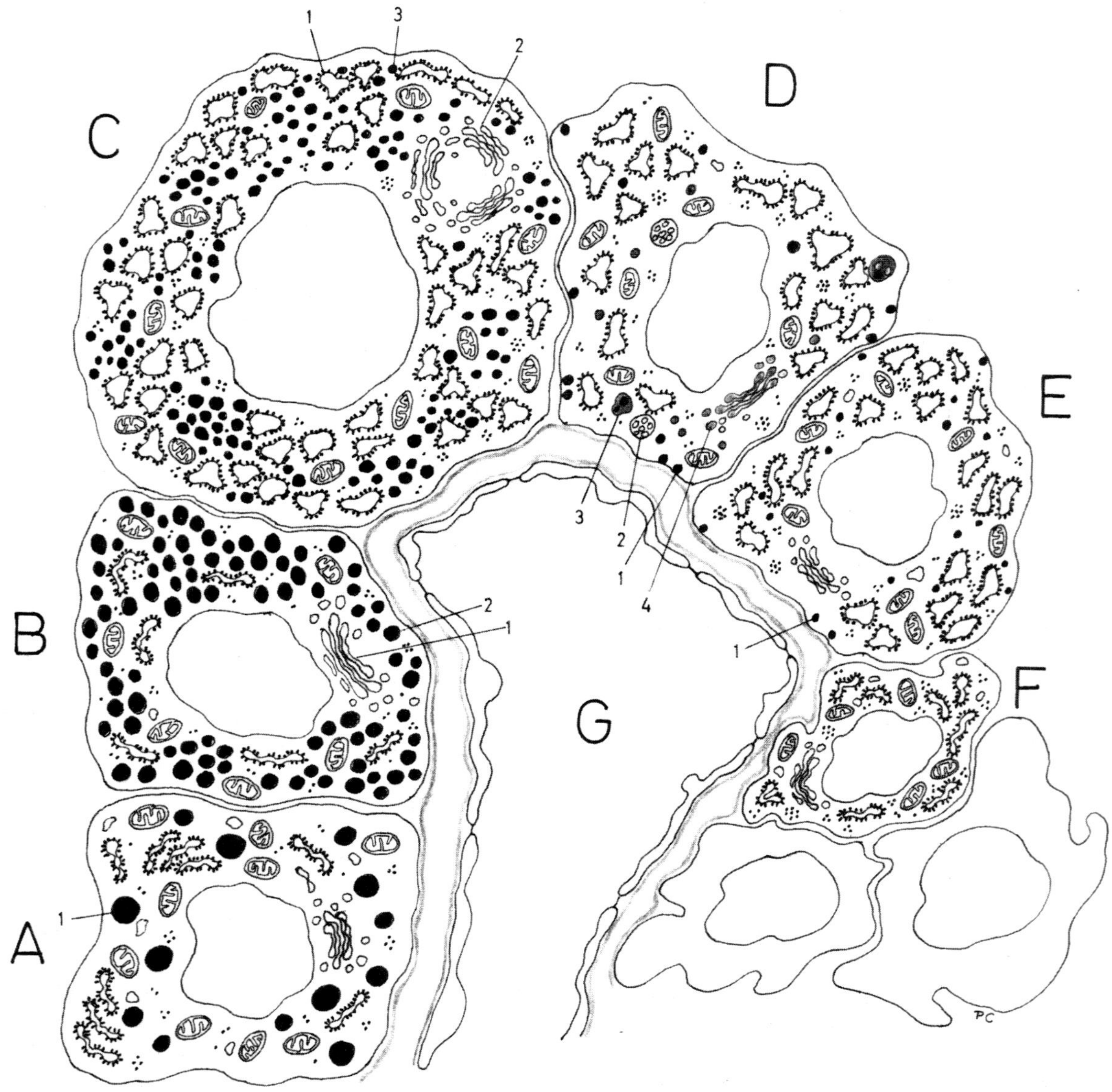

Plate 52

tissue, and (b) fluorescent anti-somatotrophin antibodies attach to the cytoplasm of these cells (as seen with the L/M). The fact that the granule number of somatotrophs is stable has been taken to indicate that growth hormone is produced and released continuously. Growth hormone releasing factor from the hypothalamus greatly stimulates somatotrophin release, Golgi activity and multivesicular body formation in these cells.

(4) Gonadotrophs (Plate 52, Fig. C)

These large cells are characterised by (a) an extensive RER system with usually dilated cisternae[1], (b) a very prominent "spherical" Golgi[2], (c) numerous 1000–2000 Å thick membrane-bound secretion granules[3] (FSH and LH), (d) moderate numbers of free ribosomes and mitochondria. FSH and LH have been identified with the secretion granules of gonadotrophs because they can be localised in this granule fraction.

The FSH produced by gonadotrophs stimulates ovarian follicle maturation in the female and spermatogenesis in the male, while LH stimulates estrogen production and ovulation in the female gonad and Leydig cells in the male. Since estrogen inhibits LH secretion by gonadotrophs through a negative feedback, it is understandable that castration (the removal of negative feedback) increases the activity of these cells, as manifested by an enormous dilatation of their RER cisternae and the appearance of a moderately dense material in them (the development of vacuolated "castration cells" as seen with the L/M). LH-releasing factor from the hypothalamus causes release of secretion granules from these cells.

(5) Corticotrophs (Plate 52, Fig. D)

These cells have the same general structure as the gonadotrophs but (a) they are smaller, (b) their Golgi is smaller and not spherical, (c) their 1500–2000 Å thick, membrane-bound secretion granules (ACTH) are relatively few and located mostly marginally[1] (close to the cell PM), and (d) they tend to exhibit some multivesicular bodies[2] and lysosomes[3]. Both ACTH and Melanocyte Stimulating Hormone (MSH) have been recently identified in the marginal granules of these cells by means of peroxidase-labelled anti-ACTH and anti-MSH antibodies.

The structure of corticotrophs (extensive RER, few and marginal granules) suggests a rapid turnover of secretion: The ACTH granules visibly arise within the Golgi as "immature' granules of low density[4], mature (become more dense) and move towards the cell PM where they are released by emiocytosis. ATCH stimulates the adrenal cortex to produce corticosteroids (*e.g.* hydrocortisone) which inhibit corticotroph secretion of ACTH by negative feedback; it is thus understandable that adrenalectomy (the removal of negative feedback) stimulates RNA synthesis ([^{3}H] adenine uptake), enormously dilates the RER cisternae and causes the appearance of low density material in them ("spongy cell"creation) while corticosteroid treatment causes an involution of RER, Golgi and cell size and increases the lysosome numbers of corticotrophs.

(6) Thyrotrophs (Plate 52, Fig. E)

The structure of these cells is similar to that of the corticotrophs, but their mostly marginal secretion granules[1] (thyrotrophic hormone) are 1000–1500 Å thick. Here too, the structure suggests a rapid secretion turnover.

Thyrotrophic hormone (TSH) stimulates the thyroid to produce thyroxine which inhibits TSH secretion by thyrotrophs through negative feedback, as in the case of the corticosteroid-ACTH and gonadal hormone-gonadotrophin relationships already described. For this reason thyroidectomy or propylthiouracil treatment (which inhibits thyroxin production) induces a great dilatation of the RER cisternae of thyrotrophs. Hypothalamic TSH-releasing factor stimulates exocytosis of TSH granules.

(7) Small, granule-free cells ("chromophobes") (Plate 52, Fig. F)

These are smaller than all granule containing cells, they have an irregular profile, and contain moderate numbers of the basic organelles. They appear to be undifferentiated reserve cells that can turn into granulated (hormone secreting) cells, or granulated cells in a resting phase of a secretory cycle.

(8) Follicular cells

These are cells of variable occurrence that form follicles, like those of the thyroid. They are of irregular shape, are bound to one another through junctional complexes, exhibit microvilli and cilia at their surface that faces the follicular lumen, and have a general cytoplasmic organelle profile similar to that of corticotrophs or thyrotrophs. Their function is uncertain at present, but there are indications that they may produce ACTH.

(9) Stellate cells

In addition to chromophobes there is another type of cell without secretory granules, the stellate (star shaped) cells. These are characterised by long processes, bundles of filaments and microtubules and abundant glycogen granules. They are attached to one another through desmosomes and form a framework in the meshes of which

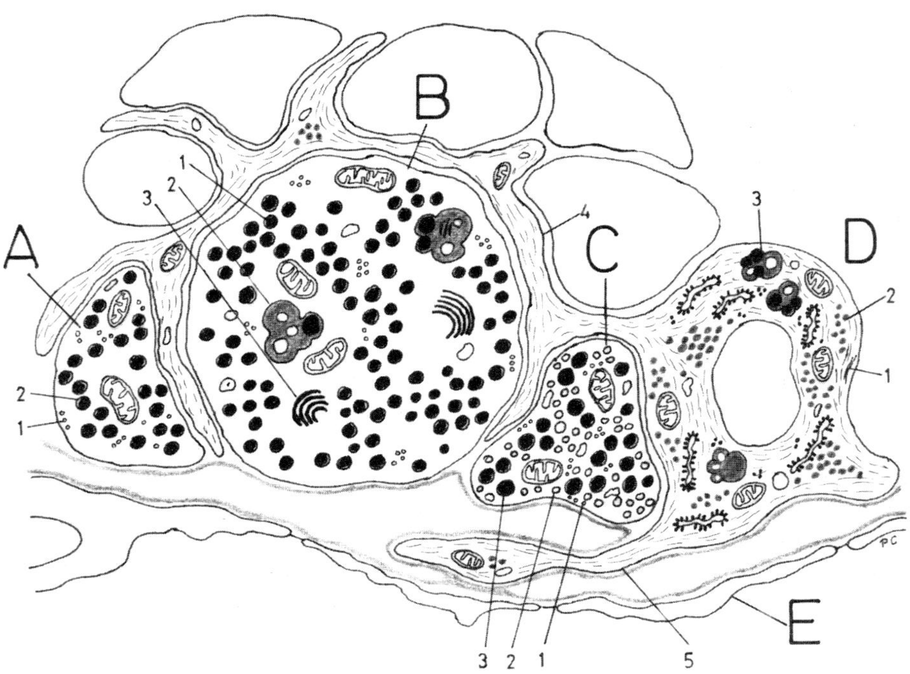

Plate 53

lie all the other cells; they are considered to be supporting cells.

(10) Capillaries (sinusoids) (Plate 52, Fig. G)

As in all endocrine glands, these have perforations sealed with thin diaphragms, a very thin cytoplasm and a BM. Their structure seems to facilitate rapid entry and exit of hormones.

III. POSTERIOR PITUITARY

(1) General

This gland contains the axons and terminals of neurosecretory neurons which are situated in the hypothalamus of the brain and which secrete the polypeptide hormones pitressin and oxytocin into the blood. Pitressin causes smooth muscle contraction, preserves body water by inhibiting urine formation (increasing tubular reabsorption) and raises the blood pressure, while oxytocin causes contraction of uterine smooth muscle during delivery. The gland consists of (a) axons of the hypothalamic neurons, (b) localised expansions of these axons at irregular intervals, the "Hering bodies", (c) terminals of these axons, (d) modified glia cells ("pituicytes") between the above structures, and (e) sinusoid thin-walled capillaries with diaphragm-sealed perforations (Fig. E), as in all endocrine glands. The sum total of the axons in the posterior pituitary constitutes part of the "hypothalamo-hypophyseal tract".

(2) Cell bodies of the neurons of the hypothalamo-hypophyseal tract

These hypothalamic neurons exhibit the basic structure common to all neurons but manufacture, in addition, membrane-bound dense 1200–2000 Å thick neurosecretory granules that first become visible in their Golgi; the granules, which represent pitressin and oxytocin (proven immunocytochemically), travel down the axons of these neurons into their terminals in the posterior pituitary glands, where they are released into the bloodstream.

(3) Axons of the hypothalamo-hypophyseal tract (Plate 53, Fig. A)

They have the structure common to all unmyelinated axons, conspicuous microtubules[1] and, in addition, numerous dense 1200–2000 Å neurosecretory granules[2] which are on their way to the axon terminals.

(4) Hering bodies (Plate 53, Fig. B)

These are localised expansions of the hypothalamo-hypophyseal axons, teeming with 1200–2000 Å neurosecretory granules[1], lysosome-lipofuscin bodies[2], and multilamellar lipoprotein structures[3] (the "zebra" or "shaslik" bodies). The role of the Hering bodies is unknown; they are currently considered local axonal swellings caused perhaps by axonal kinks or other obstructions to axonal flow; the multilamellar lipoprotein structures may represent unsequestered organelle debris and there is evidence that some of them may be extruded into the brain ventricles across their ependymal lining.

(5) Axon terminals of the hypothalamic neurons (Plate 53, Fig. C)

These terminals exhibit (a) mitochondria, (b) microtubules[1], (c) numerous 400 Å clear synaptic type vesicles[2], (d) a few larger smooth vesicles, and (e) many membrane bound 1200–2000 Å neurosecretory granules[3].

The dense neurosecretory granules of the axon terminals, like those of the axons and the neurons from which they originate, represent pitressin and oxytocin, since (a) the gland content of these hormones correlates well with the gland content of these granules and (b) these hormones are located in the 1200–2000 Å granule fraction upon fractional ultracentrifugation. Dehydration of the body causes massive release (and disappearance) of these dense granules from the neurosecretory axon terminals of the posterior pituitary gland. Their release mechanism is uncertain; it probably involves molecular diffusion of the polypeptide hormones out of their enclosing envelopes, through the cell PM, two basement membranes and capillary diaphragms into the blood stream, since neurosecretory granules have never been seen in the extracellular space. It is thought that some axon terminals secrete their hormones into capillaries that reach anterior pituitary cells.

(6) Pituicytes (Plate 53, Fig. D)

These are glial type cells which exhibit the basic organelles plus (a) appreciable microfilaments[1], (b) clusters of glycogen granules[2], (c) several lysosome-lipofuscin bodies[3], and (d) long processes[4] that meander between axons and axon terminals and envelop the Hering bodies, often terminating in the periendothelial space[5]. Their function is not yet established.

IV. PARS INTERMEDIA OF THE PITUITARY GLAND

In many vertebrates (*e.g.* the cat) the pituitary contains, in addition to the anterior and posterior parts, a minor but distinct layer of cells between the two, the "intermediate part". This consists of (a) a tangle of two types of epithelial cells (large and small granule contain-

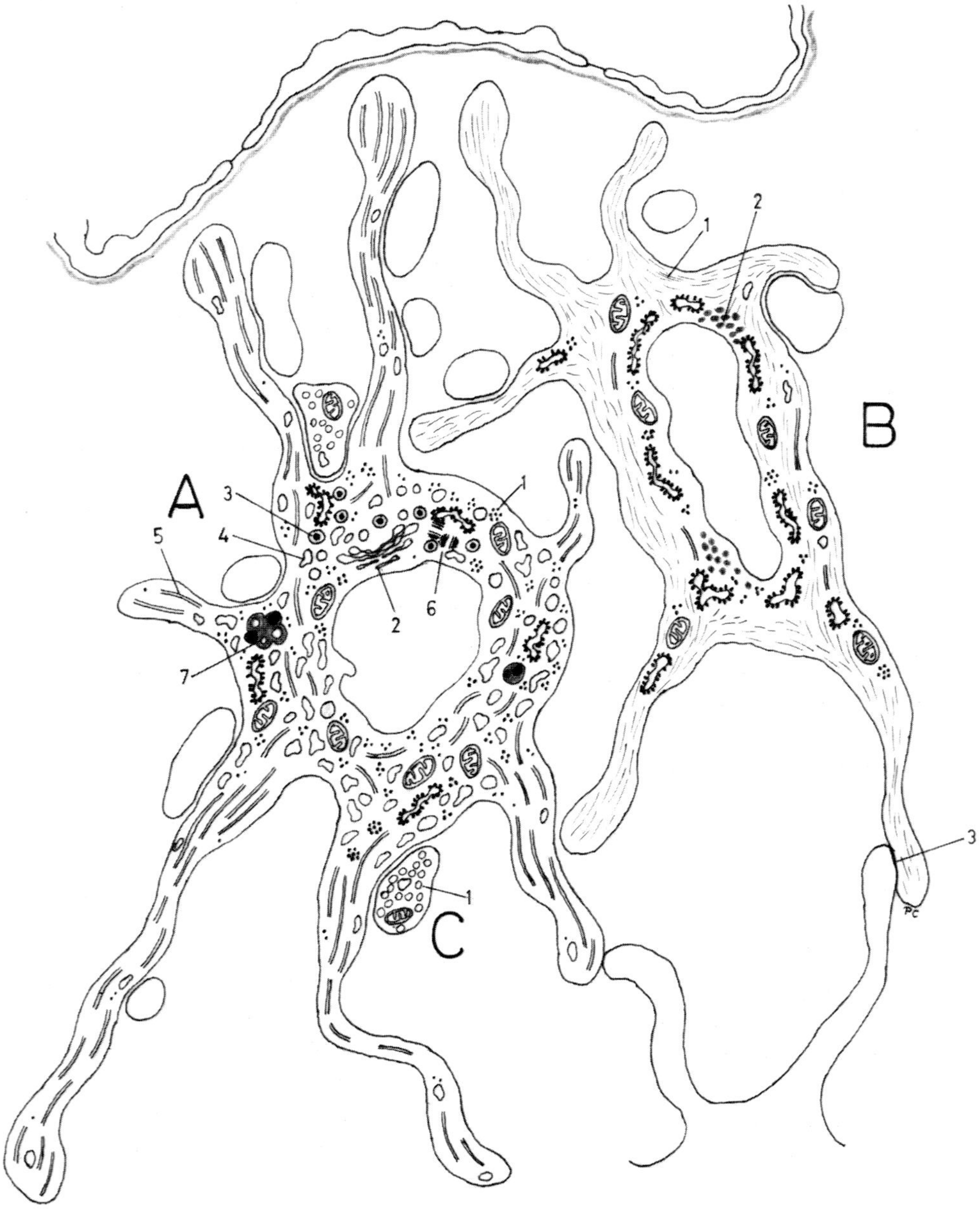

Plate 54

ing cells), (b) unmyelinated axons and axon terminals of three types: cholinergic (*i.e.* with small clear vesicles), adrenergic (*i.e.* with small cored vesicles) and peptidergic (*i.e.* terminals of the polypeptide-secreting or neurosecretory type, with both small clear and large cored vesicles), and (c) glial type cells surrounding the axons. ACTH has been recently identified immunocytochemically in the RER and granules of pars intermedia cells.

V. PINEAL GLAND

(1) General

The pineal is an organ that has a still unsettled function in mammals. It consists of (a) cords or nests of pinealocytes with several processes (the main cell type), (b) interstitial (glia) cells, also with several processes, and (c) capillaries with diaphragm-sealed perforations.

(2) Pinealocytes (Plate 54, Fig. A)

These cells exhibit (a) numerous ribosomes[1], (b) a few RER cisternae, (c) a distinct Golgi[2], (d) cored vesicles[3], 1000–1500 Å thick, that contain catecholes or indoleamines in their dense cores and an OsO_4-ZnI_2 staining material (an acidic protein) in the clear space between the envelopes and cores, (e) an extensive SER[4], (f) numerous 220–300 Å wide microtubules[5], (g) several mitochondria, (h) often prominent centrioles[6], (j) a few lipid droplets and lysosome-lipofuscin bodies[7], and (k) occasional cilia and nucleus-associated annulate lamellae. Both "dark" and "light" pinealocyte varieties have been reported.

The pineal is metabolically very active, displaying a marked uptake of aminoacids and phosphorus. It contains much serotonin and melatonin (5-hydroxy-indole) which seem to be contained in the cored vesicles of the pinealocytes, as shown by histochemical techniques; melatonin is produced from serotonin by the action of a pinealocyte transferase. In lower vertebrates (lizards, amphibia, fish) this organ is a photoreceptor outpouching of the brain – much like the retina – that translates photic stimuli into nervous impulses and sends them to other parts of the brain. In mammals, however, the pineal has so far been identified with the following functions: (a) mammalian melatonin will aggregate melanin around the nuclei of amphibian skin melanocytes and thus produce blanching, *i.e.* a brightening of skin color (an antagonistic effect to that of melanophore expand ing hormones); (b) the whole pineal has anti-gonadotrophic effects, since pinealectomy or pineal destruction by disease causes precocious puberty and increased gonadal weights, whereas pineal extracts produce opposite results; furthermore, melatonin has been recently shown to inhibit LH secretion and ovulation. (c) light exposure (*e.g.* in rats) reduces pineal mass, pinealocyte size and pinealocyte transferase activity whereas exposure to darkness (or blinding) stimulates the pineal and causes testicular regression. Thus photic stimuli may be received by the pineal through the optic pathway and translated there into skin melanocyte or gonadotrophic control.

(3) Interstitial (glia) cells (Plate 54, Fig. B)

These are apparently modified astrocytes characterised by (a) numerous 50–60 Å thick microfilaments[1], (b) a few microtubules, (c) some glycogen granules[2], (d) moderate amounts of ribosomes and RER, (e) mitochondria with denser matrix than those of the pinealocytes, and (f) frequent tight junctions[3] with neighbouring interstitial cells. The function of the interstitial cells is unknown.

(4) Axons (Plate 54, Fig. C)

Several unmyelinated axons establish contact with pinealocytes (and with interstitial cells); some of them possess numerous synaptic vesicles[1] (Fig. C), and are therefore axon terminals; they possibly transmit photic stimuli to pinealocytes or receive impulses form the latter which they relay to other parts of the brain.

VI. THYROID GLAND

(1) General (Plate 55)

The cells of the thyroid (Fig. A) form the walls of hollow spheres or "follicles" into the interior of which they secrete "colloid", a precursor form of the hormones thyroxine and tri-iodothyronine. The follicles are surrounded by capillaries with diaphragm-sealed fenestrations (Fig. B) into which the active hormones are secreted by the follicular epithelial (thyroid) cells. Attached to the thyroid follicles in mammals are the cells of another endocrine system, the calcitonin-producing "parafollicular" cells (Fig. C). Thyroxine and tri-iodothyronine increase the rate of oxidations in the body and thus influence a wide variety of processes and tissues (*e.g.* growth, intellect, skin and heart).

(2) Follicular epithelial cell (Plate 55, Fig. A)

This cell is characterised by (a) an extensive RER with dilated cisternae[1] that contain a low density flocculo-granular material[2], (b) a fair number of ribosomes, (c) a conspicuous Golgi[3], (d) numerous apical small vesicles filled with a moderately dense homogeneous material,

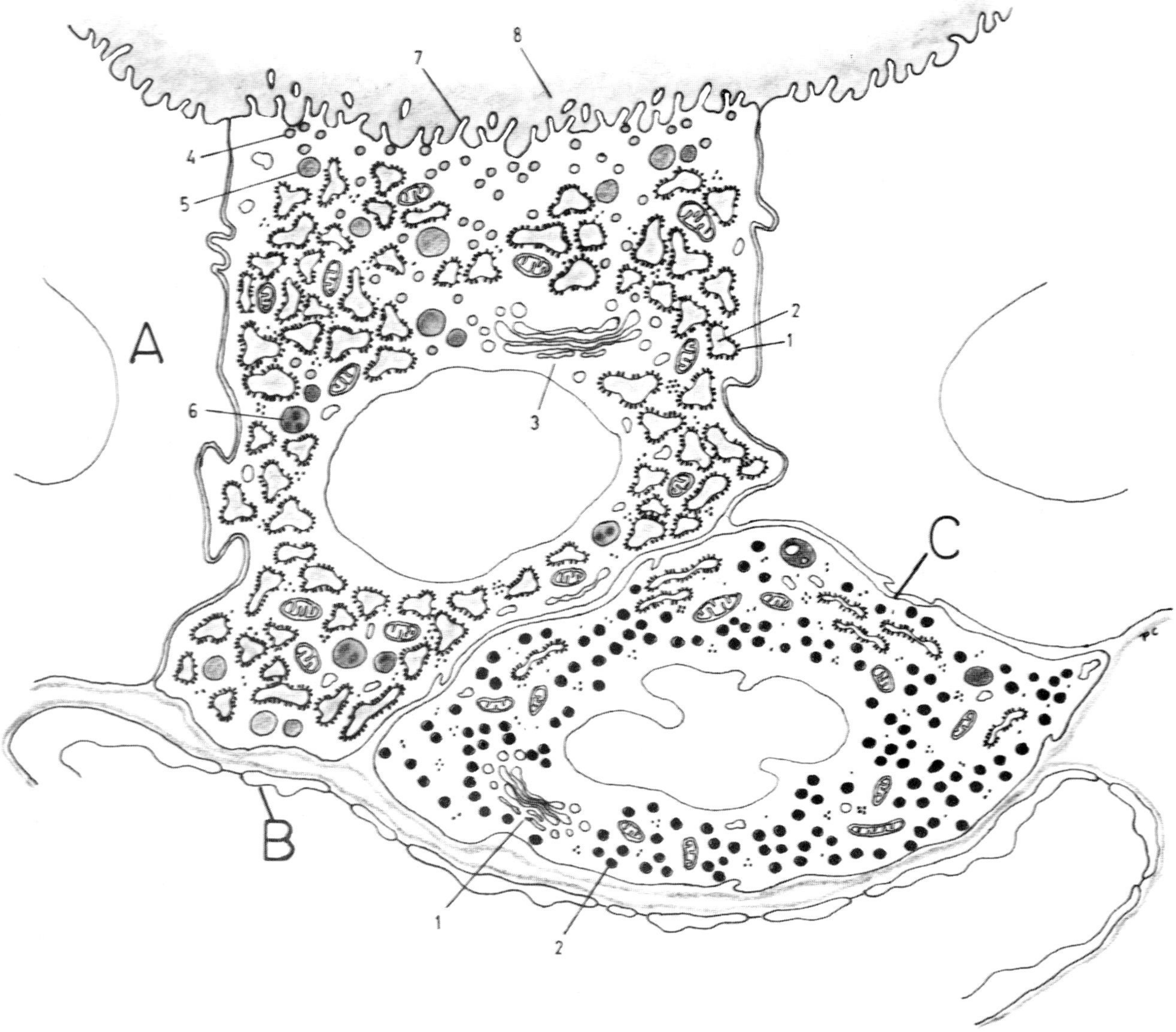

Plate 55

the intracellular "colloid vesicles"[4] (the E/M equivalent of the L/M PAS-positive material), (e) an appreciable number of Golgi-derived lysosomes[5], (f) several compound bodies containing both lysosomal enzymes and colloid[6] and apparently arising from the fusion of lysosomes with colloid vesicles (autophagolysosomes), (g) a fair mitochondrial population, and (h) apical microvilli[7], tight junctions and desmosomes at their lateral boundaries and a BM. The follicular lumen above the epithelial cells is filled with a moderately dense extracellular colloid[8].

In their active form, both thyroxine and the more potent tri-iodothyronine represent iodinated amino acid derivatives whose manufacture proceeds along the following stages: (a) both hormones are first synthesized within the ribosomes in an iodine-free, protein-bound form, the "iodine-free thyroglobuline", (b) carbohydrate is added to the iodine-free thyroglobuline first in the RER (mannose) and then in the Golgi (galactose) turning it into a glucoprotein (colloid), (c) this iodine-free glucoprotein is carried from the Golgi to the apical cell surface within the small colloid vesicles and released into the follicle lumen through an unknown mechanism (possibly emiocytosis), (d) the glucoprotein (colloid) is then mostly iodinated in the lumen according to *in vivo* autoradiographic studies utilising ^{125}I (although recent observations with isolated thyroid cells suggest that some intracellular iodination is also possible), (e) the iodinated glucoprotein (colloid) is then absorbed from the lumen through a pinocytosis-like mechanism into small apical vesicles which do not appear different from those carrying iodine-free glycoprotein and which migrate towards the cell base, (f) the small vesicles carrying iodinated glycoprotein fuse with lysosomes to form compound bodies; (g) the lysosomal proteolytic enzymes split off the active iodinated hormones thyroxine and tri-iodothyronine from the iodinated glycoprotein, and (h) the two active hormones are released from the cell base through an unknown mechanism and cross into the capillary lumen below. According to the above account, the small apical vesicles represent a mixture of secretory vesicles carrying iodine-free colloid to the lumen and absorptive vesicles carrying iodinated colloid from the lumen.

The thyroid-stimulating hormone (TSH) of the pituitary (a) increases pinocytosis and phagocytosis of colloid and the number of small apical vesicles, (b) it induces the movement of lysosomes towards the cell apex, and (c) it increases lysosomal thyroglobulin-hydrolysing (proteolytic) activity and active hormone release. By contrast, the removal of TSH from the scene through either hypophysectomy or thyroxine (which inhibits TSH secretion by negative feedback) causes the disappearance of the colloid vesicles.

When ^{131}I is given intravenously, it is picked up and held by the thyroid epithelium where its radiation has profound effects within 2–3 days: it causes a disappearance of microvilli and apical vesicles, a partial detachment of ribosomes from the RER cisternae, and a proliferation of lysosomes and segresomes.

VII. CALCITONIN-SECRETING (PARAFOLLICULAR) CELLS (Plate 55, Fig. C)

These cells are wedged between the bases of the follicular epithelial cells. They exhibit (a) a moderate number of ribosomes and RER cisternae, (b) a conspicuous Golgi[1] that may display prosecretory granules in certain species, (c) numerous 1000–2000 Å vesicles with dense contents (membrane bound granules)[2] which are apparently secreted by emiocytosis, (d) a moderate number of mitochondria that are smaller and have a denser matrix than those of the follicular epithelial (thyroid) cells, and (e) a generally smooth profile and a BM on their capillary side.

The dense contents of the 1000–2000 Å vesicles represent calcitonin which is secreted into the underlying capillaries. Calcitonin depresses the blood calcium level and its secretion is stimulated by high calcium levels. Thus a short lasting elevation of blood calcium (caused *e.g.* by vitamin D) will increase the number of polyribosomes and the Golgi size and diminish the number of secretory granules (and the calcitonin content) of the parafollicular cells because it stimulates calcitonin synthesis and release, while a prolonged calcium elevation (*e.g.* after parathyroid hormone) will greatly increase the number of parafollicular cells as well.

In lower vertebrates (*e.g.* frogs) calcitonin is produced by the ultimobranchial bodies which respond to hypercalcemia in the same manner as the mammalian parafollicular cells.

Recently, a mutant strain of mice has been discovered (grey-lethal, microphthalmic) that exhibits congenital hyperplasia of parafollicular cells, low blood calcium and congenital osteopetrosis, *i.e.* increased mineralisation of bone. A congenitally increased secretion of calcitonin may be responsible for the increased movement of calcium from the blood into the bone.

VIII. PARATHYROID

(1) General (Plate 56)

The parathyroid produces a polypeptide hormone that raises the blood calcium level by moving calcium from the bone into the blood (with the accompaniment of

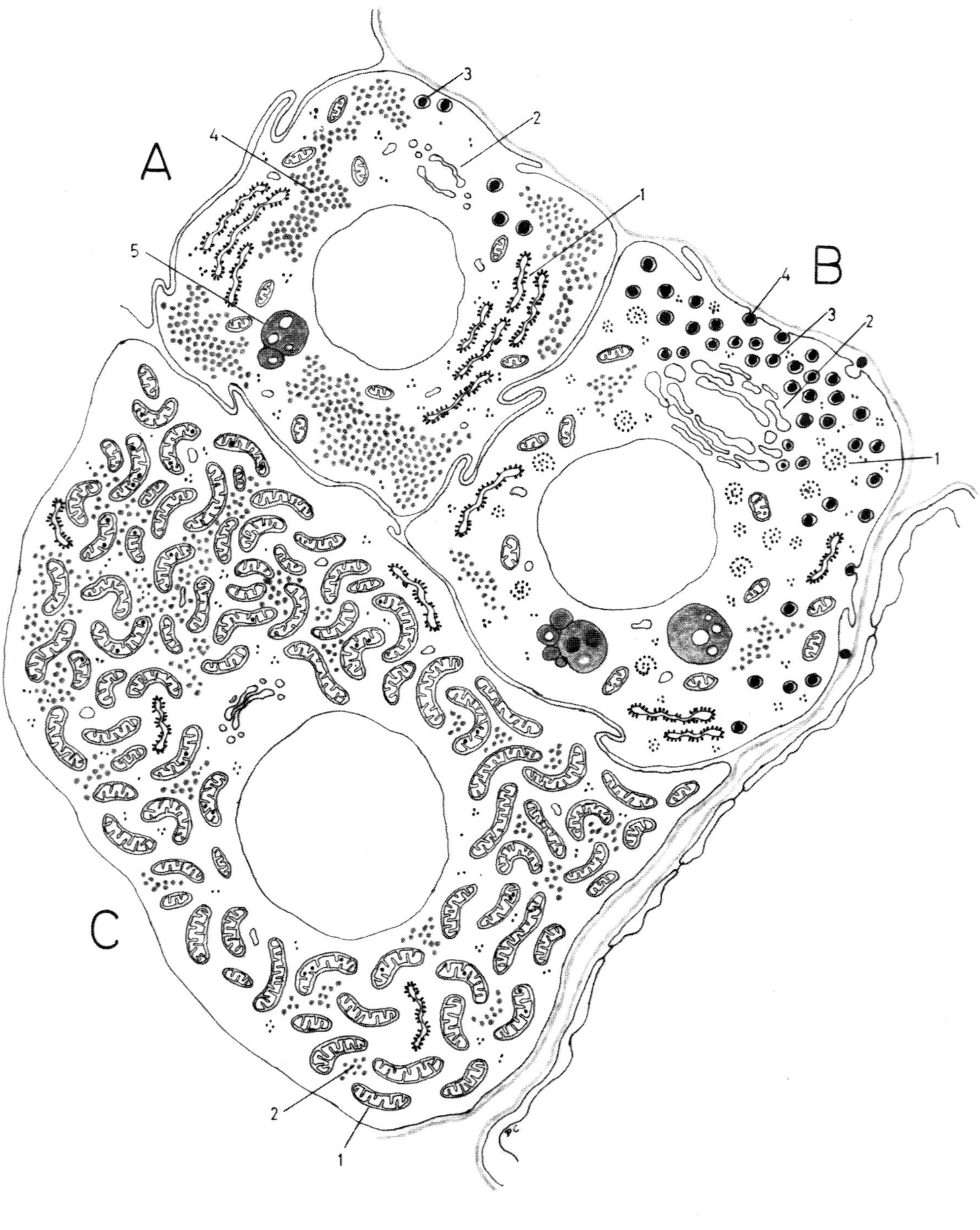

Plate 56

increased osteoclastic activity). It consists of resting (Fig. A) and active (Fig. B) chief cells, of oxyphil cells (Fig. C) and fenestrated capillaries with diaphragms that receive its hormone (Fig. D). The resting cells correspond to the "light" or "clear" and the active cells to the "dark" cells seen with the L/M.

(2) Chief cell–resting (Plate 56, Fig. A)

This cell is characterised by (a) relatively few ribosomes, an appreciable RER[1], and a distinct Golgi[2], (b) a few membrane bound 1500–2000 Å thick secretory granules[3], (c) large pools of glycogen granules[4] (which account for the large clear cytoplasmic areas in the glycogen-extracted tissues seen with the L/M), (d) occasional lipofuscin corpuscles[5], (e) interlocking boundaries, desmosomes joining it to neighbouring cells and a BM on its capillary side.

This cell manufactures and releases parathyroid hormone at a slow rate. The hormone is contained in the dense cores of the secretory granules.

(3) Chief cell–active (Plate 56, Fig. B)

Compared to the resting stage, the active stage of chief cells exhibits (a) greatly increased numbers of ribosomes[1], mostly in the form of polysomes and cochleosomes, (b) a greatly enlarged Golgi[2], (c) much more numerous secretory granules[3] which develop from the Golgi and are released through emiocytosis[4], (d) less RER cisternae, and (e) severely depleted glycogen stores.

The active chief cell increases both the synthesis and the release of parathyroid hormone in response to low blood calcium levels, no matter how induced (*e.g.* by low calcium diet *in vivo* or by low calcium concentrations in tissue culture media), or to high blood phosphate levels, and it is inhibited by high blood calcium levels (*e.g.* after a high calcium diet or vitamin D). Very prolonged stimulation of the chief cells, however, may lead to their complete degranulation, when they release their hormone faster than they synthesize it.

(4) Oxyphil cells (Plate 56, Fig. C)

These cells possess (a) moderate numbers of ribosomes and only very few RER cisternae, (b) a small Golgi, (c) an enormous number of elongated mitochondria with numerous cristae[1], and (d) great amounts of glycogen granules[2] scattered among the mitochondria. They appear very acidophilic to the L/M because of their low ribosome–RER content and their extremely high mitochondrial content.

The function of the oxyphil cells is unknown. They exist in only some species and in man where their numbers increase greatly after puberty.

IX. ADRENAL GLAND

(1) General

The adrenal consists of the cortex (a mesodermal tissue) and the medulla (an ectodermal-neural tissue). The cortex secretes a mixture of steroid hormones that preserve body sodium and water (mineralocorticoids), control carbohydrate metabolism (glucocorticoids) and some sex functions. The medulla secretes catecholamines (epinephrine and norepinephrine) that increase heart action, blood pressure and blood sugar levels. Groups of medulla-like cells are also scattered in the connective tissue of various body regions, constituting the "chromaffine system".

(2) Adrenal cortex (Plate 57, Fig. A)

The cortex consists of the following three zones, in sequence from without to within: (a) zona glomerulosa, (b) zona fasciculata, and (c) zona reticularis. The glomerulosa seems to secrete primarily mineralocorticoroids, the fasciculata glucocorticoids and the reticularis sex steroids. The cells of all three zones exhibit a similar structure with certain regional variations. Typical cells of the middle and lower cortical layers (which constitute the bulk of this gland) are characterised by (a) moderate ribosome numbers, (b) several stacks of RER cisternae (in man)[1], a distinct Golgi[2], (d) a very extensive system of SER branching tubules and vesicles[3] which are often connected to RER cisternae[4], (e) abundant lipid droplets with crenated profiles[5] that are often surrounded or contacted by SER tubules[6], (f) moderate numbers of mitochondria with lamellar[7] (ordinary shelf-like), concentric[8] or tubular-vesical[9] cristae depending on species and cortical region, (g) several lysosome-lipofuscin complexes[10] that probably represent autophagosomes and increase with age, (h) a few microvilli[11] and coated pinocytosis-type vesicles[12] at their free surfaces. They are flanked by perforated capillaries[13] from which they are separated by usually one but sometimes two BMs and an intervening pericapillary fibroblast-type cell[14]. On rare occasions cilia grow out of the glomerulosa cells.

As one moves from the glomerulosa to the reticularis one encounters the following gradual modifications of cortical cell structure: (a) the ribosome number drops, (b) the lipid droplets content first rises and then declines, (c) the lipofuscin corpuscle number rises sharply to the point where these structures may fill up to one third of the cell volume, and (d) the shape of the mitochondrial cristae changes (*e.g.* from lamellar to vesicular

A

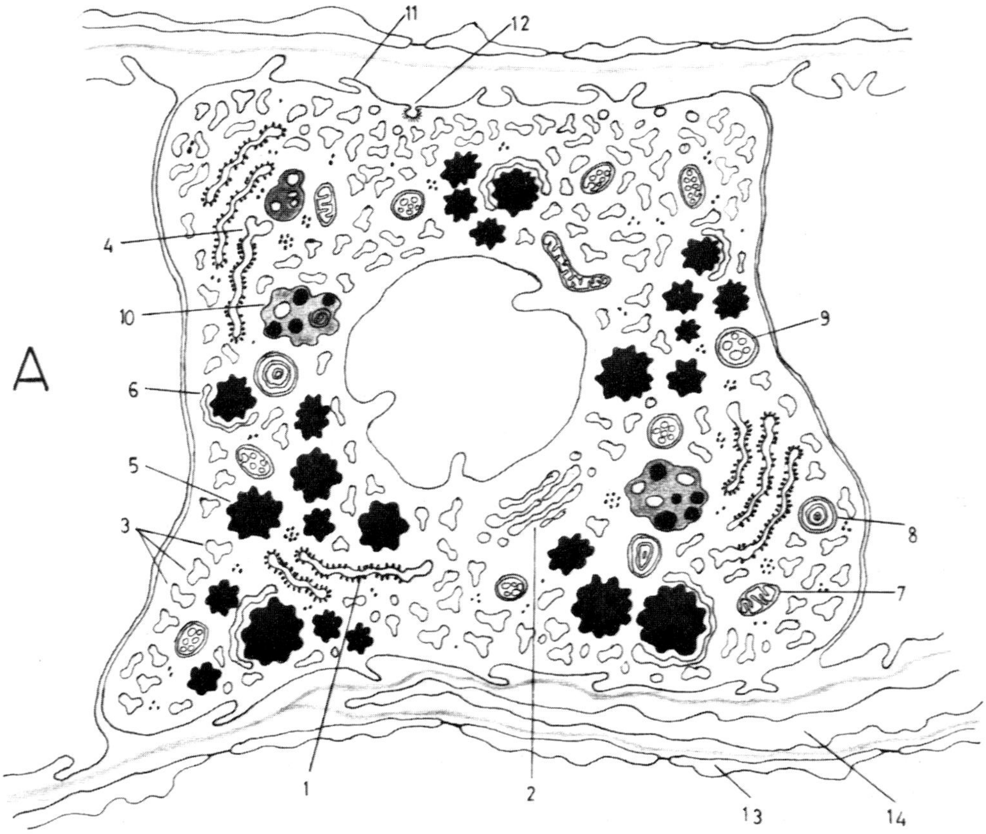

B

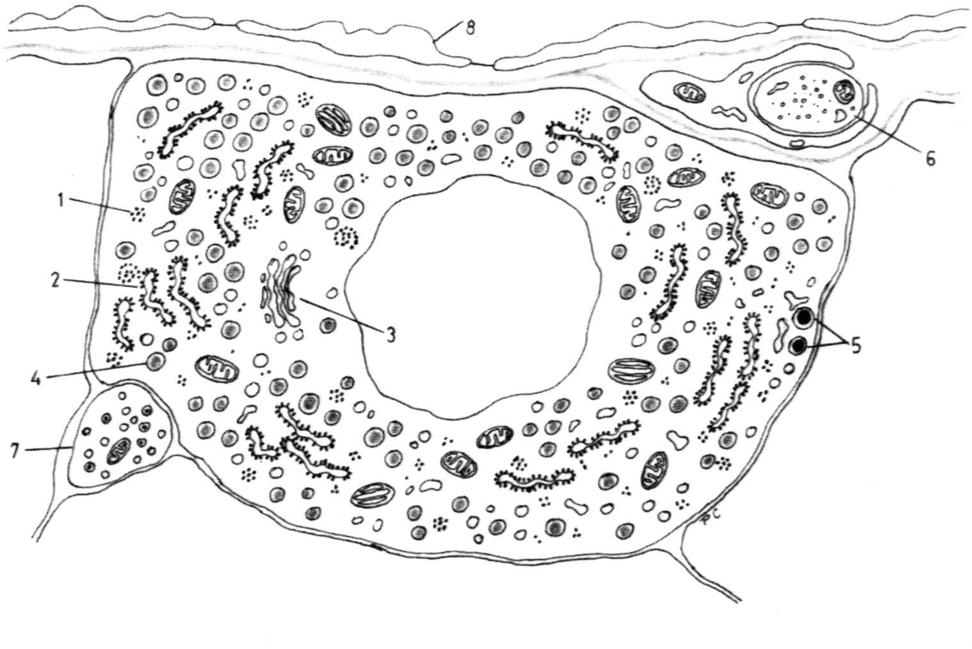

Plate 57

in man or dog, and from tubular to lamellar to concentric to vesicular in mice). Often, the nuclei in the zona fasciculata develop an inner fibrous lamina.

It is thought that the hormonal steroids are synthesised by the close cooperation of the SER and the mitochondria. Thus *e.g.*, according to present concepts, the synthesis of aldosterone involves the following sequences: (a) synthesis of cholesterol from acetate or larger building blocks in the SER, (b) transformation of cholesterol into pregnenolone in mitochondria, (c) transformation of pregnenolone into progesterone and then DOCA in the SER, and (d) transformation of DOCA into corticosterone and then aldosterone in mitochondria. Upon completion, the steroids are thought to be coupled to protein in the RER and to be finally released as highly dispersed molecules, since no secretion granule or emiocytosis is visible in these cells. The role of the lipid droplets in this process is not yet clear; they may supply ready building blocks (*e.g.* cholesterol) for rapid steroid synthesis or they may represent stores of the steroid hormones; either hypothesis would fit the fact that they rapidly dwindle under conditions of markedly increased hormonal release and synthesis.

Agents and procedures that stimulate cortical secretion (*e.g.* ACTH and, more so, sodium-deficient diet) cause an expansion of the SER, while those that inhibit steroid secretion either produce a decline of the SER (*e.g.* the negative feedback effect of corticosterone) or provoke the development of gigantic but degenerating mitochondria with accumulations of lipids and myelin figures in their matrix (*e.g.* hypophysectomy).

(3) *Adrenal medulla* (Plate 57, Fig. B)

The cells of the adrenal medulla are distinguished by (a) fairly numerous ribosomes and polyribosomes[1] and RER cisternae[2], (b) a conspicuous Golgi[3], (c) very numerous 1500–3000 Å thick cored vesicles of two types: some with light or moderately dense cores[4] representing epinephrine and some with very dense cores[5] representing norepinephrine (which forms a precipitate following glutaraldehyde fixation), and (d) a moderate number of mitochondria whose cristae are lamellar (transverse or longitudinal). Frequently axons are seen between these cells or between the cells and the capillaries[6], and also axon terminals[7] with clear (300 Å) and cored (500 Å) synaptic vesicles land on the medullary cells. The free smooth surface of these cells is separated from the perforated capillaries[8] by usually one, but occasionally two BMs and a pericapillary cell.

In some mammals (*e.g.* man, monkey, rabbit, guinea-pig) there is one cell type with 2 types of granules (light epinephrine and dense norepinephrine) while in others (*e.g.* rat) there are 2 cell types, one with exclusively epinephrine, the other with exclusively norepinephrine granules. In man most granules are of the epinephrine while in monkey most are of the norepinephrine type.

The catecholamine granules have been shown to appear first in the Golgi vesicles (with autoradiography following [^{3}H] Dopa administration and other techniques). Their release through emiocytosis has been documented in the hamster but additional release mechanisms involving rupture of the granule envelopes and molecular diffusion in fine dispersion have also been proposed. The presence of appreciable amounts of nucleotide phosphatases in the perigranular matrix and the PM of the medullary cells has been thought to facilitate the release of catecholamines, since the latter seem to be bound to nucleotides within the cytoplasm.

Catecholamine granules can be visibly released by nervous impulses (through the axon terminals that synapse with the medullary cells), by reserpine and by insulin, among other things.

In several locations of the body close to or within sympathetic plexuses and ganglia (*e.g.* in the "paraganglia" within the suprarenal plexus) there has been described a medulla-like *chromaffine tissue* which consists of (a) "type I" (actual chromaffine) cells with cored, presumably catecholamine-containing 2000–4000 Å thick vesicles, and (b) "type II" (enveloping) cells without cored vesicles. The function and relationship of chromaffine tissue to sympathetic neurons and to the adrenal medulla is not clear at the moment; perhaps it represents extra-adrenal medullary tissue.

X. ISLETS OF LANGERHANS

(1) *General* (Plate 58)

The islets produce two protein hormones that contribute to the regulation of carbohydrate metabolism: (a) insulin, which depresses blood sugar by promoting its entry into cells and utilization, and (b) glucagon, which raises blood sugar levels. The islet cells are arranged in cords and lined by BMs on their free sides and they face perforated capillaries (Fig. F). Four cell types are recognised in these cords: (a) α-cells (which produce glucagon), (b) β-cells (which produce insulin), (c) C-cells (of uncertain function), and (d) δ-cells (also of uncertain function).

(2) *α-Cells* (Plate 58, Fig. A)

These cells are characterised by (a) moderate numbers of ribosomes, RER cisternae and a small Golgi, (b) numerous secretory vesicles with very dense round cores[1] (in most species) and a low density material between the cores and the envelopes, mostly on their capillary side, and (c) several long, slender mitochondria.

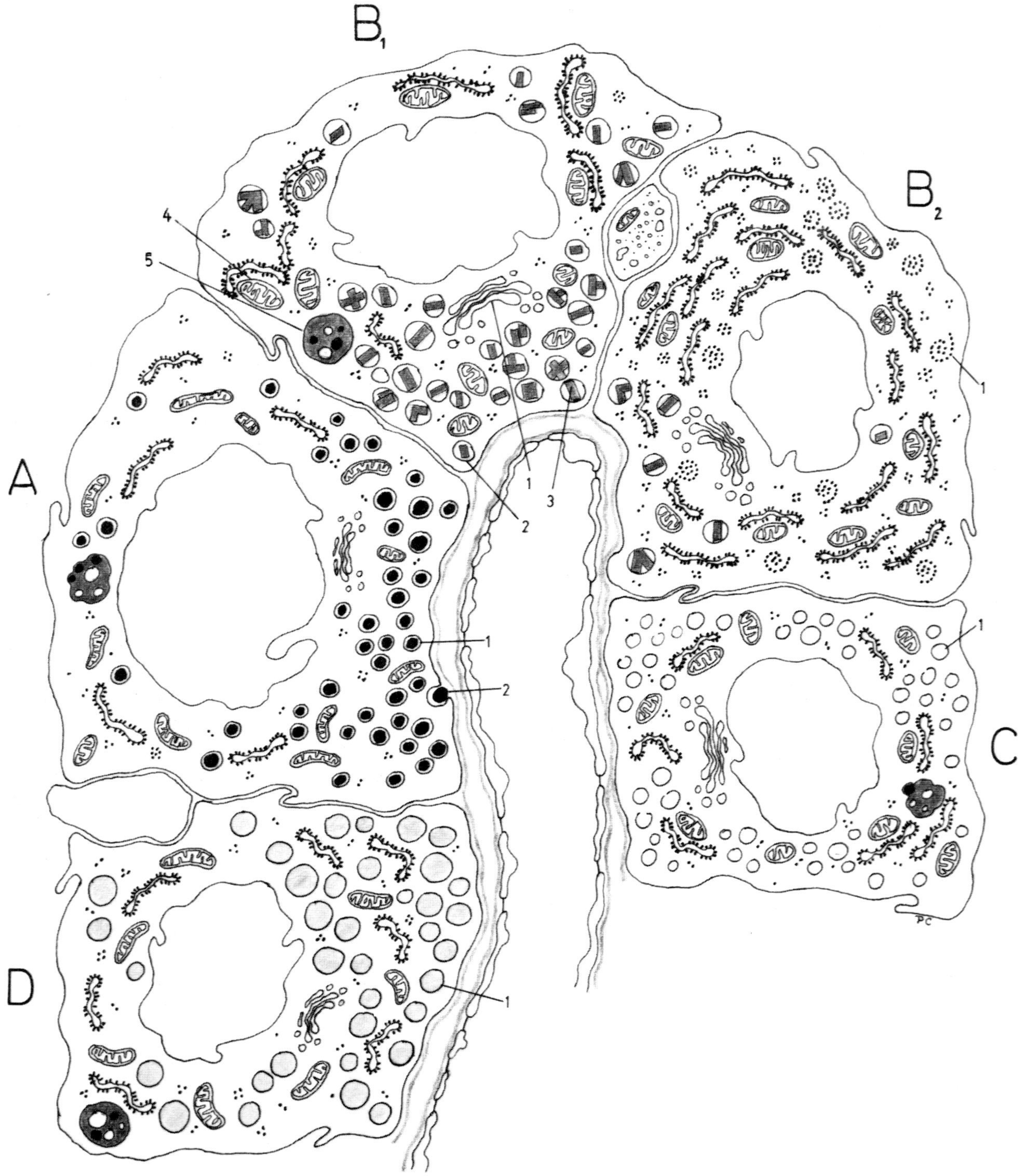

Plate 58

The cores of the secretory vesicles represent glucagon which is released by emiocytosis[2], as observed in the rabbit. Glucagon granules are visibly released in response to low blood sugar, high blood insulin levels or electrical sympathetic stimulation, leading to increased glucagon levels in pancreatic vein blood. Recently, cobalt chloride ($CoCl_2$) has been found to have a specific toxicity for α-cells and has been used as an experimental tool for their study.

(3) β-Cells (Plate 58, Figs. B_1 and B_2)

The "resting" β-cell (Fig. B_1) exhibits (a) a moderate number of ribosomes and RER cisternae, (b) a prominent Golgi[1] (more conspicuous than in α-cells), (c) numerous secretory vesicles[2] each containing 1–3 moderately dense, rectangular cores[3] with crystalloid substructure, embedded in a low density material, in man, dog, cat and bat (and different core structure in other species), (d) a moderate number of mitochondria, which are larger than those of α-cells, are closely associated with RER cisternae[4], and occasionally contain hexagonal arrays of closely packed tubules (the "multitubular inclusions"), (e) occasional lysosomes[5], and (f) occasional centriole-associated cilia. Often axons (Fig. E) are seen between β- or between β- and α-cells and sometimes axon terminals with synaptic vesicles seem in close (synaptic) contact with the α- and β-cells.

The crystalloid cores of the secretory vesicles contain insulin, as has been shown with anti-insulin antibodies; there is some evidence, supported by autoradiographic studies of labeled amino-acid uptake, that they develop from the accumulation of at first only slightly dense material in RER cisternae, followed by separation of the bulbous cisternal ends to yield secretory vesicles whose contents condense and crystallise. The release mechanism of the secretory granules is unknown; since the insulin crystalloids have not yet been seen outside cells, it has been proposed that insulin molecules move out of their envelope in fine dispersion (or are dissolved in the cytoplasmic matrix after rupture of that envelope) and then cross the β-cell PM passively or actively to reach the pericapillary space. Insulin release is triggered by high blood sugar levels, certain antagonistic hormones (*e.g.* glucocorticoids), nervous stimuli and possibly sodium ion entry into β-cells. Drugs of the sulfonylurea group (*e.g.* tolazamide) trigger a dramatic release of insulin (visible as a complete degranulation of β-cells) and stimulate its resynthesis.

Soon after vigorous release and depletion of insulin granules (Fig. B_2), the β-cell greatly increases the number of its ribosomes[1] (particularly in the form of polysomes and cochleosomes) and RER cisternae in order to resynthesize that hormone, which seems to first appear as a slightly dense (hazy) amorphous precursor material in the distended RER cisternae.

The significance of the multitubular inclusions occasionally encountered within β-cell mitochondria is unknown; similar crystalloid inclusions are sometimes seen in the mitochondria of a wide variety of other normal tissues.

Following 95% extirpation of the pancreas, β-cells start immediately regenerating from the centro-acinar and small duct cells of the pancreatic remnant; regeneration, however, gradually decreases and stops altogether within 6–8 weeks, at which time diabetes sets in due to insulin deficiency. Diabetes can also be produced by alloxan and streptozotocin which have specific cytotoxic effects on β-cells.

(4) C-Cells (Plate 58, Fig. C)

The general structure of these cells is similar to that of β-cells with the exception that they possess numerous "empty" (clear) vesicles[1] instead of cored ones, and some of them seem ruptured (perhaps due to artefact). The function of the C-cells is uncertain; it is not known whether they represent a stage in the secretory cycle of β-cells, damaged β-cells or an independent cell type.

(5) δ-Cells (Plate 58, Fig. D)

The general structure of δ-cells is similar to that of α-cells with the exception that their secretory vesicles[1] are larger than those of α-cells and are completely filled by a material of moderate to low density. As in the case of the C-cells, the function of the δ-cells is still debatable. Some believe that they constitute an independent cell species, while others think that they are altered α-cells – the latter theory being supported by the occasional finding of cells of a transitional type between α and δ (*i.e.* cells with both types of secretory granules).

XI. GASTROINTESTINAL HORMONES

Presumably endocrine cells with vesicles containing spheroid cores of variable density and size are scattered throughout the epithelial lining of the alimentary canal and have only begun to be explored with the E/M. The following types and functions have been tentatively identified so far:

(A) In the gastric mucosa: (a) *enterochromaffine cells* producing serotonin (already described as "argentaffine" cells in the section on stomach), (b) *enterochromaffine cells* producing a 5-hydroxyindole, (c) *"G"-cells* that produce gastrin (a hormone which stimulates HCl secretion by parietal cells), (d) cells resembling the pancreatic

α-cells which possibly secrete glucagon, and (e) *granulated cells* of unknown function.

(B) In the intestinal (notably duodenal) mucosa: (a) *enterochromaffine cells* producing serotonin, (b) *peptidergic cells with small granules* that probably manufacture secretin (a hormone which stimulates exocrine pancreas secretion), and (c) *peptidergic cells with large granules* that probably secrete pancreozymin (another hormone which stimulates exocrine pancreas secretion).

Chapter 14

Skin

I. GENERAL (Plate 59)

The skin insulates and protects the body from adverse environmental influences and from the loss of valuable components, and it contributes to its thermoregulation. It consists of a keratinised squamous stratified epithelium, the epidermis, and of an underlying dense fibrous tissue layer, the dermis. The epidermis (Fig. K) is, in turn, composed of the following four layers (strata) from inside out: stratum basale[1], stratum spinosum[2], stratum granulosum[3], and stratum corneum[4]. The accessory skin structures, all of which develop from invaginations of the epidermis, are: (a) keratinised outgrowths that conserve heat (hair), provide weapons (nails), or facilitate flight (feathers), (b) lipid producing sebaceous glands, (c) sweat glands of a small "eccrine" type and of a large "apocrine" type, and (d) the milk producing mammary glands. In the adjacent drawing of the ultrastructure of the epidermis, the number of cell layers of the stratum spinosum, granulosum and corneum has been arbitrarily contracted below normal for reasons of space.

II. EPIDERMIS

(1) Stratum basale

(A) Undifferentiated basal cells (Plate 59, Fig. A)

These cells are characterised by (a) numerous ribosomes[1], (b) only few RER cisternae and SER sacs and a moderate mitochondrial population, (c) numerous bundles of 50–70 Å microfilaments, the "tonofilaments"[2], which consist of the sulfated protein keratin and mostly radiate out of desmosome sites, (d) numerous desmosome junctions[3] with adjacent cells, and "hemidesmosome" densities[4] connected through short extracellular filaments to a BM basally.

The undifferentiated basal cells seem to divide to (a) reproduce themselves, and (b) turn into keratinocytes and stratum spinosum cells. When they proliferate to clothe a wound area they develop lysosomes, many glycogen granules and phagocytic potential (they will pick up and carry into their lysosomes intravenously injected particles such as thorotrast).

(B) Keratinocytes (Plate 59, Fig. B)

Keratinocytes constitute the majority of the stratum basale cells. They have the same basic structure as the undifferentiated basal cells but, in addition, exhibit (a) more RER cisternae[1], (b) a distinct Golgi, (c) pinocytotic vesicles[2] basally, (d) premelanosomes[3] and melanosomes[4], under certain circumstances, and (e) a few lipid droplets[5]. They differentiate into cells of the next higher layer (stratum spinosum) and they can produce melanin in the manner described under the next heading.

(C) Melanocytes (Plate 59, Fig. C)

Melanocytes correspond to the "clear" cells of the L/M. They are characterised by (a) moderate numbers of ribosomes, RER cisternae, SER sacs and mitochondria, (b) a distinct Golgi, (c) no tonofilaments, desmosomes or hemidesmosomes, (d) appreciable numbers of premelanosomes[1], melanosomes[2] and melanin granules[3], (e) usually conspicuous centrioles, (f) cytoplasmic processes[4] sent up into the stratum spinosum (hence their designation as "dendritic" cells of the epidermis).

These cells seem to be of neural origin and to have invaded the epidermis secondarily – they may be modified Schwann cells. Melanin granules are produced in melanocytes in the following stages (Figs. H_1–H_5): (a) ribosomes produce an enzymatic protein (tyrosinase) which is introduced into *ca.* 500 Å wide Golgi saccules where it is coupled to phospholipids; (b) the phospholipid-protein containing saccules grow in size to the *ca.* 0.5 μ wide "intermediate vesicles" and begin to develop an internal granular substructure (Fig. H_1); (c) the intermediate vesicles assume an oval shape (about $0.7 \times 0.3\ \mu$) and the enzymatic phospholipoprotein in them is arranged in parallel beaded strings – the "premelanosome" stage (Fig. H_2), which resembles the yolk platelet of the ovum, another phospholipoprotein-containing orgenelle; (d) melanin appears in the oval vesicles, whose contents condense into a dense lamellar

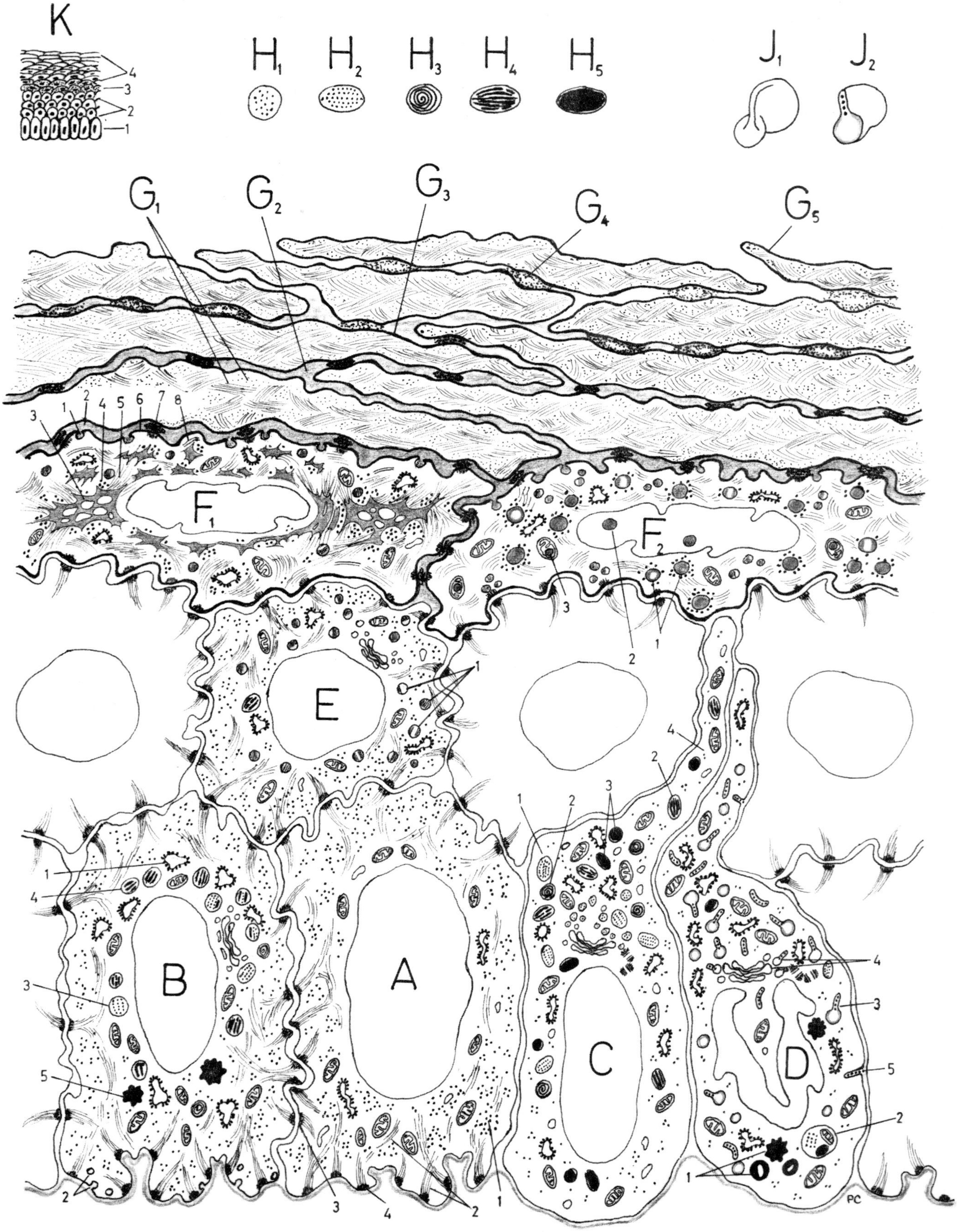

Plate 59

structure with the appearance of a spiral in cross-section (Fig. H_3) and of thick parallel streaks in longitudinal section (Fig. H_4) – the "melanosome" stage; (e) the tyrosinase activity disappears, the melanin persists and the contents of the oval vesicle condense even further to a dense homogeneous mass – the final "melanin granule" stage (Fig. H_5). During this evolutionary sequence, melanin relates to tyrosinase as hemoglobin relates to ribosomes during erythrocyte maturation.

The function of melanin seems to be to absorb the ultraviolet radiation that bombards the skin and thus to protect the epidermal and underlying cells from it; prolonged exposure of the skin to strong sunlight (and therefore ultraviolet light) stimulates an increased production of melanin granules in the epidermis, hence a darkening of the skin color (tanning). The presence of prominent centrioles in melanocytes suggests a high turnover of these cells, possibly in connection with their repeated response to external radiation. The melanocytes of albinos cannot produce any melanosomes, they can only manufacture premelanosomes – hence albinos are unable to tan when exposed to strong sunlight and suffer burns from it.

(D) Langerhans cells (Plate 59, Fig. D)

These cells, which can sometimes also be found in the dermis, exhibit a similar basic structure to that of melanocytes (and therefore appear as "clear, dendritic cells" when seen with the L/M), with the following differences: (a) they usually possess very few or no premelanosomes or melanosomes, (b) they contain several dense or lucent lipid droplets[1] and occasionally autophagosomes[2], (c) their nucleus is deeply indented, and (d) they are filled with numerous tennis-racket shaped smooth vesicles, the "Langerhans granules"[3]. The latter (Fig. J_1) consist of flattened sacs with a beaded central lamella of a periodicity of *ca.* 90 Å and expanded spherical ends with mostly lucent contents whose section presents the image of a tennis racket (Fig. J_2); they arise within the Golgi system[4] and may travel to the cell surface, fuse with the PM, break open[5] and release their contents into the extracellular space.

The function of the Langerhans cells is obscure. They were once considered degenerating, "worn out" melanocytes because of their occasional low melanosome content, but they are now viewed as very active secretory cells with an unknown secretion. The presence of lipid inclusions and of a high SER/RER ratio suggests their possible involvement in steroid metabolism, perhaps in the activation of sterols into vitamin D-like compounds with the help of ultraviolet light.

(2) Stratum spinosum (Plate 59, Fig. E)

The stratum spinosum cells have a structure which is similar to that of the undifferentiated basal cells with the following differences: (a) they exhibit occasional melanosomes (in man), and (b) they develop an appreciable number of membrane-bound granules of variable density and lamellar substructure, the so-called "lamellar" granules or "membrane coating" granules[1] (the latter designation referring to their function in the next higher epidermal layers). These cells differentiate into those of the overlying stratum granulosum.

(3) Stratum granulosum

(A) In man (Plate 59, Fig. F_1)

The cells of this layer have a basic structure that is similar to that of the underlying stratum spinosum, with the following additions: (a) their membrane-coating granules are visibly discharged through emiocytosis[1] into the intercellular space where they form a thick, moderately dense coat[2] over the PMs of their own and adjacent cells, (b) irregular, moderately dense and mostly reticular masses of keratohyalin[3] appear in their cytoplasm in close association with pools of ribosomes[4] and tonofilaments[5], (c) a very dense, *ca.* 100 Å thick "peripheral band" develops directly underneath and attaches to their entire PM so that the inner leaflet of the latter seems to thicken to *ca.* 125 Å and the whole PM to *ca.* 175 Å[6], (d) their tonofilaments disengage from their desmosomes, (e) the intercellular clefts of their desmosomal junctions with other cells (notably those of higher layers) become completely filled with a dense material[7], and (f) several *ca.* 220 Å thick microtubules[8] appear in them. The membrane-coating granules are membrane-enclosed stacks of discs, like rolls of coins in pouches, each disc consisting of a dense plate coated on either side by a translucent material; when the membrane-coating granules are discharged into the intercellular space, their discs disperse, fuse with and thicken the outer leaflet of the PM of the stratum corneum cells, while the inner leaflet is thickened by the apposition of a dense material (keratohyalin?) on its cytoplasmic face.

The stratum granulosum cells are the forerunners of the completely keratinised stratum corneum above them. Their thickened PM represents one of the changes preparatory to keratinisation and becomes impervious and resistant to several strong chemicals. The function of keratohyalin is still unknown; it may provide material for either the PM thickening or the great proliferation of tonofilaments that takes place during keratinisation. The microtubules seem to facilitate the maintenance of a flattened cell shape.

(B) In rodents (Plate 59, Fig. F_2)

The structure here is the same as in man, with the exception of the keratohyalin which assumes the shape of large, variably dense globules[1] and occurs, apart from

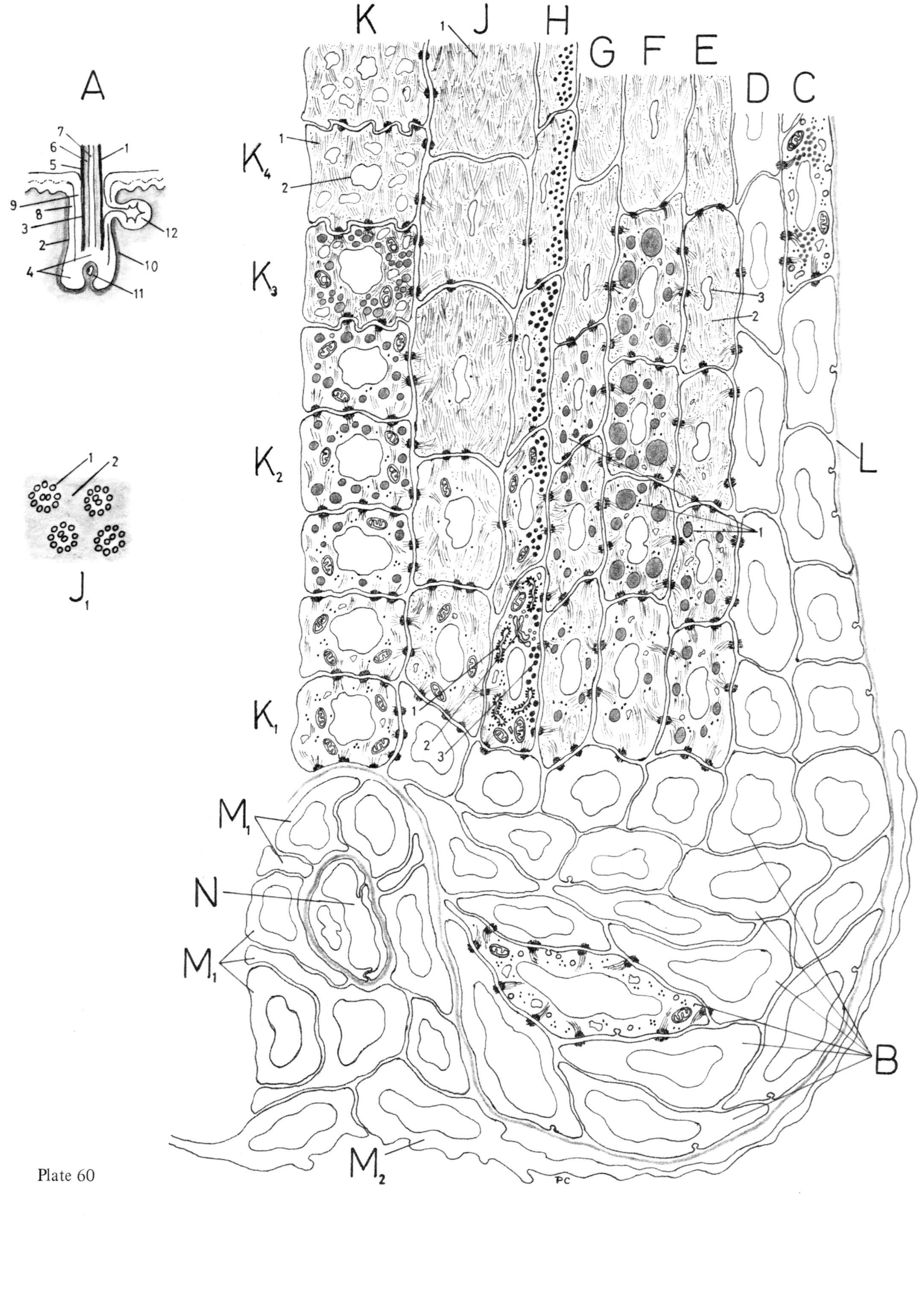

Plate 60

the cytoplasm, also in the nucleus[2] and possibly even in mitochondria[3].

(4) Stratum corneum (Plate 59, Figs. G_1–G_5)

The cells of this layer are turned into completely keratinised "squames" through the development of the following features: (a) their nucleus and almost all their organelles disappear, through an as yet unstudied regression mechanism, (b) their cytoplasm becomes filled with 50–70 Å tonofilaments (Fig. G_1), stacked in bundles of alternating directions, scaffold-wise, (c) their PM is still covered by the amorphous coat produced by the membrane-coating granules (Fig. G_2) in the previous stage, (d) their PM under its coat remains 175 Å thick (Fig. G_3) although sometimes its outer leaflet becomes invisible and it then appears to consist of only one 125 Å thick leaflet, and (e) the dense extracellular material in their desmosomes increases in amount, becomes granular and finally is split (Fig. G_4), allowing the uppermost squames to detach from the epidermis and exfoliate (Fig. G_5). The tonofilament bundles in the deepest cell layer of the stratum corneum are sometime very loosely packed, creating many large open matrix spaces and giving this layer a light (lucid) appearance under the L/M, hence the occasional description of a thin "stratum lucidum" between the stratum granulosum and the stratum corneum.

The function of the stratum corneum in man and higher vertebrates is to prevent most environmental materials (gases, water, chemicals, bacteria) from penetrating into the body interior and, conversely, to prevent the escape of valuable body materials and cells into the external environment. It owes its insulating properties to its multiple layers of flat cell derivatives or "squames" with their external coats, their extraordinarily thick PM, and their massive tonofilament (keratin) content. One of the physiological responses of the skin to any prolonged mechanical, thermal, radiation or chemical stress is to greatly thicken its stratum corneum through the proliferation of its layers of keratinised squames. For further details on keratin see Sect. III, Hair.

III. HAIR

(1) General (Plate 60, Fig. A)

A single hair shaft represents a rod of keratinising epithelial tissue[1] that grows out of the bottom of an epidermal pouch[2] (the hair follicle or epithelial root sheath); the part of the hair that is contained within the hair follicle is its root[3] and the region of the follicle from which it grows is its matrix[4]. The hair shaft consists, from without inwards, of (a) the cuticle of the cortex[5], (b) the cortex[6], and (c) the medulla[7]. The epithelial root sheath, on the other hand, consists of (a) the external root sheath[8] (which corresponds to the epidermal stratum basale and spinosum) and (b) the internal root sheath[9] (which corresponds to the stratum granulosum and corneum); the latter, in turn, is made up of the following layers, from without inwards: (a) Henle's layer, (b) Huxley's layer and (c) the cuticle of the internal root sheath. Connective tissue condenses around the epithelial root sheath to form the fibrous root sheath[10] and, along with several capillaries, it pushes into the bottom of the hair follicle to reach the matrix, forming a fibrous papilla[11]. A sebaceous gland often develops as a lateral outpouching[12] of a hair follicle. In several mammals, hair goes through cyclic phases; during each regressive ("catagen") phase, the collagen of the fibrous root sheath is completely phagocytised by macrophages and replaced by new collagen during the expansive ("anagen") phase.

(2) Matrix (Plate 60, Fig. B)

The cells of this hair part are undifferentiated, with a high nucleus/cytoplasm ratio. They contain moderate numbers of ribosomes, large smooth vesicles, small pinocytotic vesicles, mitochondria and tonofilaments. They are bound to one another through desmosomes, and the most peripheral of them rest on a BM (Fig. L). They proliferate and differentiate into cells of the overlying parts (external and internal root sheath and hair root).

(3) External root sheath (Plate 60, Figs. C–D)

The cells of this layer have the same structure as those of the matrix, with the addition of appreciable pools of glycogen granules[1].

(4) Internal root sheath (Plate 60, Figs. E–G)

The cells here are characterised by the following developments: (a) they manufacture an increasing number of tonofilaments with increasing distance from the matrix, (b) they produce numerous globules of trichohyalin[1] (a dense keratohyalin-like material) which are of intermediate size in the outer (Henle) layer (Fig. E), largest in the middle (Huxley) layer (Fig. F), and smallest in the inner (internal root sheath cuticle) layer (Fig. G), and (c) they rapidly lose all basic organelles except tonofilaments[2], and their nuclei gradually shrink[3] and disappear with increasing distance from the matrix.

(5) Hair root (Plate 60, Figs. H–K)

(A) Cuticle of cortex (Fig. H)

The lowest cells of this layer exhibit an appreciable

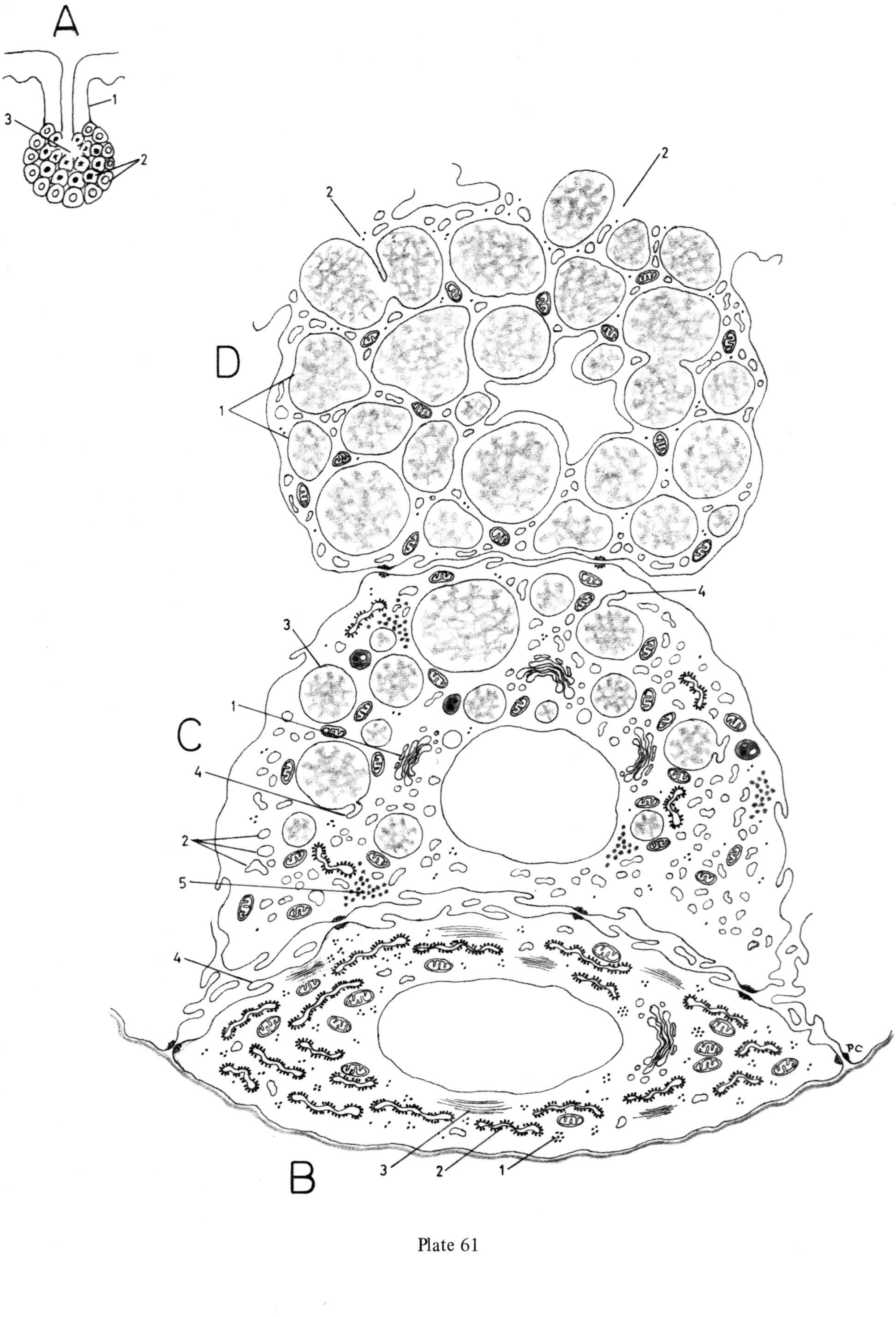

Plate 61

RER[1] and Golgi system[2] and produce numerous small dense granules of unidentified material[3] which migrate to their outer side (facing the cuticle of the internal root sheath), as well as appreciable tonofilament numbers. With increasing distance from the matrix, the nuclei and the basic organelles of these cells gradually disappear.

(B) Cortex (Fig. J)

With increasing distance from the matrix, the cells of this layer develop an increasing amount of tonofilaments and gradually lose the rest of their organelles and their nuclei; they become sacs filled with roughly 80 Å thick tonofilaments[1] and a low density amorphous matrix. Seen at very high magnification, *i.e.* 1,000,000 × or more (Fig. J_1), each tonofilament here has been reported to consist of a bundle of 11 roughly 20 Å thick "protofilaments"[1] in cilium-like (9 + 2) arrangement, embedded in an amorphous binding material[2].

(C) Medulla (Figs. K_1–K_4)

The most basal cells of the medulla are quite similar to those of the matrix (Fig. K_1) but as they move up they develop the following features: (a) at first they manufacture trichohyalin globules (Fig. K_2), (b) at a higher level they acquire large smooth vesicles in addition to the globules (Fig. K_3), (c) at a still higher level the globules disappear while the vesicles persist (Fig. K_4), and (d) their tonofilament content steadily increases[1] while their nuclei[2] and other organelles gradually disappear.

(6) The connective tissue papilla (Plate 60, Figs. M–N)

This part consists of a group of fibroblasts (Figs. M_1–M_2) that surround one or more capillaries of the unperforated type (Fig. N); some of the fibroblasts send out long processes that hug the BM of the hair matrix (Fig. M_2). Through its capillaries, the papilla supplies oxygen and nutrients to the region of maximal hair growth (the matrix).

IV. SEBACEOUS GLANDS

(1) General (Plate 61, Fig. A)

These glands produce a lipid material (sebum) that forms a water-repellent film on the surface of skin and hair. They have a short duct[1] and the wall of their secretory portion is several cell layers thick[2]. Their secretion is of the holocrine type, *i.e.* sebum is released into the duct through the disintegration[3] of the cells that produce it. As the cells proliferate and mature, they move from the periphery to the center of the secretory portion and they produce increasing amounts of lipid; simultaneously, their nuclei become progressively more pycnotic (smaller and denser). In most cases, the ducts of the sebaceous glands open into the side of hair follicles, but in certain skin areas they reach the skin surface directly.

(2) Secretory portion cells

(A) Basal cells (Plate 61, Fig. B)

These are relatively undifferentiated cells with (a) numerous ribosomes[1], RER cisternae[2] and a conspicuous Golgi, (b) moderate numbers of smooth vesicles and mitochondria, (c) a few bundles of tonofilaments[3], and (d) microvilli[4] and desmosomes on their upper and a BM on their lower surface. They correspond to the undifferentiated basal cells of the epidermis and, like the latter, they proliferate and differentiate into cells of the next higher layer.

(B) Intermediate cells (Plate 61, Fig. C)

These cells are characterised by (a) a drop in the number of ribosomes and RER cisternae, (b) the development of extensive, multiple Golgi systems[1] and a prominent SER[2], *i.e.* large numbers of smooth vesicles, (c) the emergence of many membrane-bound lipid globules[3] with moderately dense, mottled contents, several of them connected with the smooth vesicles[4], (d) several lysosomes, (e) several groups of glycogen granules[5], and (f) often whorly-lamellar inclusions with granular cores in the nuclei.

The lipid globules apparently arise within the vesicles of the SER, as indicated by their frequent connections with the latter. The significance of the nuclear inclusions is unknown.

(C) Superficial cells (Plate 61, Fig. D)

The structure of these cells is similar to that of the intermediate cells, but the following changes have occured: (a) the lipid globules have proliferated to an enormous number[1], occupying most of the intracellular space and reducing the rest of the cytoplasm to thin strands between them, (b) the nucleus shrinks greatly, it chromatin condenses and its profile is molded to the surrounding lipid globules and (c) the superficial PM breaks at several sites[2], releasing lipid globules and the rest of the cytoplasm into the duct lumen.

The sebaceous gland cells secrete their primarily lipid cytoplasmic contents by disintegrating. They present several structural and physiological analogies to steroid producing endocrine glands such as the adrenal cortex, the corpus luteum and the Leydig cells; they synthesize lipids in association with a prominent SER and their secretion appears to be controlled by several endocrine factors: it seems to be stimulated by androgen and luteotrophic hormone and to be inhibited by estrogens.

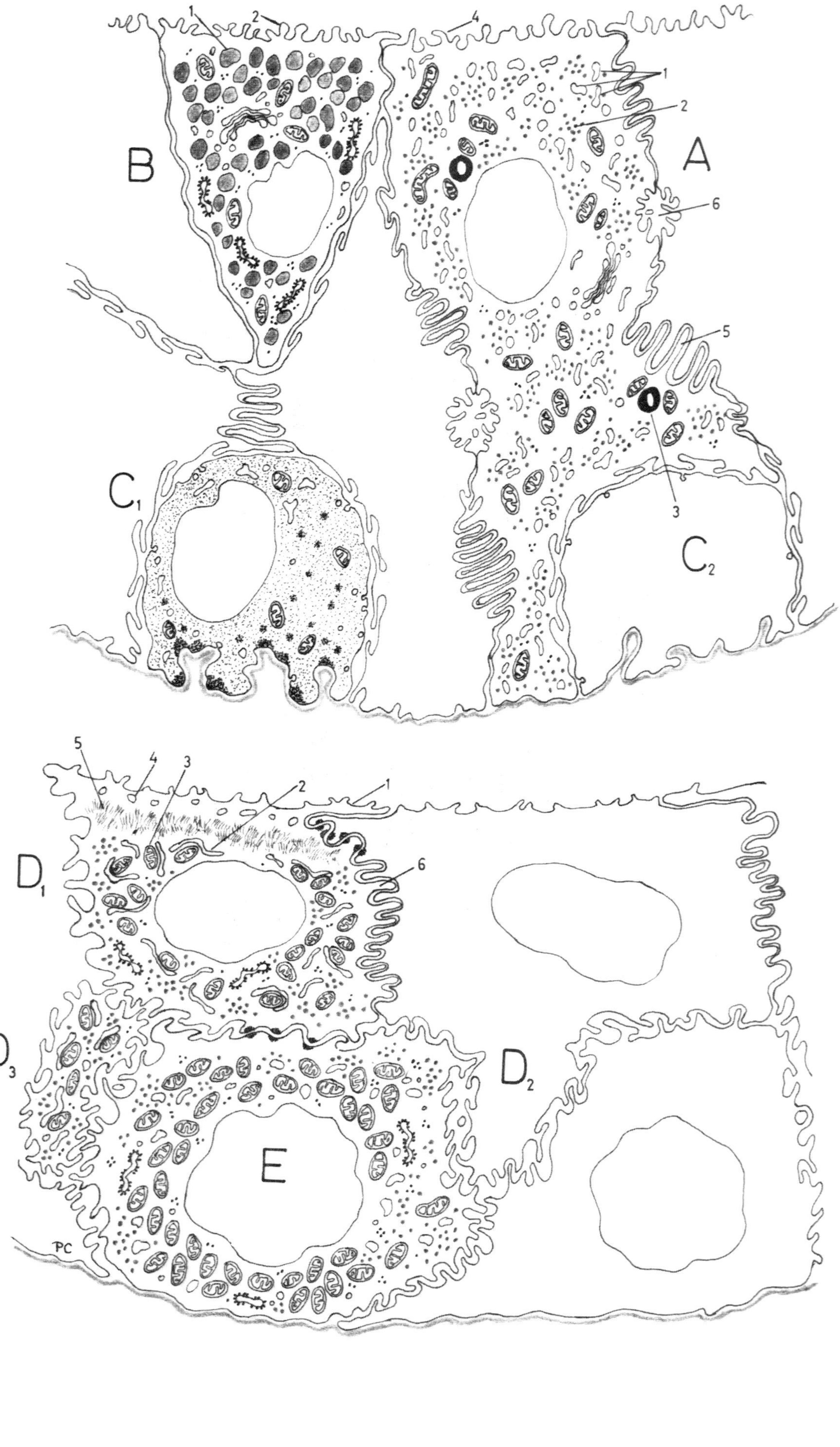

Plate 62

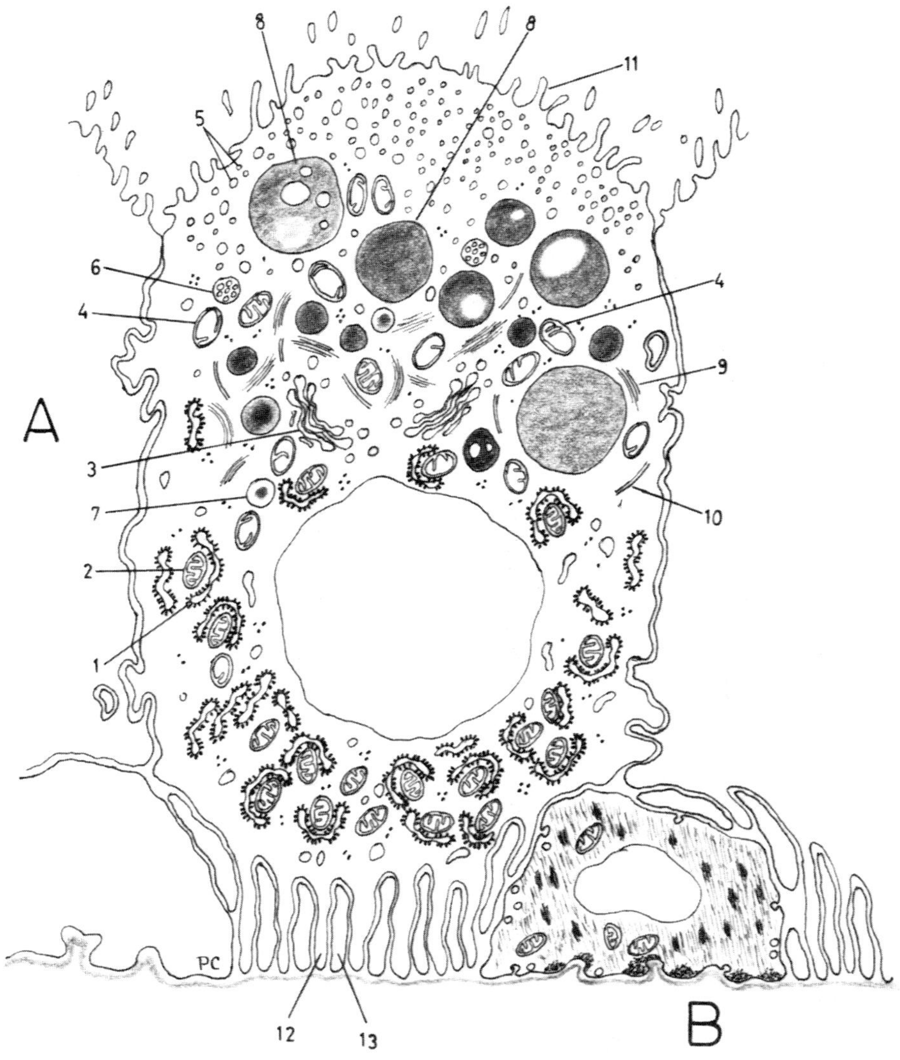

Plate 63

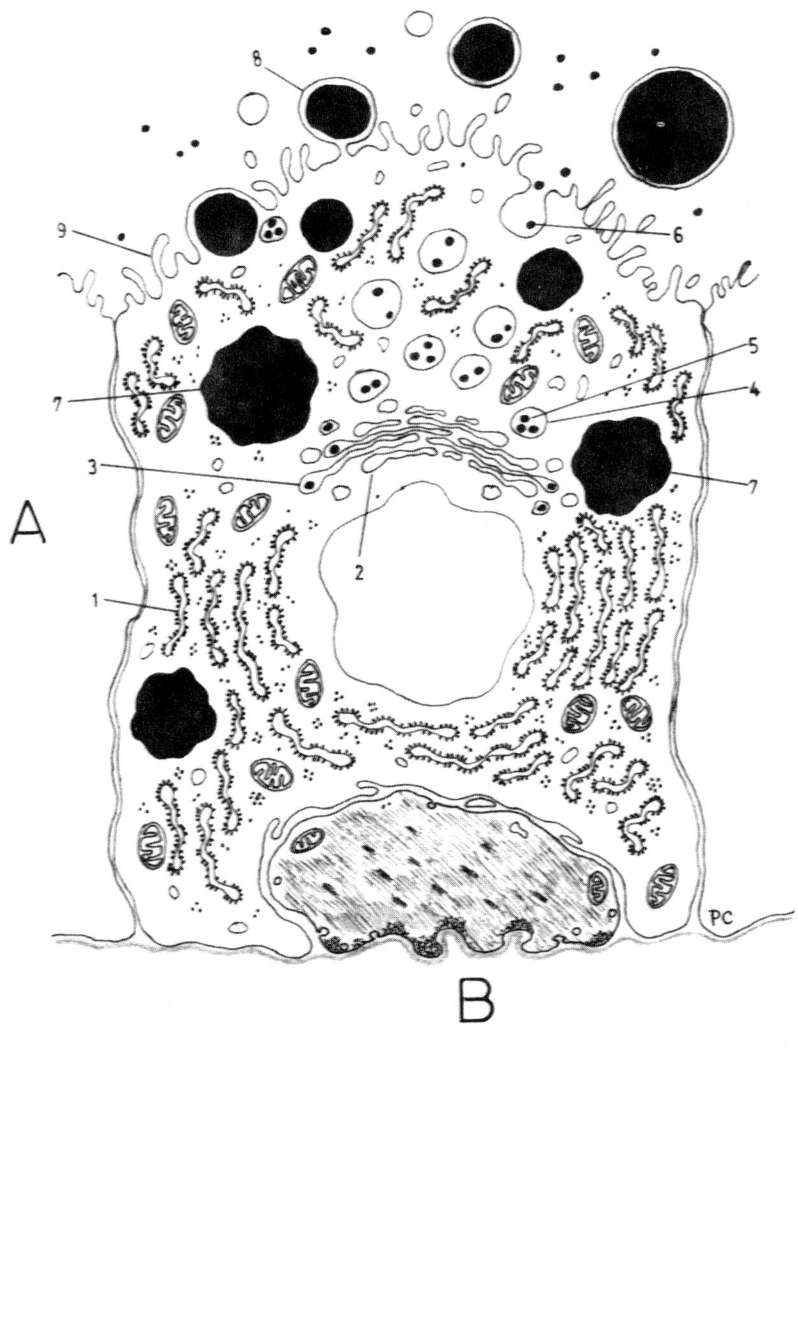

Plate 64

(3) Duct cells

The wall of the duct is 2–4 layers thick. Its cells combine the features of epidermal keratinising and sebaceous cells since they represent a transition between the two. They thus contain both keratin (tonofilaments and keratohyalin) and lipid globules.

V. SMALL "ECCRINE" SWEAT GLANDS

(1) General

These are long tubular glands whose secretory portion is coiled (the secretory coil) and whose duct loses its walls as it penetrates through the stratum corneum to reach the epidermis surface. The evaporation of their watery secretion cools the body.

(2) Secretory coil cells

(A) Clear cells (Plate 62, Fig. A)

Most cells of the secretory portion belong to this type. They are characterised by (a) only few ribosomes, few or no RER cisternae, and a distinct Golgi, (b) an extensive SER in the form of numerous round or flattened smooth vesicles[1], (c) appreciable numbers of mitochondria and glycogen granules[2], (d) a few lipid globules of tranlucent texture[3], (e) short apical microvilli[4] and long lateral microvilli which interlock extensively with those of adjacent cells[5], (f) intercellular canaliculi lined by microvilli[6], tight junctions sealing both the canaliculi and the upper ends of the intercellular clefts and a basal BM.

These cells manufacture sweat, a concentrated aqueous solution of NaCl, from blood plasma (through the tissue fluid). Electrolytes and H_2O from the tissue fluid reach the lateral interlocking surfaces of the secretory cells by seeping through the unsealed basal parts of their intercellular clefts; they are probably absorbed there by the cells under energy expenditure, as indicated (a) by the strong ATP-ase activity exhibited by these interlocking PMs and (b) by the fact that both the ability to sweat and the intricate lateral interlockings develop together at about the 10th post-natal day. The mechanism of sweat release into the gland lumen is still unknown and possibly related to the prominent SER of the secretory cells.

(B) Dark cells (Plate 62, Fig. B)

These are mucus-producing cells with dense glycoprotein granules[1] and surface microvilli[2], similar in structure to the gastric mucoid cells. The function of the mucus which they secrete into the gland lumen is unknown.

(C) Myoepithelial cells (Plate 62, Figs. C_1–C_2)

They have the same structure and function as the myoepithelial cells of salivary glands, *i.e.* they are smooth muscle cells that help to expel the secretion of the sweat glands by contracting and squeezing the secretory coils of the latter.

(3) Duct-intradermal segment

(A) Superficial cells (Plate 62, Fig. D_1)

Their general structure is similar to that of the secretory clear cells, with the following differences: (a) their apical microvilli are more rudimentary and the ends of their apical surfaces form long shelve-like processes[1] that overhang their neighbouring cells, (b) most of their prominent SER consists of flattened sacs[2] that are often closely associated with mitochondria[3], except for a row of round vesicles[4] under their apical surface, (c) they exhibit several RER cisternae, (d) they possess an apical mat of tonofilaments[5] (a "terminal web"), (e) multiple desmosomes and interlocking microvilli[6] join them to one another and to the underlying basal cells, and (f) they often send large, villous-fringed processes down below into the deeper layer (Figs. D_2–D_3). The function of these cells is considered together with those of the basal cells in the next heading.

(B) Basal cells (Plate 62, Fig. E)

Their structure is similar to that of the superficial cells with the following differences: (a) they possess even more numerous mitochondria, (b) they exhibit no terminal web, (c) their entire SER consists of round or oval smooth vesicles, and (d) they are underlaid by a BM.

The function of the sweat gland ducts seems to be not only to convey sweat to the skin surface but also to reabsorb Na^+ ions from this fluid and transport them back into the blood stream (into the capillaries below the BM). The occurrence of such a reabsorption process is suggested by microcannulation studies which show lower Na^+ concentrations in the lumen of the duct than in the lumen of the secretory coil; its mechanism is unknown but appears to be energy-consuming, as indicated by the high mitochondrial concentrations in the basal cells.

(4) Duct-intraepidermal (terminal) segment

The wall of the part of the intra-epidermal sweat duct that goes through the lower epidermis (*i.e.* the stratum basale, spinosum and granulosum) consists of a single layer of cells that are similar to the superficial cells of the intradermal segment of the duct and, in addition, exhibit numerous dense lysosomes. The part of the duct that goes through the stratum corneum has no cellular wall of its own – it is just a spiralling tunnel through the corneum.

VI. LARGE "APOCRINE" SWEAT GLANDS

(1) General

The secretory portions of this variety of sweat glands, unlike those of the small eccrine ones, have an alveolar shape with a relatively large lumen. They are far less numerous than the small sweat glands and their function is not yet quite settled.

(2) Secretory cells (Plate 63, Fig. A)

These are characterised by (a) a fair number of ribosomes and numerous RER cisternae[1], most of them closely associated with mitochondria[2], (b) prominent and multiple Golgi systems[3], (c) numerous mitochondria, many of them associated with RER cisternae, and several others (particularly the apical ones) with few or no cristae[4], (d) numerous small vesicles apically[5] and a moderate number of larger vesicles throughout the rest of the cytoplasm, (e) a few multivesicular bodies[6] and microbodies[7] and annulate lamellae, (f) a considerable number of lysosomes, some of them very large and very dense[8], (g) several bundles of tonofilaments[9] and microtubules[10] criss-crossing in the central cytoplasm region, (h) numerous short microvilli[11] on the luminal surface, (i) several long basal processes[12] that interdigitate extensively with the corresponding processes of adjacent cells[13] and exhibit marked ATP-ase activity, and (j) tight junctions apically and a BM basally.

These cells have been traditionally assumed to produce ordinary sweat, like those of the small eccrine glands, but their structural peculiarities suggest additional or different functions. Perhaps they secrete certain sex-identifying or other odorous chemicals. Neither the production nor the release mechanism of their secretion has yet been established.

(3) Myoepithelial cells (Plate 63, Fig. B)

They are smooth muscle cells, contracting to expell secretion, as in the case of the salivary and other skin glands.

(4) Duct cells

They are similar to the duct cells of the small eccrine glands.

VII. MAMMARY GLAND

(1) General

The mammary gland produces milk for the nutrition of the newborn. It is a compound gland whose ducts are few and whose secretory portions are rudimentary and inactive in the absence of pregnancy or lactation. When, however, a need for milk is anticipated or present, the duct tree proliferates enormously and the secretory acini enlarge and start producing milk, under appropriate hormonal stimulation.

(2) Secretory acini

(A) Active secretory cells (Plate 64, Fig. A)

These cells exhibit (a) numerous ribosomes and RER cisternae[1] in stacks, (b) a very large Golgi system[2], some of whose flattened sacs and vesicles contain small dense protein granules[3], (c) numerous relatively large vesicles[4] containing one or more dense protein granules[5] (similar to those found in the Golgi) that are released into the lumen by emiocytosis[6], (d) a moderate number of mitochondria, (e) several large lipid globules[7] that are apparently not bound by a membrane and seem to be released into the gland lumen together with a very thin cytoplasmic rim[8] through a pinching-off ("apocrine") process, and (f) numerous short microvilli[9] apically, tight junctions laterally and a basal BM.

The secretory cells manufacture and release the two main organic components of milk that mix in the lumen: protein and lipid. The protein component (casein) is synthesized in the RER, moves to the Golgi where it becomes visible in the form of small dense granules, then aggregates in the large secretory vesicles and is finally released through emiocytosis. The lipid component is represented by the large lipid droplets that apparently materialize free in the cytoplasmic matrix and grow in size, moving towards the apical PM which they push out before pinching off. The secretion of both components is stimulated by the luteotrophic hormone (prolactin) of the anterior pituitary.

During the involution of this gland that follows enforced cessation of lactation (weaning), there is a dramatic proliferation of lysosomes and cytosegresomes (autophagosomes) and several cells slough off into the lumen.

(B) Myoepithelial cells (Plate 64, Fig. B)

These are smooth muscle cells that seem to squeeze out secretion as in the case of certain other glands.

(3) Duct cells

Their structure in the initial segments of the ducts is similar to that of the secretory cells (indicating secretory potential) while in the terminal segments of the ducts it becomes epidermis-like. Duct cells are stimulated to proliferate by estrogen.

Chapter 15

Sensory Organs

I. EYE

(1) General (Plate 65, Fig. A)

The eye is a hollow sphere whose anterior wall[1] (the cornea) is transparent to allow the entry of light, while the rest of its wall consists of three layers (the hard sclera[2], the dark choroid[3] and the mostly photosensitive retina[4]). Anteriorly, the choroid with its thinned retinal lining forms a diaphragm[5] (the iris) with an aperture[6] (the pupil) and behind it a bulging mass with finger-like processes (the ciliary body[7] with the ciliary processes[8]). Behind the iris, and suspended from the ciliary processes through a suspensory ligament[9] (the zonula) is the transparent lens[10] which focusses the incoming light on the retina. The space between the lens and the cornea is filled by a thin fluid (the aqueous humor) which is produced by the ciliary processes and is drained into a channel at the corner between iris and cornea[11] (the canal of Schlemm) across a loose collagenic diaphragm, the pectinate ligament[12]. The space behind the lens and its suspensory ligament is filled by a more viscous, jelly-like material, the vitreous body, which consists of a framework of collagen-like fibers ("vitrosin") permeated by hyaluronate and soluble proteins.

The *lens* arises from an embryonic ball, which is surrounded by a capsule[13] and whose anterior wall consists of cuboidal epithelium cells[14] while its posterior wall cells elongate greatly to form long prismatic "lens fibers" that obliterate its cavity; in adult life, the nuclei of most lens cells of the posterior wall disappear except for a few that survive at the margins[15] and seem to constitute growth and regeneration areas for this structure. The *cornea* consists of avascular and transparent dense fibrous tissue[16] (the substantia propria) that is lined externally by a stratified squamous (Bowman's) epithelium[17] and internally by a single layer of flattened cells, Descemet's endothelium[18]. Bowman's epithelium continues beyond the cornea as a columnar stratified epithelium[19] to line the conjunctival sacs (the spaces between the eye balls and the eye lids) which receive the watery secretion of the *lacrimal glands*. The *sclera* consists of opaque dense fibrous tissue which is continuous with the substantia propria of the cornea. The *choroid* represents loose areolar connective tissue with many vessels[20] and pigment-containing cells (melanophores); its anterior expansions also contain smooth muscle: the meridional[21] and sphincteric[22] components of the ciliary muscle (which control the state of stretch and thus the curvature and focal distance of the lens) and the dilator[23] and sphincter[24] muscles in the iris (which control the diameter of the pupil). Finally, the *retina* consists of (a) a layer of photosensitive "rod" and "cone" cells[25], (b) two connector neuron layers[26], the axons of the second layer converging towards a hole in the posterior sclera to form the optic nerve which takes the visual impulses to the brain, and (c) a pigment cell epithelium[27] that separates the rod and cone cells from the choroid. At a point close to the ciliary body[28] (the ora serrata), the retina is reduced to two cell layers (a pigmented[29] and a non-pigmented[30] or "ciliary" epithelium) and ceases to function as a photosensitive tissue; beyond the ora serrata the two residual retinal layers go on to line the ciliary processes and – after the non-pigmented one acquires pigment – the posterior iris surface[31].

(2) Lens (Plate 65, Fig. B)

The structure of the embryonic nucleated lens cells and their adult nucleated remnants indicates very active protein synthesis. The anuclear cells or "lens fibers" that make up the bulk of the adult lens are characterised by (a) numerous polyribosomes[1] but relatively rare RER cisternae and mitochondria, (b) numerous microtubules[2] that run parallel to the long fiber axis, (c) extensive fusions of adjacent PMs[3], (d) marked interdigitations[4] and PM thickening of adjacent capsular ends, and (e) appreciable numbers of dense bodies[5] in their capsular ends; the capsule[6] that surrounds the lens corresponds to a BM, consists of a fibrillar and an amorphous low density component and contains carbohydrates and protein.

The few marginal anterior lens cells that retain their nuclei seem to proliferate, move around the equator to

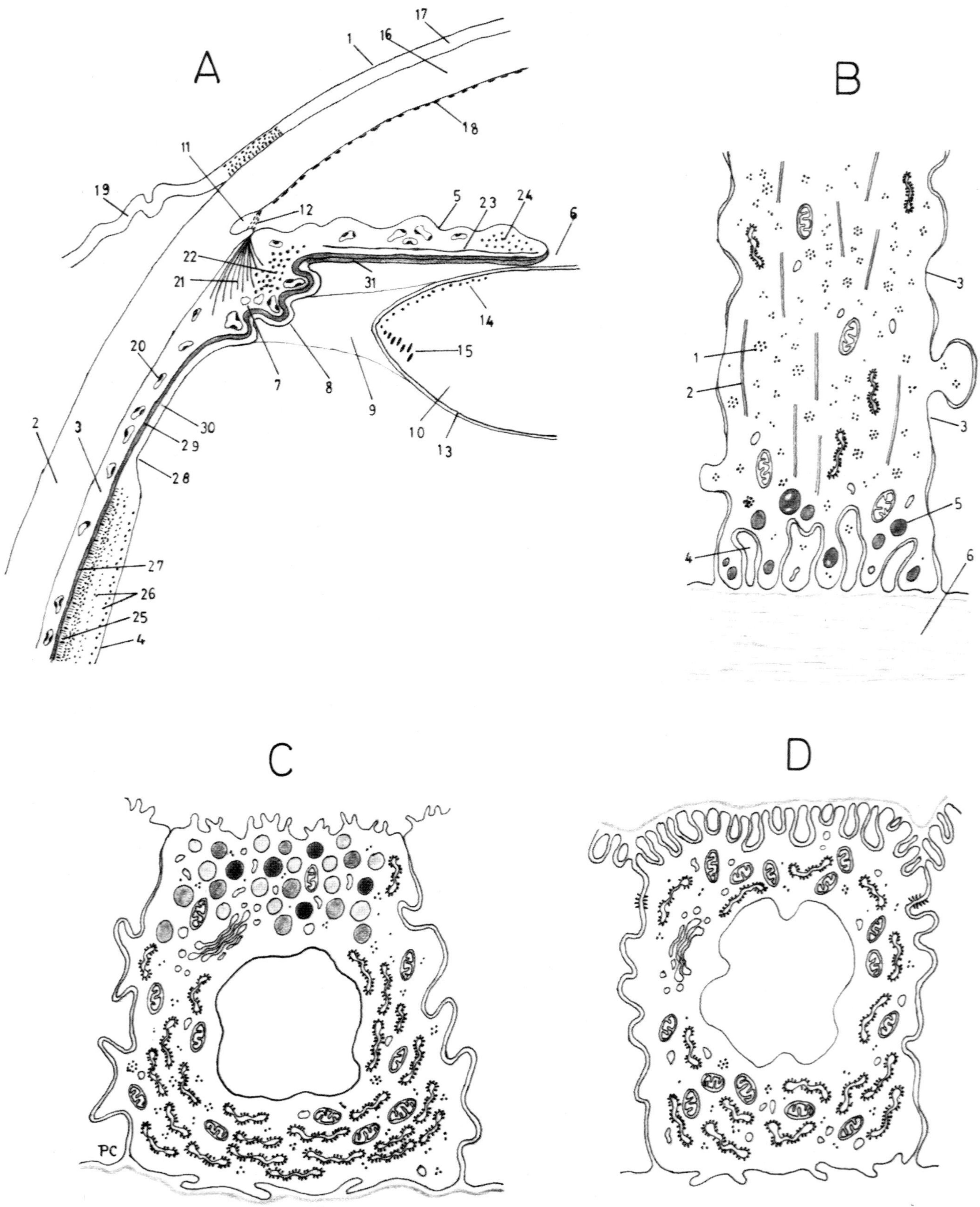
A
1
2
3
4
5
6
7
8
9
10
11
12
13
14
15
16
17
18
19
20
21
22
23
24
25
26
27
28
29
30
31
B
1
2
3
4
5
6
C
PC
D

Plate 65

the back and differentiate into new lens fibers, thus contributing to a slow growth of the lens by lateral apposition throughout life. Despite the loss of their nuclei (through envelope fragmentation and lysis), the lens fibers appear to persist for life and to produce protein continuously, probably through an unusually stable type of cytoplasmic RNA; the proteins produced by the lens polyribosomes evidently represent the soluble α-, β- and γ-"crystallines" (or specific transparent proteins of the matrix of lens fibers) as well as the capsule protein. The mechanism of the formation of the capsule is obscure and perhaps involves secretion of the dense bodies in the capsular ends of the lens fibers. As the lens ages it often tends to become more opaque and more rigid and it loses the ability to change its curvature and focal length, apparently due to the accumulation of an insoluble protein at the expense of γ-crystalline. Derangements of calcium-phosphorus metabolism (as in parathyroid disease) and of carbohydrate metabolism (as in diabetes) also affect the elasticity and the transparency of the lens, although the mechanism of these effects, like that of ageing, requires further study. In the case of diabetes, it has been recently proposed that clouding develops because glucose is turned within the lens fibers into sorbitol, a compound that cannot get out of cells and therefore accumulates, causing osmotic lens edema.

(3) Cornea

Bowman's *squamous stratified epithelium* is similar to the epidermis except for the fact that it does not possess any melanoblasts and its cells do not keratinise; it is supported by a very thick BM (Bowman's membrane) that separates it from the substantia propria and consists of a feltwork of *ca.* 200 Å wide banded collagen fibrils of ordinary periodicity embedded in an amorphous glycoprotein component. The *substantia propria* is composed of dense fibrous tissue with (a) regularly stacked, *ca.* 200 Å wide collagen fibrils of ordinary periodicity, in layers of alternating direction, (b) an amorphous glycoprotein ground substance containing chondroitin sulfate and keratosulfate, and (c) fibroblasts aligned parallel to the corneal surface. Finally, *Descemet's endothelium* consists of flat cells that exhibit moderate numbers of ribosomes, RER cisternae and mitochondria and are joined to one another through tight junctions and appreciable interlocking of their lateral surfaces; its BM, like that of Bowman's epithelium, is composed of glycoprotein and collagen fibrils but the latter are arranged in a regular hexonal pattern and exhibit an unusual periodicity of *ca.* 1100 Å.

The cornea seems to be transparent because it contains no vessels and because it loses water continuously; it becomes opaque when it develops edema. It is apparently oxygenated and nourished by diffusion of fluid from the aqueous humor behind it (through an absorptive function of Descemet's endothelium) and from the conjunctival and scleral vessels near its rim (the limbic vessels). Various metabolic derangements affect its structure: Prolonged hypercholesterolemia can lead to marked lipid deposits within the marginal substantia propria, and marked vitamin A deficiency produces corneal opaqueness through a still unsettled mechanism.

The cells of the cornea have unusual phagocytic abilities. Thus, unlike fibroblasts elsewhere in the body, corneal fibroblasts will phagocytise foreign particles (*e.g.* ink, silver, protein, myelin) injected into the substantia propria, and the epithelial cells may contain ferritin in phagosomal sacs as well as free in the matrix.

(4) Lacrimal gland (Plate 65, Fig. C)

The structure of this gland is very similar to that of the predominantly serous salivary glands. Its secretory cells are distinguished by an extensive RER and numerous large variable density secretion granules, and they are surrounded by myoepithelial cells. They secrete the tears, a watery fluid that contains the bacteriostatic enzyme lysozyme and electrolytes and functions to (a) keep the outer corneal surface wet, and (b) prevent bacterial colonisation on the same surface.

Lacrimal secretion is known to be under nervous control. It is inhibited by parasympathetic denervation and axon terminals of cholinergic type have been seen to approach secretory and myoepithelial cells to within 200 Å of their surface, but no true synaptic junctions (with parasynaptic densities) have yet been documented.

A remarkable sexual dimorphism of this gland has been observed in the rat: the secretory acini of the female are small, have many intercellular canaliculi, no nuclear inclusions and are always serviced by perforated capillaries, while those of the male are large, have only a few intercellular canaliculi, numerous nuclear inclusions and are usually supplied by capillaries of the continuous endothelium type.

(5) Sclera

This is composed of ordinary dense fibrous tissue identical with that of ligaments and tendons. It provides a rigid structural framework for the eyeball.

(6) Choroid, ciliary body and iris

These structures consist of very vascular areolar tissue which is rich in melanophores (highly branched fibroblast-like cells containing numerous premelanosomes and melanosomes) and capillaries with multiple diaphragm-sealed perforations. The myocytes of the ciliary body and the iris are innervated by axon terminals of both the

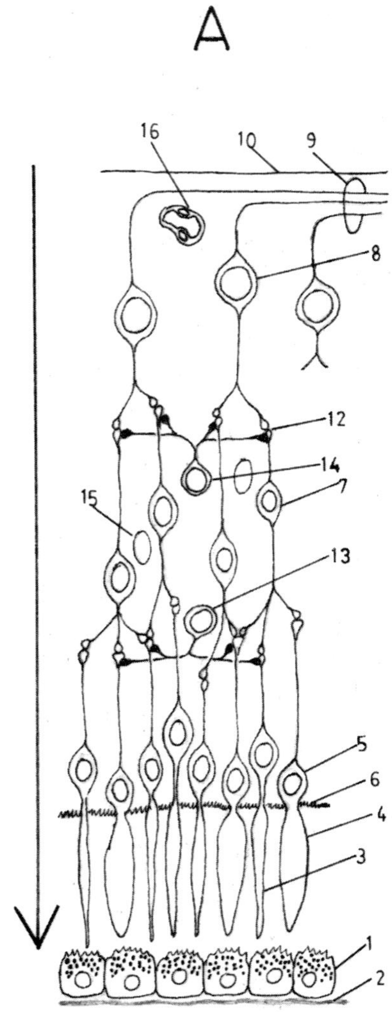

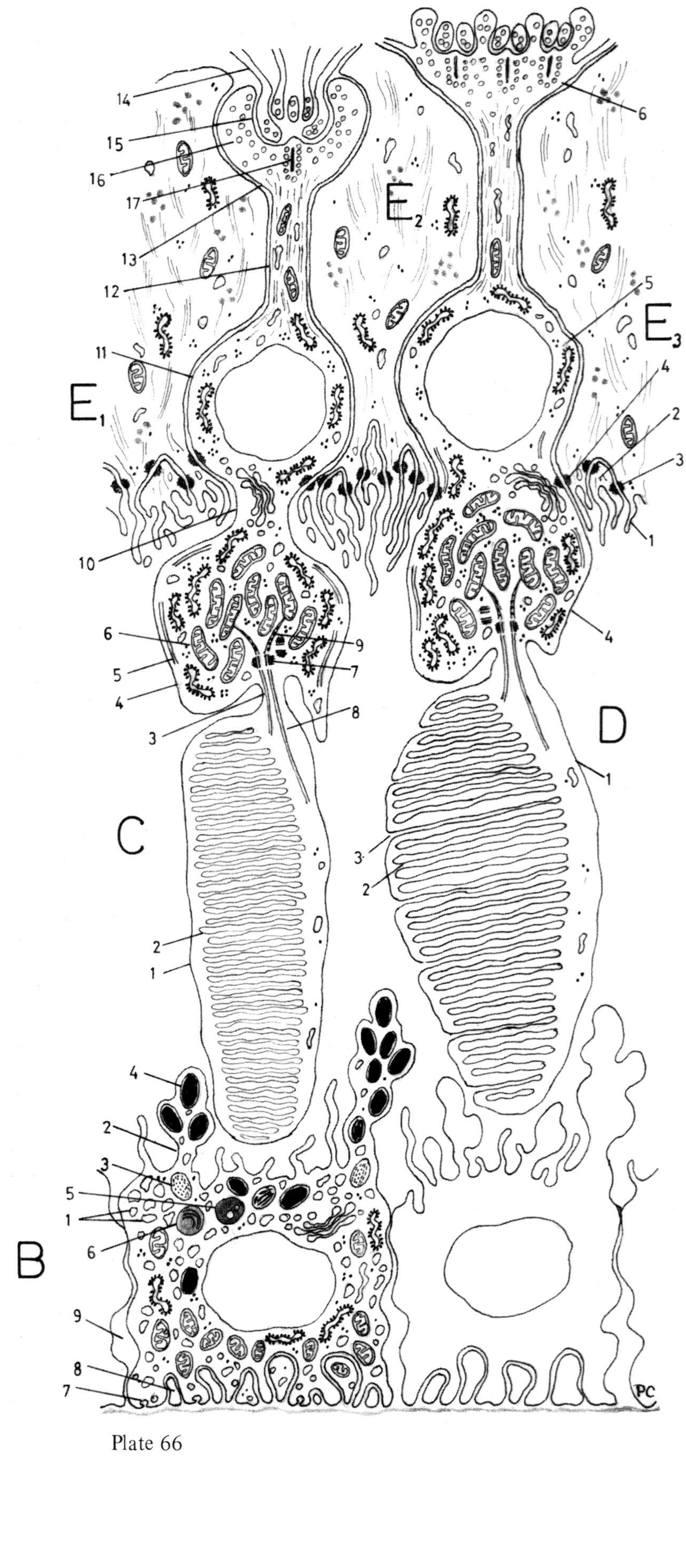

Plate 66

cholinergic and the adrenergic type: terminals with clear synaptic vesicles seem to contact myocytes of the pupillary sphincter, while terminals with clear and cored vesicles appear to abut on the dilator of the pupil myocytes – some of the latter reportedly containing pigment granules.

The ciliary body is covered by a double epithelial lining which consists of a superficial, non-pigmented "ciliary" epithelium and a deep pigmented epithelium. The non-pigmented "ciliary" epithelial layer (Plate 65, Fig. D), is characterised by (a) the absence of melanosomes, (b) extensively interdigitating *superficial* processes, and (c) a superficial rather than a basal BM and junctional complexes; its features indicate it is involved in intensive fluid transport, presumably for the production of aqueous humor. By contrast, the pigmented basal epithelial layer, which probably also participates in the production of aqueous humor, is characterised by (a) the presence of melanosomes, (b) extensively interdigitating *basal* processes, and (c) a basal BM; it is described more fully in the next section (Plate 66, Fig. B). The reverse structural polarity of the above two epithelial layers is easily understood if one considers their embryological origin, *i.e.* the development of the optic cup from an invagination of the optic vesicle.

Apart from the contractile properties of its anterior formations, the choroid provides (a) a dark screen that absorbs excess photons and prevents their reflection (which would confuse the photoreceptors) (b) oxygen and nutrients for the outer retina layers and materials for the manufacture of the aqueous humor through its rich vasculature. There are certain congenital defects associated with an absence of melanin producing enzymes from the choroid (albinism).

(7) Retina

(A) General (Plate 66, Fig. A)

The outer limit of the retina is formed by a row of pigment epithelium cells[1] which are separated from the underlying choroid by a membrane (Bruch's)[2] that consists of the following 5 layers: (a) the BM of the pigment epithelium, (b) an inner collagen layer, (c) an elastic layer, (d) an outer collagen layer, and (e) the BM of the closest subepithelial capillaries. Facing the pigment epithelium is a row of photoreceptor cells with long rod[3] or cone[4] shaped processes whose nuclei[5] lie above a dense sieve-like line, the external limiting membrane[6]. The light, penetrating into the retina from above (moving in the direction of the arrow) hits the photosensitive tips of the rod and cone cells and initiates in the latter impulses which are transmitted through bipolar connector neurons[7] to large neurons[8], the so-called ganglion cells; the combined centripetal axons of the latter form the optic nerve[9] which leaves the eye ball to carry the visual impulses to the brain. At its upper limit, the retina is demarcated against the vitreous body by the inner limiting membrane[10]. Apart from the main "vertical" synapses between photoreceptor and bipolar[11] and between bipolar and ganglion cells[12] there are also appreciable "horizontal" connections between the central processes of the photoreceptor and the bipolar cells; these horizontal connections are effected by the "horizontal"[13] and "amacrine"[14] connector neurons, respectively. The space between the pigment epithelium and the external limiting membrane is filled with a glycoprotein-rich fluid of fibrillogranular E/M structure; conversely, the entire space between neurons from the external to the internal limiting membrane is occupied by the watery cytoplasm of glia cells, the so-called Müller cells, whose nuclei[15] are encountered at random intervals. Capillaries occur only in the inner zone of the retina[16].

(B) Pigment epithelium cells (Plate 66, Fig. B)

These are characterised by (a) few ribosomes and RER cisternae, (b) an extensive SER[1], a distinct Golgi and appreciable numbers of mostly basal mitochondria, (c) numerous apical processes[2] that surround the tips of the rods and cones, (d) numerous premelanosomes[3] and melanin granules[4] that move into the apical processes, (e) several lysosomes[5] and phagolysosomes[6] ("myeloid bodies"), (f) several pinocytotic vesicles[7], (g) marked interdigitations[8] with the basal processes of adjacent cells, and (h) junctional complexes with neighbouring cells as well as often dilated intercellular clefts[9].

The pigment epithelium cells seem to have the following functions: (a) their melanin granules respond to illumination by migrating into their apical processes towards the rods and cones to protect these photoreceptors from excessive light and to increase their visual discrimination (a photo-mechanical response), (b) they transport fluids and ions (especially chlorides) from the choroid capillaries into the space between the rods and cones and contribute part of the glycoproteins found in the above space, and (c) they phagocytise debris arising in their neighbourhood, notably parts of rod outer segments (the "multilamellar" phagosomal inclusions) which are perhaps shed frequently as part of a continuous wearing out and renewal process. It has also been speculated that they may respond to illumination by generating impulses which travel across tight junctions along the entire length of the pigment epithelium to reach the iris muscles. Finally, in certain lower vertebrates, the pigment epithelium can apparently become the source of regeneration of a whole new retina, when the latter is removed experimentally – a phenomenon that is less surprising than it seems when the embryological kinship of the two structures is kept in mind.

(C) Rod cells (Plate 66, Fig. C)

The photoreceptor part of a rod cell is a long, cylindrical process, the "outer segment"[1], which contains a stack of flattened saccules[2] that carry the photosensitive pigment rhodopsin on their 35 Å thick membranes and enclose *ca.* 80 Å wide spaces. The outer segment is connected by means of a very thin neck[3] to an organelle-rich paranuclear mass of cytoplasm, the "inner segment"[4], that is distinguished by (a) an appreciable number of ribosomes and RER cisternae, (b) a distinct Golgi, (c) several peripheral microtubules[5], (d) numerous mitochondria[6], and (e) a centriole[7] from which a 9 + 0 type cilium[8] grows into the outer segment and banded rootlets[9] exhibiting ATPase activity grow towards the mitochondria. The inner segment, in turn, connects by means of a constriction[10] (the "outer rod fiber") with the pericaryon[11] of the rod cell; from the pericaryon, an axon[12] (the "inner rod fiber") leads to a synaptic body[13] in which the visual impulses of the rod cell are transmitted to several small dendritic processes of bipolar cells. In the main type of synaptic body which is illustrated here, four bipolar cell dendritic processes[14] dip into a cup-like depression[15] of the end bulb of the rod cell axon, two on each side of an incomplete partition; the axon end bulb contains many clear synaptic vesicles[16] and a synaptic ribbon[17] in its presynaptic cytoplasm, the dense plate of the latter possibly representing an organiser (RNA?) for the rapid synthesis of vesicles close to the synaptic cleft. One of the interesting but still unexplained features of this and other synapses of sensory organs is that synaptic vesicles can be found on both sides of the synaptic cleft (not only on the presynaptic side, as in ordinary synapses elsewhere). Direct contacts between adjacent photoreceptor cells have also been described, but it is not known whether they represent functional synapses.

Rods collect light under twilight conditions, *i.e.* they expedite "black and white" vision at low illumination levels – many nocturnal birds possess only rods in their retinae. When rhodopsin is illuminated, it is rapidly transformed into an unstable compound that breaks down into a protein (scotopsin) and a carotenoid (vitamin A aldehyde or retinene); this breakdown somehow releases ions that initiate depolarisation wave (an impulse) in the rod cell. It is thought that protein and vitamin A recombine after illumination to form new rhodopsin in readiness for the next photonic stimulation. It is very probable, however, that both the protein and the vitamin A are gradually lost in the repeated photochemical reactions and have to be replaced by local synthesis and dietary supply, respectively. The above assumption is supported (a) by the autoradiographic evidence that protein is continuously synthesized in the inner segment and migrates from there into the outer segment, moving from RER to Golgi to basal discs, and (b) by the fact that unless vitamin A is continuously supplied by the diet, night blindness ensues. Apart from their main photoreceptor function, rod cells apparently also contribute (through their Golgi) a polysaccharide secretion to the glucoprotein fluid that fills the space between rods and cones. Finally, the cilium that grows from their centriole seems to be a vestige of a motor apparatus which in lower species moves the rods in response to illumination stimuli.

(D) Cone cells (Plate 66, Fig. D)

They are similar to rod cells, except for the following differences: (a) their outer segments[1] are appreciably wider, (b) their saccule membranes[2] are thicker (*ca.* 50 Å), often communicate with the extracellular space[3] and are charged with photopsin, a photosensitive pigment that is different from rhodopsin, (c) the cytoplasmic portions between their inner segments[4] and pericarya[5] are much less constricted, and (d) the end bulbs[6] of their axons are triangular, wider and synapse with more bipolar neuron dendrites than those of the rod cell axons. Recent freeze-etch studies have shown that gap junctions with a 20–40 Å wide synaptic gap exist between distal rod and cone axons, and that the two synapsing membranes exhibit rows of 100–120 Å intramembranous particles in perfect register with one another, in these junctions.

The photochemical processes here appear to be basically similar to those that occur in rod cells but are still largely under debate; there may be three types of cones with selective sensitivities for red, green and blue light, respectively. The Golgi and the cilium of the cone cells seem to function as in rod cells.

(E) Müller cells (retinal glia cells) (Plate 66, Figs. E_1–E_3)

These fill all spaces between the retinal cells above the inner segments of the rod and cone cells, each Müller cell apparently enveloping through cytoplasmic expansions 10–15 cell bodies of rod and cone cells. . They are characterised (Fig. E_3) by (a) a low density matrix with only a few microfilaments, ribosomes, mitochondria and tubular SER vesicles but abundant glycogen granules, (b) numerous long microvilli[1] at their termination just above the inner segment level of the rod and cone cells, (c) extensive interdigitations[2] between the villous terminations of adjacent cells, and (d) numerous desmosomes between their interdigitating villous processes[3] and between the latter and the adjacent rod and cone cells[4]. The series of desmosomes at the basal (outer) ends of the Müller cells constitute the "external limiting membrane", while their upper (inner) terminations constitute the "internal limiting membrane" of low magnifications. The function of these cells, like that of glia cells elsewhere, seems to be insulation and metabolic servicing of the retinal neurons.

(F) Bipolar connector neurons and ganglion cells

These are like neurons elsewhere. In the synapses between them, the presynaptic axon terminals of the bipolar neurons possess synaptic ribbons and synaptic vesicles, but the postsynaptic axon terminals of the ganglion cells also possess synaptic vesicles, a finding which suggests the possibility of occasional retrograde firing of impulses (from the ganglion cells towards the bipolar neurons).

II. EAR–VESTIBULAR

(1) General (Plate 67, Fig. A)

This part of the inner ear houses the sense of position in space and of movement (acceleration or retardation). It has five functional units (the three cristae ampullares of the semicircular canals, the macula of the saccule and the macula of the utricle) all of which exhibit an essentially similar structure with the following features: Sensory hair cells[1] attached to a jelly-like mass[2] (the "cupola" in the case of the cristae ampullares and the "otolithic membrane" in the case of the maculae) are interspersed among supporting cells[3] on the surface of a connective tissue hill[4] that grows out of the wall of a membranous sac[5] (part of the membranous labyrinth); the sac is filled with fluid (endolymph) and is surrounded by fluid (exolymph). Movements of the head cause movements of the endolymph and the cupolae and otolithic membranes and thus elicit impulses in the hair cells which are picked up by nerve terminals[6]. There are two types of hair cells.

(2) Hair cells

(A) Type I hair cell (Plate 67, Fig. B)

This cell is characterised by (a) a long cilium[1] growing out of a basal body[2] (occasionally accompanied by a centriole at right angles), containing 9 outer and 2 central tubule pairs in non-mammals but 9 outer and 1 central dense fiber in mammals, (b) several variably long villus-like processes[3] ("sensory hair") with multiple thin central filaments[4] that are rooted in a terminal web[5], (c) a jelly-like mass of translucent glycoprotein[6] without (cupola) or with (otolithic membrane) $CaCo_3$ crystalloids, to which the cilium and hair are attached in a still obscure manner, (d) appreciable numbers of ribosomes but only a few RER cisternae, (e) prominent, multiple Golgi[7] (f) an extensive SER[8] (mostly larger vesicles), (g) numerous mitochondria[9] (mostly apically), (h) a synaptic ribbon[10] at the base, facing the cup-like nerve terminal, (i) desmosomes[11] joining it to the adjacent supporting cells and multiple tight junctions[12] attaching it to the surrounding nerve terminal. The afferent axon terminal (Fig. C) that synapses with the hair cell has the shape of a cup in which the latter is embedded; the synaptic cleft between the tight junctions[1] is *ca.* 300 Å wide and the axon terminal exhibits (a) clear synaptic[2] and larger vesicles, (b) several mitochondria (some with longitudinal cristae[3]), and (c) microtubules.

Movements of the head cause movements of the endolymph and the cupolae or otolithic membranes, stimulating the sensory hair and initiating impulses in hair cells in a still uncertain manner; the impulses are possibly transmitted to the afferent nerve terminals electrically (through the tight junctions) and carried by the latter to the brain.

(B) Type II hair cell

This is similar to the type I cell, with the difference that (a) its SER vesicles are mostly smaller than in type I, and (b) it is contacted synaptically by several small bulb-like axon terminals rather than by one big cup-like terminal. Most of the synapsing nerve terminals seem to be of the afferent type (with clear vesicles), but some of them contain cored as well as clear vesicles and are thought to be efferent. The functional difference between type I and II hair cells in unknown at the present time.

(3) Supporting cells

(A) Central or "light" cells (at the top of the hill) (Plate 67, Fig. D)

These are pseudostratified cells with the following characteristics: (a) a few apical microvilli[1], (b) a marked terminal web[2], (c) numerous microtubules[3], (d) multiple prominent Golgi systems[4], (e) numerous membrane limited dense granules[5], and (f) several mitochondria. Their function is unknown.

(B) Peripheral or "dark" cells (at the slope of the hill) (Plate 67, Fig. E)

These are similar to the more centrally placed supporting cells but, unlike the former, they exhibit (a) extensive lateral infoldings and basal interdigitations, (b) a dense cytoplasmic matrix, and (c) low density granules.

They may be involved in the transport of ions between blood and endolymph and in the manufacture of sulfated polysaccharides for the endolymph.

(4) Endolymphatic sac

This is a reservoir of endolymph that is connected to both the utricle and the saccule. Its epithelial lining resembles – with some variations – the supporting epithelium of the vestibular ear which was just described.

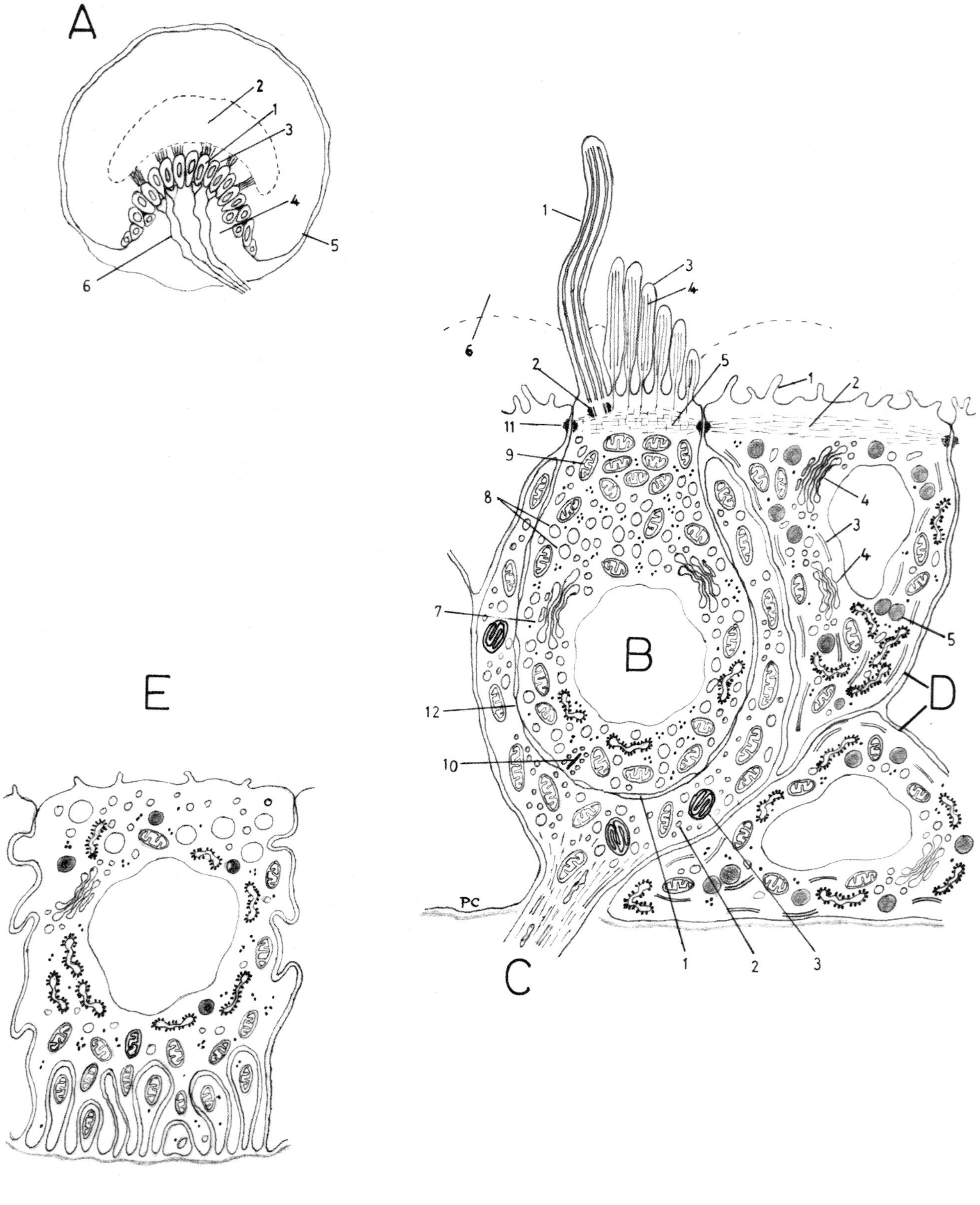

Plate 67

III. EAR–COCHLEAR

(1) General (Plate 68, Fig. A)

The cochlear ear houses the sensory apparatus for hearing, which originates in the organ of Corti. The latter is a cellular mound, containing sensory hair cells[1] nesting within cup-shaped depressions of supporting cells[2]; it runs along the entire length of the floor of a membranous tube of roughly triangular cross-section, the cochlear duct[3] (a part of the membranous labyrinth). The cochlear duct is filled with endolymph, it sits on a mat of taut, regularly oriented collagen fibers, the basilar membrane[4], and has a thin roof, the Reissner membrane[5]; jutting from a triangular cell mass[6] within the narrow side of the cochlear duct (the limbus) is an amorphous jelly-like mass, the tectorial membrane[7], which seems to be produced by a row of "interdental" cells[8] and attaches to the hair of the sensory cells; at its wide side, the cochlear duct wall thickens to double layer of outer clear[9] and inner dark[10] cells with capillaries[11] in between, the stria vascularis. Within the organ of Corti, two rows of tall, narrow cells (the outer[12] and inner[13] "pillar" cells) lean against one another to form a tunnel[14]. Three rows of sensory hair cells are situated on the outer and one row on the inner side of the tunnel; all hair cells are lodged in cup-shaped depressions of specialised supporting cells, the "phalangeal" cells, and they are synaptically contacted by the end bulbs[15] of mostly afferent axons[16] of the cochlear ganglion cells[17] that go between pillar cells and through phalangeal cells to reach them.

Air vibrations are transmitted through the external auditory meatus to the eardrum that consists of 3 layers: (a) an outer epidermis-like epithelium, (b) an inner single cell layer of extremely flat cells, and (c) a middle layer of protein fibers of an unusual amino acid composition, different from that of both collagen and elastin. From the eardrum, the vibrations pass through a chain of three middle ear ossicles to an exolymph-filled space above and below the cochlear duct (the scala vestibuli and scala tympani); the exolymph vibrations are transmitted through an as yet obscure mechanism to the hair cells of the Corti organ where they initiate impulses which are picked up by the peripheral axons of the cochlear ganglion cells and carried through their central axons (the cochlear nerve) to the brain.

(2) Corti–outer hair cells (Plate 68, Fig. B)

The outer hair cells are characterised by (a) peculiar apical processes[1] with internal filaments[2] that are embedded in the translucent tectorial membrane, (b) appreciable numbers of mostly apical RER cisternae[3] and ribosomes, (c) a fair number of smooth round vesicles[4] and chains of smooth sub-surface cisternae[5] along their lateral margins, (d) numerous mitochondria basally[6] and laterally[7], (e) several dense lipid-like inclusions apically[8], (f) synaptic ribbons[9] and subsynaptic cisternae[10] basally, and (g) zonulae adherentes attaching them to adjacent supporting cells. Several axon terminals synapse with the basal surface of these cells; most contain clear synaptic vesicles (Fig. C) and are afferent, but some contain clear and cored vesicles (Fig. D) and are considered efferent. The part of the hair cell cytoplasm facing the afferent axon terminals exhibits synaptic vesicles and ribbons, while that facing the efferent terminals displays subsurface cisternae.

In some obscure way, the mechanical vibrations from the exolymph are transmitted to the hair cells and are transduced there in an equally obscure manner into impulses which are picked up by the underlying afferent axon terminals. The role of the apical dense bodies, the lateral chains of SER cisternae and the alleged efferent axon terminals is unknown.

(3) Supporting cells (Plate 68)

Both the phalangeal (Fig. E) and the pillar cells (Fig. F) are attached firmly to the underlying basilar membrane[1] through hemidesmosomes[2]. They exhibit a relatively undifferentiated cytoplasm, with the exception of extraordinarily numerous microtubules[3] that run in thick bundles across the entire cell bodies from the apical zonulae[4] adherentes to the basal hemidesmosomes. Their function is obscure; it is not known whether they provide purely structural support for the hair cells with their microtubule bundles, or whether they transmit exolymph-induced vibrations of the basilar membrane to the hair cells through their apical zonulae adherentes. A "nursing role" seems unlikely in view of the exposure of both supporting and hair cells to the same fluids.

(4) Corti–inner hair cells

These are generally similar to the outer hair cells but (a) their numerous smooth round vesicles are smaller, (b) they possess no lateral chains of flattened SER cisternae or dense apical bodies, and (c) they exhibit a much smaller number of RER cisternae.

(5) Tectorial membrane

This apparently amorphous mass consists of a keratin-like protein and exhibits an orderly fibrillar structure at high magnification.

(6) Interdental cells

These cells possess an appreciable RER and a distinct

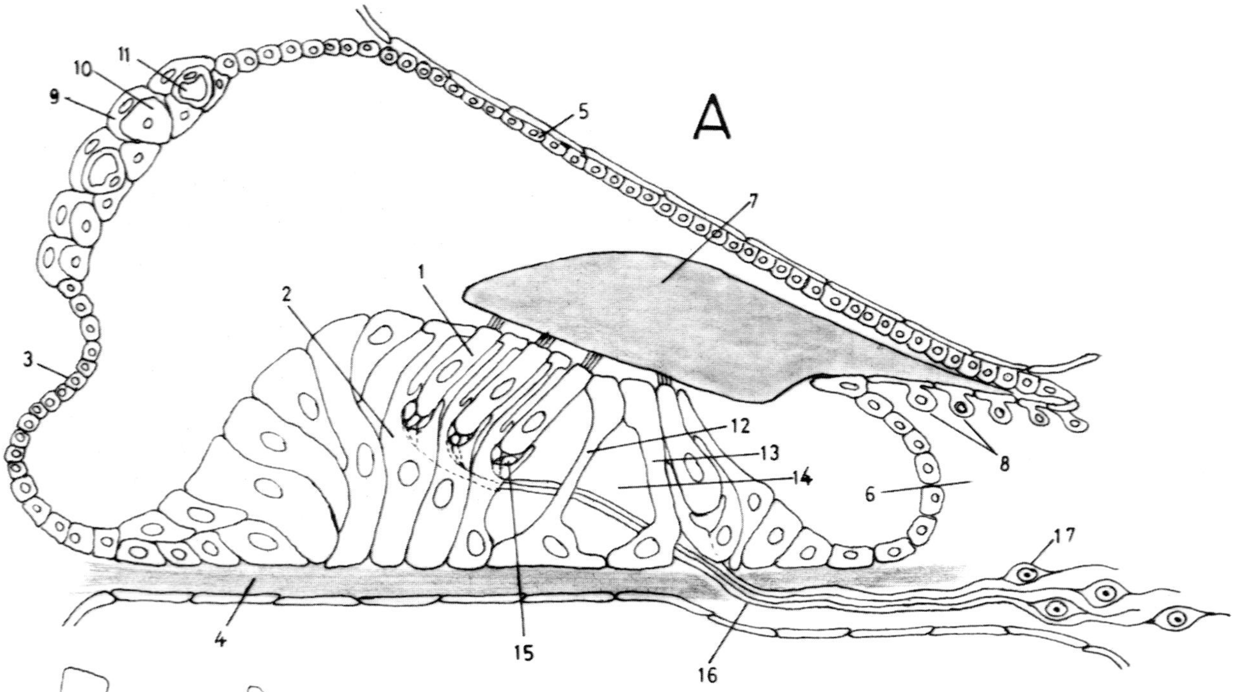
A
1
2
3
4
5
6
7
8
9
10
11
12
13
14
15
16
17

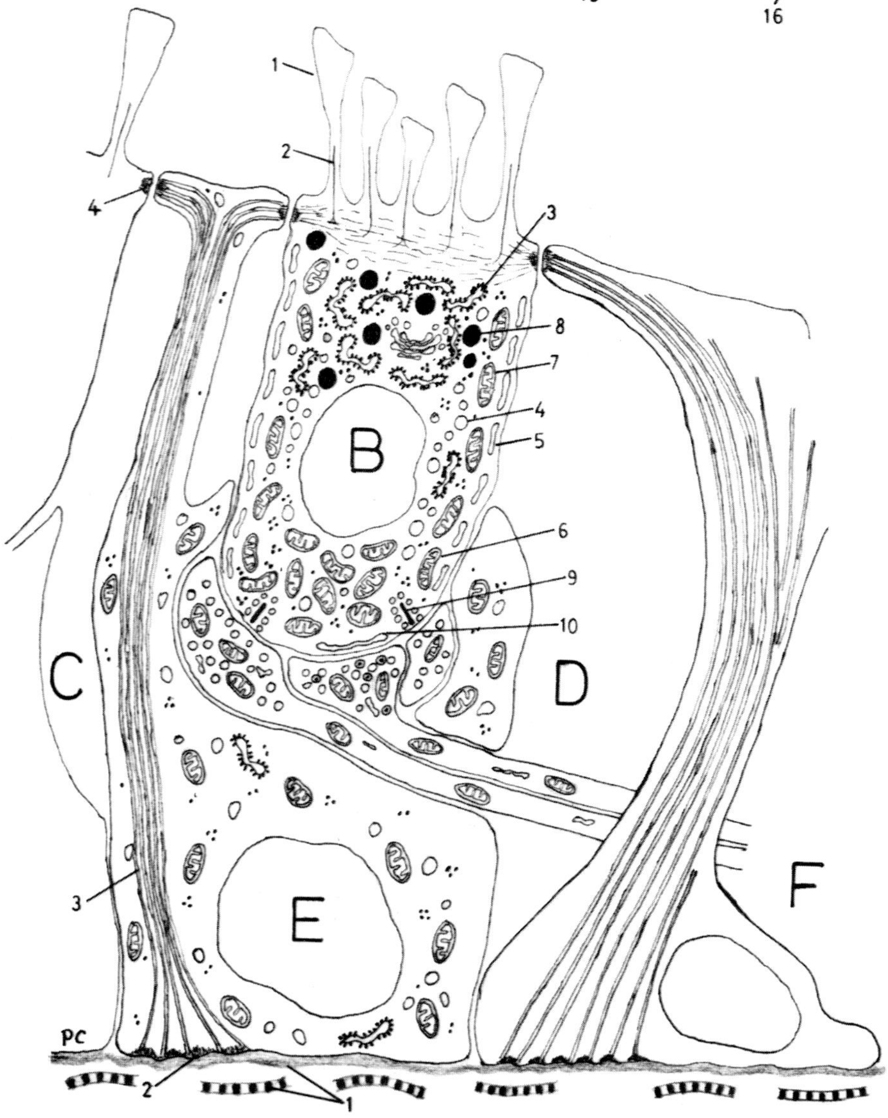
B
C
D
E
F
1
2
3
4
5
6
7
8
9
10
PC

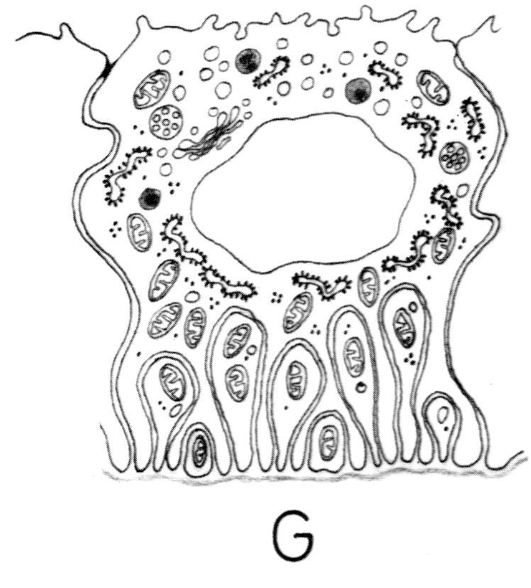
G

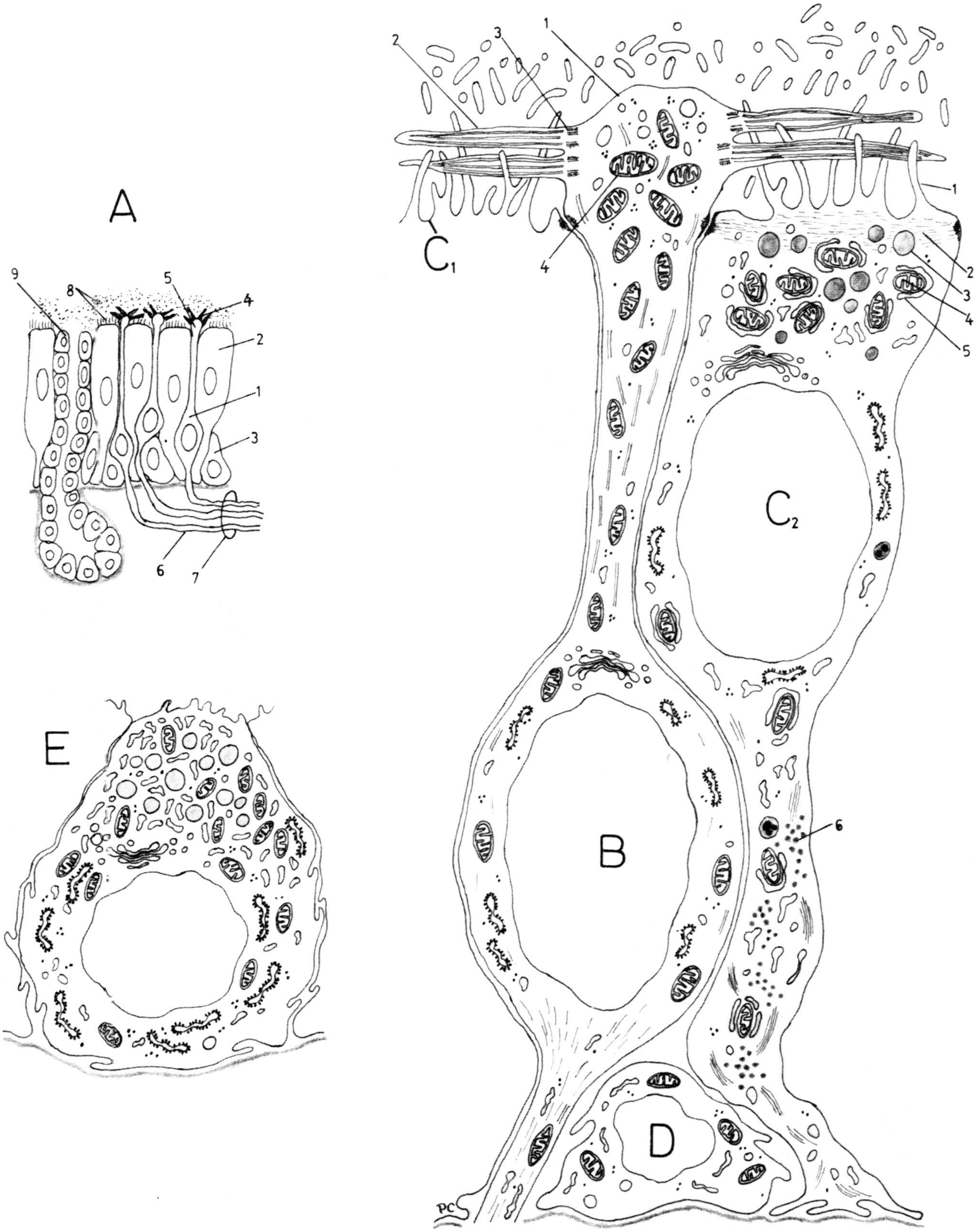

Plate 69

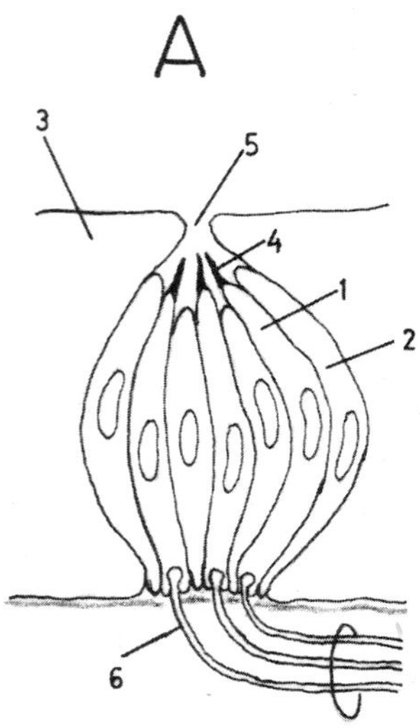

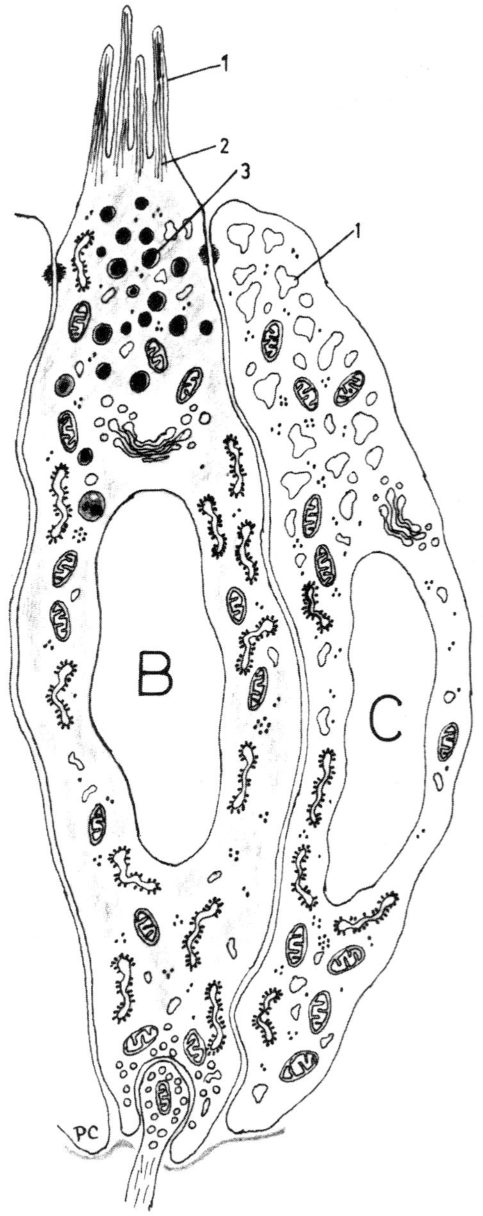

Plate 70

Golgi; their apices flare out and interdigitate extensively with one another. Interdental cells seem to secrete the tectorial membrane.

(7) Stria vascularis

The outer clear cells have an undifferentiated structure with only few mitochondria and send out several processes that interdigitate with the inner dark cells; the latter exhibit numerous mitochondria and coated vesicles and basal interdigitations reminiscent of kidney tubules (Fig. G, Plate 68). It is thought that the cells of this area produce and/or reabsorb endolymph from the capillaries that run among them. Frequently, an intermediate cell layer is interposed between inner and outer cells, its structure resembling that of the former.

(8) Reissner membrane

It consists of an outer layer of extremely thin mesothelium-type cells and an inner layer of more cytoplasm-rich cells. The latter develop numerous plump microvilli on their lower (endolymphatic) surface reminiscent of ependymal cells in the choroid plexus, while their opposite surface exhibits numerous interdigitations; they are probably involved in water and electrolyte transport between perilymph and endolymph.

IV. OLFACTORY EPITHELIUM

(1) General (Plate 69, Fig. A)

The olfactory epithelium that lines the uppermost recesses of the nasal cavities consists of olfactory sensory cells[1], supporting cells[2] and basal[3] cells which are underlaid by a BM. The olfactory sensory cells are modified bipolar neurons whose peripheral processes carry several cilia[4] on their bulbous ends[5] while their central axons[6] band together to form bundles of the olfactory nerve[7]; the apical surfaces of the tall supporting cells form a forest of branching microvilli[8] that surround the ciliated end bulbs of the olfactory cell processes. Several small tubular Bowman's glands[9] discharge their secretion on the surface of this epithelium.

(2) Olfactory sensory cells (Plate 69, Fig. B)

Their apical end bulb[1] possesses (a) several cilia[2] of the 9 + 2 type that tend to run parallel to the epithelial surface and are attached to basal corpuscles[3], (b) numerous large mitochondria[4], and (c) several ribosomes, microtubules and smooth vesicles. The manner in which chemical stimuli elicit impulses and, therefore, "odor sensation" in them is still obscure. Recent research, however, suggests that the identification of myriads of compounds by these cells is a stereochemical process whereby molecules of different size, shape and electrical charge "fit" different receptors on the PM of the apical end bulbs and (or) their cilia; there appear to be seven basic receptor types that recognize as many basic molecular configurations and elicit seven "primary odor sensations", all other olfactory sensations being combinations of the primary seven.

(3) Supporting cells (Plate 69, Figs. C_1–C_2)

They are characterised by (a) numerous relatively long and branching apical microvilli[1] that form a forest in which the endbulbs and the cilia of the sensory cells are buried, (b) a terminal web[2], (c) several vesicles and dense bodies[3] (apparently dense mucous droplets), (d) numerous small mitochondria[4] wrapped in flattened SER sacs[5], (e) basal glycogen[6], and (f) zonulae adherentes joining them to the sensory cells. One of their functions is apparently to secrete mucus which together with the secretion of Bowman's glands covers the apical surfaces of the sensory cells. They may also play an auxiliary role in the perception of olfactory stimuli.

(4) Basal cells (Plate 69, Fig. D)

These are undifferentiated cells and probably function as a reserve for the replacement of sensory cells, as indicated by the occasional documentation of mitoses in them, by the existence of transitional cells between the former and the latter in young animals and by recent reports of regeneration of neuroepithelial from basal cells under certain conditions. Regeneration of sensory cells, however, has also been observed to proceed from the duct cells of Bowman's glands, after destruction of the olfactory epithelium by $ZnSO_4$.

(5) Bowman's glands (Plate 69, Fig. E)

The main or "dark" cell types of their secretory portions are characterised by a luxurious SER; they produce a watery secretion that possibly contains glycolipids and provides a solvent for the molecules that stimulate the olfactory sensory cells. A "light" cell variant has also been described.

V. TASTE BUDS

(1) General (Plate 70, Fig. A)

A taste bud consists of a cluster of elongated sensory taste receptor cells[1] and supporting cells[2] that are arranged parallel to one another and are embedded within the squamous stratified epithelium[3] lining a certain area of the tongue. The apical ends of the taste cells carry thin hair-like processes[4] that converge into a small pit[5] (filled with an amorphous dense neutral mucopolysaccharide material) which communicates with the mouth cavity; the receptor cells respond to the various chemicals that reach them by generating impulses which are picked up by afferent axon terminals[6] embedded in pits of their basal ends (the glossopharyngeal nerve rootlets) and carried to the brain. The location of synaptic vesicles in the receptor cell-axon synapses seems to vary with the species; in frogs and carps, the synaptic vesicles are in the receptor cell cytoplasm mostly, while in other animals the reverse seems to be true.

(2) Taste receptor (dark) cells (Plate 70, Fig. B)

The long apical process (hair) of each taste cell proves to represent a group of several long microvilli[1] with filamentous cores[2] while its cytoplasm is distinguished by a dense matrix and numerous mostly apical granules[3] which are produced in the RER, concentrated in the Golgi and secreted into the taste pit. The chemoreceptor mechanism that generates impulses in the taste cells is still under debate.

(3) Supporting (light) cells (Plate 70, Fig. C)

These are characterised by a lucent, watery matrix and numerous usually dilated SER vesicles[1]. Some of them seem to be contacted synaptically by axon terminals too. Their function is unsettled. Recently, it was proposed that these light cells are the real sensory receptors while the dark cells with the granules and the microvilli have a supporting function. Additional research is evidently needed in this area.

VI. PACINIAN CORPUSCLES (DEEP PRESSURE RECEPTORS)

A Pacinian corpuscle consists of a myelinated peripheral (afferent) axon with an endbulb that contains numerous mitochondria and some synaptic-type vesicles, surrounded by concentric shells of collagen ("lamellae") with attached flat mesenchymal (endothelium-like) cells, which are more crowded centrally than peripherally; the spaces between the lamellae are filled with tissue fluid. When pressure is applied to a Pacinian corpuscle it elicits an impulse in its axon through an unknown mechanism, perhaps by stretching it and increasing its permeability for Na^+ ions.

Bibliography

CONTENTS

Electron microscopic histology (General textbooks & reviews)
J.A.G. Rhodin, *An Atlas of Ultrastructure*, Saunders, Philadelphia, London, 1963 - S.M. Kurtz, *Electron Microscopic Anatomy*, Academic Press, New York, London, 1964 - D.W. Fawcett, *An Atlas of Fine Structure*, Saunders, Philadelphia, London, 1966 - K.R. Porter and M.A. Bonneville, *Fine Structure of Cells and Tissues*, Lea and Febiger, Philadelphia, 1968 - E.B. Sandborn, *Cells and Tissues by Light and Electron Microscopy, Vols. 1 and 2*, Academic Press, New York, London, 1970 - T.L. Lentz, *Cell Fine Structure*, Saunders, Philadelphia, London, 1971 - J.L. Matthews and J.H. Martin, *An Atlas of Human Histology and Ultrastructure*, Lea and Febiger, Philadelphia, 1971 - M.J. Hollenberg and A.M. Erickson, J. Histochem. Cytochem., 21(1973)109

General molecular biology
J.D. Watson, *Molecular Biology of the Gene*, Benjamin, New York, Amsterdam, 1965 - J.B. Finean, *Biological Ultrastructure*, Academic Press, New York, London, 1967 - C.U.M. Smith, *Molecular Biology*, Faber and Faber, London, 1968

Membranes, natural
Structure and function (general texts and reviews) W. Fawcett, *The membranes of the cytoplasm*, Lab. Invest., 10(1961)1162 - A.S.G. Curtis, *The Cell Surface*, Logos Press and Academic Press, London, New York, 1967 - W.D. Stein, *The Movement of Molecules across Cell Membranes*, Academic Press, London, New York, 1967 - D. Branton and R.B. Park (Eds.), *Papers on Biological Membrane Structure*, Little, Brown, Boston, 1968 - J. Järnefelt (Ed.), *Regulatory Functions of Biological Membranes*, Elsevier Amsterdam, London, New York, 1968 - D.H. Northcote (Ed.), *Structure and Function of Membranes*, Brit. Med. Bull., 24(2)(1968)101 - W. Stoeckenius and D.M. Engelman, J. Cell Biol., 42(1969)613
Structure (freeze-etching) P. Pinto da Silva and D. Branton, J. Cell Biol., 45(1970)598

Intramembranous particles (freeze-etching)
V.T. Marchesi *et al.*, Proc. Nat. Acad. Sci., 69 (1972) 1445 - T.W. Tillack *et al.*, J. Exp. Med., 135(1972)1209 - D.S. Friend, Anat. Rec., 175(1973)324

Membranes, artificial
D. Chapman and D.J. Fluck, J. Cell Biol., 30(1966)1 - O.R. Anderson *et al.*, J. Ultrastruct. Res., 19(1967)600 - K.D. Dreher *et al.*, J. Ultrastruct. Res., 19(1967)586

Coats
Cytochemistry (carbohydrate and other components) - D.C. Pease, J. Ultrastruct. Res., 15(1966)555 - A. Rambourg and C.P Leblond, J. Cell Biol., 32(1967)27 - B. Monis *et al.*, Z. Zellforsch., 99(1969)64 - A. Rambourg, J. de Microscopie, 8(1969)325

Basement membranes
Structure M.H. Ross and L. Grant, Exp. Cell Res., 50-(1968)277 - A. Rambourg and C.P. Leblond, J. Ultrastruct. Res., 20(1967)306
Origin G.B. Pierce *et al.*, Amer. J. Path., 45(1964)929 - W. Linb, Morph. Jb., 111(1967)429

Junctions
Structure (general, including freeze-etch studies) S. Bullivant and W.R. Loewenstein, J. Cell Biol., 37(1968)621 - M.V.L. Bennett and J.P. Trinkaus, J. Cell Biol., 44(1970)592 - M.A. Spycher, Z. Zellforsch., 111(1970)64 - J.Z. Rosenblith and J.P. Revel, Anat. Rec., 172(1972)394
Structure (hemidesmosome) C.F. Flickinger, Anat. Rec., 168 (1970)195
Structure (septate desmosome (including freeze-cleave studies)) J. Gouranton, J. de Microscopie, 6(1967)505 - R.E. Bulger and B.F. Trump, Exp. Cell Res., 51(1968)587 - L.V. Danilova *et al.*, Z. Zellforsch., 100(1969)101 - N.S. McNutt and R.S. Weinstein, J. Cell Biol., 47(1970)666

Cilia
Structure R. Gliddon, J. Cell Science, 1(1966)439 - F.L. Renaud *et al.*, J. Cell Biol., 36(1968)79
Origin (ciliogenesis, from centrioles) D. Frisch and A.I. Farbman, Anat. Rec., 162(1968)221 - H.E. Heist and B.D. Mulvaney, J. Ultrastruct. Res., 24(1968)86 - P. Martinez Martinez and W.T. Daems, Z. Zellforsch., 87(1968)46 - V.I. Kalnins and K.R. Porter, Z. Zellforsch., 100(1969)1 - L.L. Millecchia and M.A. Rudzinska, J. Cell Biol., 46 (1970)553
Effects of chloral hydrate (deciliation) J.R. Kennedy and E. Brittingham, J. Ultrastruct. Res., 22(1968)530

Pinocytosis
Function (the pinocytotic process) H. Holter, Sci. American, 205(1961)167 - W. Stockem, Z. Zellforsch., 74(1966)372 - K.E. Wohlfarth-Bottermann and W. Stockem, Z. Zellforsch., 73(1966)444 - B. Riedel and W.O. Gross, Z. Zellforsch., 92(1968)360
Function (role of the "bristle coat" in the formation of "alveolate" vesicles) D.B. Slautterback, J. Cell Science, 2 (1967)563 - T. Kanaseki, Jap. J. Electr. Micr., 19(3) (1970)253

Phagocytosis
Function (uptake of particulate matter) M.C. Loni *et al.*, Z. Zellforsch., 76(1967)525 - H. Nakahara and G. Bevelander, J. Morph., 122(1967)139 - M.G. Wetzel and E.D. Korn, J. Cell Biol., 43(1969)90

Ribosomes
Structure E.L. Benedetti *et al.*, Lab. Invest., 15(1966)196 - N.T. Florendo, J. Cell Biol., 41(1969)335 - J.Y. Haga *et al.*, J. Cell Biol., 47 (1970)211
Function (protein synthesis) Y. Tashiro *et al.*, J. Cell Biol. - III. J. Cell Biol., 38(1968)604
Effects of hypothermia B. Byers, J. Cell Biol., 30(1966)451

Smooth endoplasmic reticulum membranes
Structure W. Hasselbach and L.G. Elfvin, J. Ultrastruct. Res., 17(1967)598 - K.S. Prezbindowski *et al.*, Exp. Cell Res., 50(1968)241
Origin (biogenesis) G. Dallner *et al.*, J. Cell Biol., 30(1966)73
Cytochemistry (enzymatic activities) P.R. Dallman *et al.*, J. Cell Biol., 41(1969)357 - J.M. Papadimitriou and P. Van Duijn, J. Cell Biol., 47(1970)84

Golgi
Structure B. Fleischer *et al.*, J. Cell Biol., 43(1969)59

Function (synthesis of complex carbohydrates) A. Rambourg *et al.*, J. Cell Biol., 40(1969)395 - J.P. Thiery, J. de Microscopie, 8(1969)689

Origin C.J. Flickinger, J. Cell Biol., 43(1969)250

Effects of medium renewal on Golgi of cultured cells B. Riedel and W.O. Gross, Z. Zellforsch., 94(1969)220

Secretion (general)

S.L. Palay, The morphology of secretion. In: S.L. Palay (Ed.), *Frontiers in Cytology*, Yale University Press, New Haven, 1958, pp. 305–342

Annulate lamellae

Structure R.G. Kessel, J. Cell Biol., 36(1968)658 - G.G. Maul, J. Cell Biol., 46(1970)604

Mitochondria

Structure H.W. Deane *et al.*, Z. Zellforsch, 75(1966)166 - Y. Shinagawa *et al.*, Exp. Cell Res., 43(1966)301 - I.S. Vaisman, Arkh. Anat. Gistol. Embriol., 51(10)(1966)31 - M. Hagopian, J. Morph., 122(1967)147 - S.K. Malhotra and R.T. Eakin, J. Cell Science., 2(1967)205 - C. Noirot-Timothee and C. Noirot, J. de Microscopie, 6(1967)87 - W. Thoenes, Morph. Jb., 111(1967)462 - D. Lloyd and A.J. Griffiths, Exp. Cell Res., 51(1968)291 - F.S. Sjöstrand and L. Barajas, J. Ultrastruct. Res., 25(1968) 121 - Y. Le Beux *et al.*, Z. Zellforsch., 99(1969)491 - J.R. Ruby *et al.*, Z. Zellforsch., 97(1969)30 - M.T. Tellez De Inon *et al.*, J. de Microscopie, 8(1969)615

Cytochemistry (digestion by enzymes) K. Deutsch and W. Krause, Jap. J. Electr. Micr., 16(2)(1967)143

Cytochemistry (lipid content) S. Fleischer *et al.*, J. Cell Biol., 32(1967)193

Cytochemistry (DNA content) F.S. Vogel, Lab. Invest., 14 (1965)1849 - F.S. Vogel and L. Kemper, Lab. Invest., 14(1965)1868 - T. Bisalputra and A.A. Bisalputra, J. Cell Biol., 33(1967)511

Function (synthesis of RNA) F.S. Vogel and L. Kemper, Exp. Cell Res., 47(1967)209 - J.J. Curgy, J. de Microscopie, 7(1968)849

Function (specific metabolic activities) C.R. Hackenbrock, J. Cell Biol., 30(1966)269 - E.C. Weinbach *et al.*, Exp. Cell Res., 46(1967)129 - C.R. Hackenbrock, J. Cell Biol., 37 (1968)345 - L. Ernster and Z. Drahota (Eds.), *Mitochondria – Structure and Function,* Academic Press, London, New York, 1969 - U. Muscatello and E. Carafoli, J. Cell Biol., 40(1969)602

Origin, regeneration and proliferation H. Klug, Z. Mikr.-Anat. Forsch., 75(1966)109 - A.A. Manina, Arkh. Anat. Gistol. Embriol., 52(3)(1967)77 - R.H. Hedley and J.ST. Wakefield, Z. Zellforsch. 87(1968)429 - M. Osumi and N. Sando, Jap. J. Electr. Micr., 18(1)(1969)47 - C. Stang-Voss and J. Staubesand, Z. Zellforsch., 111(1970)127

Effects of electromagnetic fields K.A. Zufarov and V.B. Shneivais, Arkh. Anat. Gistol. Embriol., 57(No.12) (1969)22

Effects of ruby laser microbeam Y. Tanaka, J. Cell Biol., 41(1969)424

Effects of starvation E.W. Daniels and E.P. Breyer, Z. Zellforsch., 91(1968)159

Effects of glutamine-deficiency M. Jagendorf-Elfvin and E. Elliasson, J. Cell Biol., 41(1969)905

Effects of calcium C.R. Hackenbrock and A.I. Caplan, J. Cell Biol., 42(1969)221

Effects of lead R.A. Goyer and R. Krall, J. Cell Biol., 41 (1969)393

Effects of ambient osmolarity C.D. Stoner and H.D. Sirak, J. Cell Biol., 43(1969)521

Effects of thyroid hormone L.D. Peachey and R.L. Greif, Endocrinol., 77(1965)61

Effects of cortisone D.V. Kimberg *et al.*, J. Cell Biol., 37 (1968)63

Other effects (see section on liver mitochondria, p. 218)

Chloroplasts

Structure (DNA molecule content) G. Werz and G. Kellner, J. Ultrastruct. Res., 24(1968)109

Origin (biogenesis) I. Ohad *et al.*, J. Cell Biol. 35(1967)521, 553

Lysosomes

Structure W. Schwarz, Z. Zellforsch., 73(1966)27 - H.R. Thacore and D.A. Wolff, Exp. Cell Res., 49(1968)266

Cytochemistry (enzymes) H.J. Mohr, Morph. Jb., 111(1967) 454

Function (in lytic processes) D. Brandes and E. Anton, Lab. Invest., 15(1966)987

Microbodies

D. Svoboda *et al.*, J. Cell Biol., 35(1967)127 - V.H. Black, Anat. Rec., 172(1972)271

Multivesicular bodies

Cytochemistry D.S. Friend, J. Cell Biol., 41(1969)269

Origin W. Kilarski and A. Jasinski, J. Cell Biol., 45(1970)205

Filaments

Structure F. Kallman and N.K. Wessells, J. Cell Biol., 32(1967)227 - L.T. Chen and L. Weiss, Anat. Rec., 172(1972)288 - H.L. Malech and T.L. Lentz, Anat. Rec., 175(1973)382

Structure (filaments related to ameboid movement) T.D. Pollard and S. Ito, J. Cell Biol., 46(1970)267

Relation to cell contraction B. Burnside, Anat. Rec., 172(1972)281

Relation to cell surface mobility and phagocytosis J. Overton and N. Culver, Anat. Rec., 175(1973)404

Microtubules

Structure W.A. Anderson *et al.*, Z. Zellforsch., 71(1966)1 - J.G. Gall, J. Cell Biol., 31(1966)639 - A.C. Taylor, J. Cell Biol., 28(1966)155 - L. Tilney *et al.*, J. Cell Biol., 29 (1966)77 - I.B. Tokin, Arkh. Anat. Gistol. Embriol., 51 (10)(1966)3 - O. Behnke and A. Forer, J. Cell Science, 2(1967)169 - P.R. Burton, J. Cell Biol., 44(1970)693

Immunochemical protein composition J. Alcala and A. La Velle, Anat. Rec., 172(1972)260 - A. La Velle, Anat. Rec., 175(1973)368

Functions C.A. Auclair and B. Messier, Anat. Rec., 175(1973)267 - L.G. Tilney, Fed. Am. Soc. Exp. Biol., symposium on Microtubules, Atlantic City, April 1973, In press

Development T.M. Harris, Anat. Rec., 172(1972)325

Effects of vinblastine G.E. Tyson and R.E. Bulger, Anat. Rec. 175(1973)459

Centriole

Structure A. Ross, J. Ultrastruct. Res., 23(1968)537

Effects of acriflavine on centriolar DNA M. Steinert and S.V. Assel, J. Cell Biol., 34(1967)489

Ameboid movement
S. Schafer-Danneel, Z. Zellforsch., 78(1967)441

Light-generating (photogenic) organelles
S. Yasutake *et al.*, Jap. J. Electr. Micr., 12(4)(1963)240 - V.C. Barber and P.N Dilly, Z. Zellforsch., 73(1966)286 - J.M. Bassot, Z. Zellforsch., 74(1966)474 - J.M. Strum, Anat. Rec., 164(1969)433

Electricity-generating organelles
M.N. Sheridan *et al.*, Z. Zellforsch., 74(1966)291 - R.M. Meszler, Anat. Rec., 172(1972)367

Gas-secreting organelles
D.E. Copeland, Z. Zellforsch., 93(1969)305

Glycogen inclusions
Structure α and β particles C. Biava, Lab. Invest., 12(1963) 1179 - T. Iwamasa *et al.*, Jap. J. Electr. Micr., 19(4) (1970)371
Structure (glycogen bodies (glycogen-SER complexes)) Y.J. Le Beux, *(maintenance* Zellforsch., 96(1969)325

Ferritin inclusions
G.W. Richter, Lab. Invest., 12(1963)1026

Calcium inclusions
J. Andre and E. Faure-Fremiet, J. de Microscopie, 6(1967) 391

Nucleus
Structure and function (general) A. Dalton and F. Haguenau (Eds.), *The Nucleus*, Academic Press, New York, London, 1968
Structure (general, including perichromatin and interchromatin) P.D. Sadowski and J.W. Steiner, J. Cell Biol., 37(1968)147 - A. Bererhi and K. Malkani, J. de Microscopie, 8(1969)841 - A. Monneron and W. Bernhard, J. Ultrastruct. Res., 27(1969)266 - N.G. Garcia and A.M. Garcia, Anat. Rec., 175(1973)325
Structure (nuclear envelope) W.W. Franke, J. Cell Biol., 31 (1966)619 - W.W. Franke, Z. Zellforsch., 80(1967)585 - G. Patrizi and M. Poger, J. Ultrastruct. Res., 17(1967)127 - E. Vivier, J. de Microscopie, 6(1967)371 - J.C. Weston, Z. Zellforsch., 87(1968)199 - W.W. Franke *et al.*, J. Cell Biol., 46(1970)379
Structure (nuclear pore complexes) J.G. Gall, J. Cell Biol., 32(1967)391 - E.W. Daniels *et al.*, Z. Zellforsch., 98 (1969)357 - P. Comes and W.W. Franke, Z. Zellforsch, 107(1970)240 - W.W. Franke, Z. Zellforsch., 105(1970) 405 - V. Speth and F. Wunderlich, J. Cell Biol., 47 (1970)772 - J. Scogna, Anat. Rec., 172(1972)402
Structure (inner fibrous lamina) D.W. Fawcett, Amer. J. Anat., 119(1966)129 - S.R. Kalifat *et al.*, J. de Microscopie, 5(1967)1019 - K. Mazanec, J. de Microscopie, 6 (1967)1027
Structure (inclusions other than chromatin and nucleolus) G.D. Bloom, J. Cell Biol., 35(1967)266 - E. Bucciarelli, J. Cell Biol., 30(1966)664 - D.W. Buttner and E. Horstmann, Z. Zellforsch., 77(1967)589 - A. Krishan *et al.*, J. Ultrastruct. Res., 19(1967)563 - M. Mori and T. Onoé, Jap. J. Electr. Micr., 16(2)(1967)137 - D.W. Buttner, Z. Zellforsch., 85(1968)527 - H. Norberg, Z. Zellforsch., 110 (1970)61
Cytochemistry (DNA isolation) D.K. Chattoraj *et al.*, Jap. J. Electr. Micr., 18(4)(1969)272
Cytochemistry (DNA binding by actinomycin and antibodies) K.W. Jones, J. Ultrastruct. Res., 18(1967)71 - R. Simard, J. Cell Biol., 35(1967)716
Cytochemistry (RNA in nuclear pores) P. Meutré, J. de Microscopie, 8(1969)51
Cytochemistry (RNA in perichromatin granules) H. Yamamoto *et al.*, Jap. J. Electr. Micr., 18(1)(1969)57
Cytochemistry (enzymes) G. Yasuzumi *et al.*, Jap. J. Electr. Micr., 14(4)(1965)346 - A. Vorbrodt and W. Bernhard, J. de Microscopie, 7(1968)195
Cytochemistry (inorganic cations) C.J. Tandler *et al.*, J. Cell Biol., 45(1970)355
Function (maintenance of cytoplasmic membranes) C.J. Flickinger, J. Cell Biol., 37(1968)300
Function (transport of materials from nucleus to cytoplasm) B.J. Stevens and H. Swift, J. Cell Biol., 31(1966)55 - J.C. Clerot, J. de Microscopie, 7(1968)973 - Y. Tashiro *et al.*, J. Cell Biol., 36(3)(1968)C5 - N. Hillman and R.J. Tasca, Amer. J. Anat., 126(1969)151 - A. Monneron and W. Bernhard, J. Ultrastruct. Res., 27(1969)266 - B. Scharrer and S. Wurzelman, Z. Zellforsch., 96(1969)325
Function (transport of materials from cytoplasm to nucleus) C.M. Feldherr, J. Cell Biol., 42(1969)841

Nucleolus
Structure E.D. Hay and J.B. Gurdon, J. Cell Science, 2(1967) 151
Cytochemistry (nucleic acid and protein content of nucleolar constituents) N. Paweletz *et al.*, Z. Zellforsch., 76(1967) 577 - K. Smetana *et al.*, Exp. Cell Res., 51(1968)105 - J. Recher *et al.*, J. Ultrastruct. Res., 29(1969)1 - L. Recher *et al.*, J. Cell Biol., 45(1970)479
Origin (from "nucleolar organizer" chromatin) S.G. Phillips and D.M. Phillips, J. Cell Biol., 40(1969)248
Function (RNA formation) H.C. MacGregor, J. Cell Science, 2(1967)145
Effects of heat R. Simard and W. Bernhard, J. Cell Biol., 34(1967)61
Effects of fluorouracil U. Stenram, Z. Zellforsch., 94(1969) 282
Effects of actinomycin D C.J. Flickinger, J. Ultrastruct. Res., 23(1968)260 - T. Unuma, Jap. J. Electr. Micr., 18 (1)(1969)25
Effects of various metabolic inhibitors (comprehensive review) E. Farber, *Biochemical Pathology*, Ann. Rev. Pharmacol., 11(1971)71

Nuclear division (mitotic)
Structural aspects (general) C.M. Feldherr, J. Cell Biol., 31 (1966)199 - G. Gimenez-Martin *et al.*, Exp. Cell Res., 43(1966)293 - A.L. Allenspach and L.E. Roth, J. Cell Biol., 33(1967)179 - T. Kuroiwa and N. Tanaka, Jap. J. Electr. Micr., 19(1)(1970)63
Structural aspects (chromosome kinetochores, centromeres) R.C. Buck, J. Ultrastruct. Res., 18(1967)489 - P.T. Jokelainen, J. Ultrastruct. Res., 19(1967)19
Structural aspects (centriole and mitotic spindle) M. Friedlander and J. Wahrman, J. Cell Sci., 1(1966)129 - E. Robbins *et al.*, J. Cell Biol., 36(1968)329 - E. Robbins

and G. Jentzsch, J. Cell Biol., 40(1969)678 - P.K. Hepler *et al.*, J. Cell Biol., 45(1970)438

Structural aspects (synaptinemal complexes of chromosomes) P.B. Moens, J. Cell Biol., 40(1969)542 - L.F. La Cour and B. Wells, J. Cell Sci., 6(1970)655

Structural aspects (sex chromosomes (sex vesicles)) A.J. Solari, J. Ultrastruct. Res., 27(1969)289

Effects of mitotic inhibitors B.R. Brinkley *et al.*, J. Ultrastruct. Res., 19(1967)1 - L.E. Roth, J. Cell Biol., 34 (1967)47 - A. Krishan, J. Ultrastruct. Res., 23(1968)134

Effecıs of radiation on chromosomes R.M. Humphrey and B.R. Brinkley, J. Cell Biol., 42(1969)745

Effects of ecdysone (an insect hormone) on polytene chromosomes M. Lezzi and L.I. Gilbert, J. Cell Sci., 6(1970) 615

Nuclear division (amitotic)

Structural aspects (general) I. Boll *et al.*, Z. Zellforsch., 83 (1967)1 - F.W. Pehlemann, Z. Zellforsch., 84(1968)516

Functional (nucleus constricting filament ring) J. Boddingins, Z. Zellforsch., 108(1970)59

Cytoplasmic division

Functional (role of contractile filament ring in cytoplasmic cleavage) L.G. Tilney and D. Marsland, J. Cell Biol., 42 (1969)170 - D.G. Scott and C.W. Daniel, J. Cell Biol., 45(1970)461

Effects of cytochalasin-B on the contractile ring A. Krishan and R. Ray-Chaudhuri, J. Cell Biol., 43(1969)618 - T.E. Schroeder, Z. Zellforsch., 109(1970)431

Cell fusion (fertilisation-induced)

F.J. Longo and E. Anderson, J. Ultrastruct. Res., 29(1969)86 - B. Gondos and P. Bhiraleus, Z. Zellforsch., 111(1970)149

Cell fusion (virus-induced)

E.E. Schneeberger and H. Harris, J. Cell Sci., 1(1966)401

4. CONNECTIVE TISSUES

Areolar and Dense Fibrous Tissue

Collagen

Structure L. Ornstein, J. Biophys. Biochem. Cytol., 2(1956) 297 - F. Wassermann *et al.*, Exp. Cell Res., 13(1957)407 - K.E. Wohlfarth-Bottermann and E. Kuhnke, Naturwissenschaften, 44(1957)595 - W. Schwarz, Z. Zellforsch., 48 (1958)309 - N.V. Fernando *et al.*, Exp. Molec. Path., 3 (1964)529 - B.R. Olsen, J. Ultrastruct. Res., 19(1967)432

Histochemistry F.O. Schmitt, Rev. Modern Phys., 31(1959) 349 - A.J. Hodge and F.O. Schmitt, in: M.V. Edds, Jr. (Ed.), *Macromolecular Complexes*, Ronald Press, New York, N.Y., 1961, p. 19

Development and biosynthesis M. Nishikawa, Arch. Histol. Japan, 14(1958)463 - H.J. Merker, Z. Zellforsch., 53 (1961)411 - K.R. Porter, Biophys. J., 4(1964) Suppl. 167 - R.L. Hayes and E.R. Allen, J. Cell Sci., 2(1967)419

Ageing C.D. Norschow, Exp. Molec. Path., 5(1966)350

Elastin

Structure T.K. Greenlee *et al.*, J. Cell Biol., 30(1966)59 - J.J. Taylor and V.L. Yeager, Anat. Rec., 156(1966)129 - R. Ross and P. Bornstein, J. Cell Biol., 40(1969)366

Development W.H. Fahrenbach *et al.*, Anat. Rec., 155(1966) 563 - A.J. Collet and G. Des Biens, Anat. Rec., 175 (1973)295

Microfibrils

Structure F.N. Low, Anat. Rec., 142(1962)131 - D. Haust, Amer. J. Path., 47(1965)1113 - R.G. Frederickson and F.N. Low, Amer. J. Anat., 130(1971)347 - E.C. Carlson and F.N. Low, Amer. J. Anat., 130(1971)331

Oxytalan fibers

Structure G.G. Carmichael and H.M. Fullmer, J. Cell Biol., 28 (1966)33

Amorphous ground substance

Histochemistry J.H. Yardley and G.D. Brown, Lab. Invest., 14(1965)501 - M. Schubert, Biophys. J., 4(1964)Suppl. 119 - H.H.R. Friederici, J. Ultrastruct. Res., 24(1968)269 - K. Kajikawa *et al.*, Jap. J. Electr. Micr., 19(1970)347

Fibroblasts

Structure H.Z. Movat and N.V.P. Fernando, Exp. Molec. Path., 1(1962)509 - K. Kajikawa, Jap. J. Electr. Micr., 12(1963)159 - H.S. Di Stefano, Z. Zellforsch., 72(1966) 157 - D. Reibig and K. Schippel, Morph. Jb., 111(1967) 372 - R.G.P. Pugh-Humphreys and W. Sinclair, J. Cell Sci., 6(1970)477 - J.H. Yardley *et al.*, Bull. Johns Hopk. Hosp., 106(1960)381 - J.A. Chapman, Brit. Med. Bull., 18(1962)233 - R. Ross and E.P. Benditt, J. Cell Biol., 15(1962)99 - W. Schwarz *et al.*, Z. Zellforsch., 56(1962) 107 - C.W. Castor and K.D. Muirden, Lab. Invest., 13(1964)560 - R. Ross and E.P. Benditt, J. Cell Biol., 27(1965)83 - M.E. Fedorko *et al.*, J. Cell Biol., 38(1968) 377

Development S. Fitton-Jackson, Proc. roy. Soc. London, 144B(1956)556 - F. Wassermann and L. Kubota, J. Biophys. Biochem. Cytol., 2(1956)67 - K.R. Porter and G.D. Pappas, J. Biophys. Biochem. Cytol., 5(1959)153 - K. Kajikawa, Jap. J. Electr. Micr., 10(1961)131 - T.K. Greenlee and R. Ross, J. Ultrastruct. Res., 18(1967)354 - R. Ross *et al.*, J. Cell Biol., 44(1970)645

Teratogenesis D.N. Wheatley, J. Anat., 105(1969)351

Regeneration and repair J.A. Chapman, J. Biophys. Biochem. Cytol., 9(1961)639 - R. Peach *et al.*, Amer. J. Path., 38 (1961)495 - R. Ross and E.P. Benditt, J. Biophys. Biochem. Cytol., 11(1961)677 - N.V.P. Fernando and H.Z. Movat, Lab. Invest., 12(1963)214

Effects of vitamin C deficiency R. Peach, J. Ultrastruct. Res., 6(1962)579 - R. Ross and E.P. Benditt, J. Cell Biol., 12 (1962)533 - I.A. Schafer *et al.*, J. Cell Biol., 34(1967)83

Effects of alkaloids K.G. Bensch and S.E. Malawista, J. Cell Biol., 40(1969)95
Effects of colchicine E. Stubblefield and B.R. Brinkley, J. Cell Biol., 30(1966)645

Macrophages
Structure T.J. Athanassiades *et al.*, Lab. Invest., 14(1965)409 - I. Carr *et al.*, Z. Zellforsch., 105(1970)339
Histochemistry R.J. North, J. Ultrastruct. Res., 16(1966)83
Function E. Skutelsky and D. Danon, J. Cell Biol., 43(1969) 8 - A Dumont, J. Ultrastruct. Res., 29(1969)191
Origin and giant cell formation J.S. Sutton and L. Weiss, J. Cell Biol., 28(1966)303

Mast cells
Structure N.V.P. Fernando and H.Z. Movat, Exp. Molec. Path., 2(1963)450 - A. Serafini-Fracassini *et al.*, J. Ultrastruct. Res., 28(1969)131 - T. Kobayashi *et al.*, J. Ultrastruct. Res., 23(1968)153
Histochemistry S. Schiller, Ann. N.Y. Acad. Sci., 103(1963) 199 - D. Lagunoff *et al.*, Lab. Invest., 13(1964)1331 - G.T. Gustafson and E. Pihl, Acta Path. Microbiol. Scand., 69(1967)393
Function E.P. Benditt *et al.*, Ann. N.Y. Acad. Sci., 103 (1963)179 - J.F. Riley, Ann. N.Y. Acad. Sci., 103(1963) 151 - D.E. Smith, Ann. N.Y. Acad. Sci., 103(1963)40 - J.P. Thiery, J. de Microscopie, 2(1963)549 - T. Setoguti, J. Ultrastruct. Res., 27(1969)377 - G.L. Brinkman, J. Ultrastruct. Res., 23(1968)115 - J. Padawer, J. Cell Biol., 40 (1969)747
Development and differentiation J.W. Combs, J. Cell Biol., 31(1966)563 - H. Ginsburg and D. Lagunoff, J. Cell Biol., 35(1967)685 - L. Vollrath and T. Wahlin, Z. Zellforsch., 111(1970)286 - H. Fujita *et al.*, J. Ultrastruct. Res., 28 (1969)353
Effects of microwaves E.J. Valtonen, Z. Zellforsch., 80(1967)322
Effects of compound 48/80 G.D. Bloom and O. Haegermark, Exp. Cell Res., 40(1965)637

Adipose Tissue

White
Structure H. Sheldon, in: K. Rodahl and B. Issekutz, Jr. (Eds.), *Fat as a Tissue,* McGraw-Hill, New York, 1964, p. 41 - L. Napolitano, in: A.E. Renold and G.F. Cahill, Jr. (Eds.), *Handbook of Physiology; Adipose Tissue,* American Physiological Society, Washington, D.C., 1965, p. 109 - S.W. Cushman, J. Cell Biol., 46(1970)326
Histochemistry R.J. Barnett. In: L.W. Kinsel (Ed.), *Adipose Tissue as an Organ,* Thomas, Springfield, Ill., 1962, p. 3 - D.W. McKeel and L. Jarrett, J. Cell Biol., 44(1970)417
Function F. Wasserman and T.F. McDonald, Z. Zellforsch., 59(1963)326 - J.R. Williamson, J. Cell Biol., 20(1964)57 - M. Locke and J.V. Collins, J. Cell Biol., 36(1968)453 - S.W. Cushman, J. Cell Biol., 46(1970)342
Development L. Napolitano, J. Cell Biol., 18(1963)663 - E.M. Wood, Anat. Rec., 157(1967)437
Effects of Epinephrine S.K. Murthy, Exp. Cell Res., 46(1967)155

Brown
Structure W. Bargmann *et al.*, Z. Zellforsch., 85(1968)601 - E.R. Suter, Lab. Invest., 21(1969)246
Development T. Barnard, J. Ultrastruct. Res., 29(1969)311
Function D. Picard *et al.*, Z. Zellforsch., 69(1966)260 - O. Lindberg *et al.*, J. Cell Biol., 34(1967)293 - V. Mizuhira and H. Ozawa, Jap. J. Electr. Micr., 16(2)(1967)173 - J.F. Thomson *et al.*, J. Cell Biol., 41(1969)312

Effects of cold exposure
E.R. Suter, Lab. Invest., 21(1969)259

Cartilage

Structure H. Sheldon and R.A. Robinson, J. Biophys. Biochem. Cytol., 4(1958)401 - T. Zelander, Z. Zellforsch., 49(1959)720 - K.H. Knese and A.M. Knoop, Z. Zellforsch., 54(1961)1 - A.J. Palfrey and D.V. Davies, J. Anat., 100(1966)213 - J.P. Scherft and W.T. Daems, J. Ultrastruct. Res., 19(1967)546 - R. Silberberg and M. Hasler, Arch. Path., 87(1969)502 - J.P. Scherft, J. Ultrastruct. Res., 23(1968)333 - G. Levai and I. Marx, Z. Mikr.-Anat. Forsch., 80(1969)177
Histochemistry K.H. Knese and A.M. Knoop, Z. Zellforsch., 53(1961)201 - V.J. Matukas, *et al.*, J. Cell Biol., 32(1967) 365 - J.W. Smith *et al.*, J. Cell Sci., 2(1967)129 - G. Levai and I. Marx, Z. Mikr.-Anat. Forsch., 80(1969)582 - E. Bonucci, Z. Zellforsch., 103(1970)192 - R. Eisenstein *et al.*, J. Cell Biol., 46(1970)626 - J.W. Smith, J. Cell Sci., 6(1970)843
Function H. Sheldon and F.B. Kimball, J. Cell Biol., 12 (1962)599 - D. Fewer *et al.*, J. Ultrastruct. Res., 11(1964) 166 - G.C. Godman and N. Lane, J. Cell Biol., 21(1964) 353 - V. Mizuhira and K. Morimoto, Jap. J. Electr. Micr., 14(1965)328 - H. Rohr and G. Gebert, Beitr. Path. Anat., 135(1967)92 - G.W. Cooper and D.J. Prockop, J. Cell Biol., 38(1968)523 - A.L. Horwitz and A. Dorfman, J. Cell Biol., 38(1968)358 - H. Clarke Anderson, J. Cell Biol., 41(1969)59 - G. Levai and I. Marx, Z. Mikr.-Anat. Forsch., 80(1969)203
Development R.A. Robinson and D.A. Cameron, J. Biophys. Biochem. Cytol., 2(1956)Suppl. 253 - D.A. Cameron and R.A. Robinson, J. Bone and Joint Surg., 40(1958)163 - G.C. Godman and K.R. Porter, J. Biophys. Biochem. Cytol., 8(1960)719 - S. Takuma, Arch. Oral Biol., 2 (1960)111 - J.P. Revel and E.D. Hay, Z. Zellforsch., 61 (1963)110 - M.D. Olson and F.N. Low, Amer. J. Anat., 131(1971)197
Regeneration E.D. Hay, J. Biophys. Biochem. Cytol., 4(1958)583
Regression, ageing and calcification R. Silberberg *et al.*, Amer. J. Anat., 109(1961)251 - C.H. Anderson, J. Cell Biol., 35(1967)81 - E. Bonucci, J. Ultrastruct. Res., 20 (1967)33 - R.K. Schenk *et al.*, J. Cell Biol., 34(1967)275 - M.A. Spycher *et al.*, Z. Zellforsch., 98(1969)512
Effects of papain H. Sheldon and R.A. Robinson, J. Biophys. Biochem. Cytol., 8(1960)151
Effects of lard-enriched diet R. Silberberg *et al.*, Anat. Rec., 166(1970)447
Effects of hormones R. Silberberg *et al.*, Amer. J. Path., 46 (1965)289 - R. Silberberg *et al.*, Anat. Rec., 155(1966) 577

Bone

General and osteoblasts
Structure S. Fitton-Jackson and J.T. Randall, Nature, 178 (1956)798 - F.C. McLean, Science, 127(1958)451 - C.W.M. Pratt, Anat. Rec., 136(1960)261 - R.H. Dudley

R.A. Robinson and D.A. Cameron, in: S.M. Kurtz (Ed.), *Electron Microscopic Anatomy*, Academic Press, New York, 1964, p. 315 - A. Ascenzi *et al.*, J. Ultrastruct. Res., 18(1967)605 - D.G. Silva and J.A. Hart, J. Ultrastruct. Res., 20(1967)227 - A. Boyde, Z. Zellforsch., 93(1969) 213

Function (collagen synthesis and mineralization) S. Fitton-Jackson and R.H. Smith, J. Biophys. Biochem. Cytol., 3(1957)897 - H. Sheldon and R.A. Robinson, J. Biophys. Biochem. Cytol., 3(1957)1011 - R.A. Robinson and H. Sheldon, in: R.F. Sognnaes, *Calcification in Biological Systems*, AAAS, Publication No. 64, Washington, D.C., 1960, p. 261 - M.J. Glimcher, in: M.V. Edds, Jr. (Ed.), *Macromolecular Complexes*, The Ronald Press Company, New York, 1961, p. 53 - A. Ascenzi *et al.*, J. Ultrastruct. Res., 12(1965)287 - R. Ores *et al.*, Arch. Path., 88(1969) 54 - G.W. Bernard and D.C. Pease, Amer. J. Anat., 125 (1969)271 - R.M. Frank and P. Frank, Z. Zellforsch., 99 (1969)121 - M. Weinstock and C.P. Leblond, Anat. Rec., 175(1973)466

Histochemistry D.B. Myers *et al.*, J. Ultrastruct. Res., 28 (1969)203 - S. Jande and M. Windisch-Laroche, Anat. Rec., 172(1972)335

Development S. Fitton-Jackson, Proc. Roy. Soc. London, 146B(1957)270 - K.H. Knese and A.M. Knoop, Z. Zellforsch., 48(1958)455 - R.A. Robinson and D.A. Cameron, J. Bone and Joint Surg., 40A(1958)687 - K.H. Knese and A.M. Knoop, Z. Zellforsch., 55(1961)413 - J.D. Decker, Amer. J. Anat., 118(1966)591

Effects of nutritional factors (rickets, scurvy) H. Sheldon and R.A. Robinson, Z. Zellforsch., 53(1961)685 - H. Sheldon and R.A. Robinson, Z. Zellforsch., 53(1961)671 - E. Bonucci, J. de Microscopie, 5(1966)725

Effects of parathyroid hormone D.A. Cameron *et al.*, J. Cell Biol., 33(1967)1

Technical I.L. Baird *et al.*, Anat. Rec., 159(1967)281

Osteoclasts

Structure and function B.L. Scott, J. Ultrastruct. Res., 19 (1967)417 - F. Gonzales and M.J. Karnovsky, J. Biophys. Biochem. Cytol., 9(1961)299

Development N.M. Hancox and B. Boothroyd, J. Biophys. Biochem. Cytol., 11(1961)651

Joints

Synovial membrane

General F.N. Ghadially and S. Roy, in: *Ultrastructure of Synovial Joints in Health and Disease*, Butterworth, London, 1969, p. 1

Structure J.C. Wyllie *et al.*, Lab. Invest., 13(1964)1254

Histochemistry T. Ohkura, Jap. J. Electr. Micr., 15(1966)167 - P. Barland *et al.*, J. Cell Biol., 37(1968)13

Function W.S. Adam, Lab. Invest., 15(1966)680

Hemopoietic Tissue

General

Structure of blood cells F.N. Low and J.A. Freeman, *Electron Microscopic Atlas of Normal and Leukemic Human Blood*, McGraw-Hill, New York, 1958

Relations between myeloid and lymphoid cells C.E. Ford *et al.*, Ann. N.Y. Acad. Sci., 129(1966)283 - H.S. Micklem *et al.*, Proc. Roy. Soc. Biol., 165(1966)78

Reticular cells and reticuloendothelial system

Structure L. Weiss, Ann. N.Y. Acad. Sci., 73(1958)131 - L. Weiss, Anat. Rec., 136(1960)300 (Abstract) - S.S. Han, Anat. Rec., 139(1961)235 (Abstract) - J.M. Hill *et al.*, J. Appl. Phys., 32(1961)1643 - T. Hoshino, Z. Zellforsch., 59(1963)513 - G. Pereira and E.W. Dempsey, Anat. Rec., 175(1973)409

Function E. Essner, J. Biophys. Biochem. Cytol., 7(1960)329 - T. Kluge and T. Hovig, Amer, J. Path., 54(1969)355 - J.M. Rauchwerger *et al.*, Anat. Rec., 175(1973)420

Neutrophil leukocytes

General Y. Watanabe, Jap. J. Electr. Micr., 5(1957)46 - F. Campbell, J. Morph., 123(1967)405 - L.W. McDonald and T.L. Hayes, Exp. Molec. Path., 10(1969)186

Structure (general and granules) M. Bessis and J.P. Thiery, Int. Rev. Cytol., 12(1961)199 - K.E. Fritz *et al.*, Exp. Molec. Path. 3(1964)19 - D.R. Anderson, J. Ultrastruct. Res., Suppl., 9(1966)1 - I. Watanabe *et al.*, J. Ultrastruct. Res., 20(1967)366 - W.T. Daems, J. Ultrastruct. Res., 24 (1968)343 - M. Baggiolini *et al.*, J. Cell Biol., 40(1969) 529

Structure (Auer bodies) K. Kondo *et al.*, Jap. J. Electr. Micr., 15(4)(1966)237 - N. McDuffie, J. de Microscopie, 6 (1967)321

Cytochemistry Z.A. Cohn and J.G. Hirsch, J. Exp. Med., 112 (1960)983 - R.G. Horn *et al.*, J. Appl. Phys., 34(1963) 2517 - Y. Shinagawa *et al.*, Jap. J. Electr. Micr., 15(1966) 81 - G.A. Ackerman, Lab. Invest., 19(3)(1968)290 - J.H. Hardin *et al.*, Lab. Invest., 21(1969)214 - S.S. Spicer and J.H. Hardin, Lab. Invest., 20(5)(1969)488 - M. Baggiolini *et al.*, J. Cell Biol., 45(1970)586- F. Osculati, Z. Zellforsch., 109(1970)398

Function J.M. Riddle and M.L. Barnhart, Amer. J. Path., 45(1964)805 - M. Zatti *et al.*, Brit. J. Exp. Path., 46 (1965)227 - D. Graf Keyserlingk, Exp. Cell Res., 51 (1968)79

Development G. Winqvist, J. Ultrastruct. Res., 9(1963)396 - D.F. Bainton and M.G. Farquhar, J. Cell Biol., 28(1966) 277 - M.E. Fedorko and J.G. Hirsch, J. Cell Biol., 29 (1966)307 - B.K. Wetzel *et al.*, Lab. Invest., 16(1967)349 - E.A. McCulloch, Differentiation of hemopoietic stem cells. In: *Plenary Session Papers, 12th Congress of the International Society of Hematology*, International Society of Hematology, New York, 1968, p. 260 - A. Balazs, Z. Zellforsch., 99(1969)286 - F.R. Campbell, Anat. Res., 163(1969)427

Effects of irradiation J. Hugon and M. Borgers, J. de Microscopie, 5(1966)649

Effects of freezing and thawing E.I. Terentiyeva and A.G. Fedotenkov, Arkh. Anat. Gistol. Embriol., 54(1)(1968)61

Growth in diffusion chambers R. Ross and J.W. Lillywhite, Lab. Invest., 14(1965)1568

Eosinophil leukocytes

Structure A. Faller, Z. Zellforsch., 69(1966)551 - F. Miller *et al.*, J. Cell Biol., 31(1966)349 - G. Hudson, Exp. Cell Res., 46(1967)121 - G. Hudson, J. Anat., 103(2)(1968) 337

Cytochemistry (enzymes in granules) G.T. Archer and J.G. Hirsch, J.Exp. Med., 118(1963)277 - G.T. Archer *et al.*, Biochim. Biophys. Acta, 99(1965)96 - P.M. Seeman and G.E. Palade, J. Cell Biol., 34(1967)745 - F. Miller and V. Herzog, Z. Zellforsch., 97(1969)84 - D.F. Bainton and M.G. Farquhar, J. Cell Biol., 45(1970)54

Basophil leukocytes
Structure R.W. Terry *et al.*, Lab. Invest., 21(1)(1969)65
Function B.S. Chan, Anat. Rec., 175(1973)288

Globule leukocytes
Structure J.F. Kent, Anat. Rec., 156(1966)439 - K.E. Carr, J. Anat., 101(4)(1967)793 - K.E. Carr and P. Whur, Z. Zellforsch., 86(1968)153

Lymphocytes
General (origins, life history, turnover and recirculation) N.B. Everett *et al.*, The small lymphocyte of the rat: rate of formation, extent of recirculation and circulating life span. In: *Proceedings of the 9th Congress of the International Society of Hematology*, Mexico City, 3(1962) 345 - J.R. Little *et al.*, Blood, 19(1962)236 - D.G. Osmond and N.B. Everett, Blood, 23(1964)1 - J.M. Yoffey, Annual Rev. Med., 15(1964)125 - J.M. Yoffey and D.G. Osmond, J. Anat., 99(1965)841 - M. Bennett and G. Cudkowicz, Functional and morphological characterization of stem cells: The unipotential role of "lymphocytes" of mouse marrow. In: J.M. Yoffey (Ed.), *The Lymphocyte in Immunology and Haemopoiesis* (Symp.), Arnold, London, 1967 - F. Brahim and D.G. Osmond, Proc. Canad. Fed. Biol. Soc., (1967)136 - J.L. Gowans, Int. Rev. Exp. Path., 5(1967) - D.G. Osmond, Lymphocyte production in the bone marrow: radioautographic studies in polycythaemic guinea pigs. In: J.M. Yoffey (Ed.), *The Lymphocyte in Immunology and Haemopoiesis (Symp.)*, Edward Arnold, London, 1967, pp. 120–130 - I. Törö and I. Olah, J. Ultrastruct. Res., 17 (1967)439 - M.R. Schwarz, The life history of lymphocytes (Symposium), Anat. Rec., 165(1969)105 - F. Brahim, Anat. Rec., 172(1972)276 and 175(1973)277
Structure (including Kurloff bodies) N. Granboulan, Rev. Hematol., 15(1960)52 - P.B. Berendsen and I.R. Telford, Anat. Rec., 156(1966)107 - R.A. Welsh, J. Ultrastruct. Res., 14(1966)556 - K. Smetana *et al.*, Exp. Cell Res., 52(1968)112 - R. Hebel and H.G. Liebig, Z. Zellforsch., 93(1969)232
Cytochemistry (enzymes) G. Brittinger *et al.*, J. Cell Biol., 37(1968)394
Function (including protein synthesis and immune response) S.L. Clarke, Jr., Amer. J. Anat., 119(1966)375 - R.D. Meader and D.F. Landers, Amer. J. Anat., 121(1967)763 - M.R. Schwarz, Amer. J. Anat., 121(1967)559 - J.M. Yoffey (Ed.), *The Lymphocyte in Immunology and Haemopoiesis* (Symp.), Arnold, London, 1967
Effects of phytoagglutinine G. Procicchiani *et al.*, J. Ultrastruct. Res., 22(1968)195
Effects of hydrocortisone A.L. Chapman, Anat. Rec., 142 (1962)300

Plasma cells
Structure H.Z. Movat and N.V.P. Fernando, Exp. Molec. Path., 1(1962)535 - G. Patrizi, J. de Microscopie, 7(1968) 293 - A. Weinstock, Anat. Rec., 162(1968)289 - L.J. Simar, Z. Zellforsch., 99(1969)235
Cytochemistry R.A. Welsh, Amer. J. Path., 40(1962)285
Function (immune response) H. Braunsteiner and F. Pakesch, Blood, 10(1955)650 - M.C. Bessis, Lab. Invest., 10(1961) 1040 - C.C. Clawson *et al.*, Lab. Invest., 15(1966)1830 - D. Zagury *et al.*, J. Cell Biol., 46(1970)52
Development A.M. Smith *et al.*, Anat. Rec., 167(1970)351

Macrophages derived from leukocytes
Structure and origin J.A. Chapman *et al.*, J. Cell Sci., 2(1967)371 - J.G. Howard *et al.*, Macrophage-type cells in the liver derived from thoracic duct cells during graft-vs.-host reactions. In: J.M. Yoffey (Ed.), *The Lymphocyte in Immunology and Haemopoiesis* (Symp.), Arnold, London, 1967

Lymphatic organs (general)
W. Stoeckenius, Verhandl. Deut. Ges. Pathol., 41(1958)304 - H.Z. Movat and N.V.P. Fernando, Exp. Molec. Path., 3(1964) 546 - C.C. Clawson *et al.*, Lab. Invest., 16(1967)407

Tonsils
Structure H.K. Müller-Hermelink and R. Caesar, Z. Zellforsch., 96(1969)521 - G.C. Schofield and R.N.P. Cahill, J. Anat., 105(1969)447
Cytochemistry E. Kaiserling and R. Caesar, Z. Zellforsch., 95(1969)202

Thymus (non-lymphatic cells)
Structure P. Kohnen and L. Weiss, Anat. Rec., 148(1964)29 - I. Törö *et al.*, Z. Zellforsch., 56(1965)915 - T. Ito and T. Hoshino, Z. Zellforsch., 69(1966)311 - J. Izard, J. de Microscopie, 5(1966)361 - T. Mandel, Z. Zellforsch., 92 (1968)159 - I. Törö *et al.*, Z. Zellforsch.,89(1968)241 - U.T.G. Van Haelst, Z. Zellforsch., 99(1969)198 - I. Törö *et al.*, Anat. Res., 165(1969)329 - T. Hoshino *et al.*, Jap. J. Electr. Micr. 19(3)(1970)271
Development T. Mandel, Z. Zellforsch., 89(1968)180 - T. Mandel, Z. Zellforsch., 106(1970)498
Effects of estrogen J. Izard, Z. Zellforsch., 66(1965)276

Thymus (lymphatic cells)
General V. Defendi and D. Metcalf (Eds.), *The Thymus*, The Wistar Institute Symposium, Monograph No. 2, The Wistar Institute Press, Philadelphia, 1964 - U. Van Haelst, Z. Zellforsch., 77(1967)534
Structure S.L. Clark, Jr., Amer. J. Anat., 112(1963)1 - J. Izard *et al.*, J. de Microscopie, 3(1964)69 - B.V. Gaudecker and U.K. Hinrichsen, Z. Zellforsch., 65(1965)139 - R.G. Murray *et al.*, Anat. Rec., 151(1965)17 - D.E. Bockman and W.B. Winborn, J. Morph., 121(1967)277 - P.H. Sebuwufu, J. Ultrastruct. Res., 24(1968)171 - K. Henry and V. Petts, J. Ultrastruct. Res., 27(1969)330 - C. Smith, Amer. J. Anat., 124(1969)389 - K. Abe and T. Ito, Z. Zellforsch., 110(1970)321
Function S.L. Clark, Jr., Electron microscopy of the thymus in mice of the strain 129/J. In: R.A. Good and A.E. Gabrielsen (Eds.), *The Thymus in Immunobiology*, Hoeber Medical Division, Harper and Row, New York, 1964 - R.H. Levey, Sci. Amer., 211(1964)66 - S.L. Clark, Jr., Cytological evidences of secretion in the thymus. In: G.E.W. Wolstenholme and R. Porter (Eds.), *The Thymus: Experimental and Clinical Studies* (Ciba Foundation Symposium), Little, Brown, Boston, 1966, p. 3
Development and origins B.S. Weakley *et al.*, J. Morphol., 115(1964)319 - G.A. Ackerman and R.A. Knouff, Anat. Rec., 152(1965)35 - J. Izard, Exper. Cell Res., 37(1965) 487 - F.T. Sanel, Z. Zellforsch., 83(1967)8 - T. Hoshino *et al.*, Anat. Rec., 164(1969)47 - G.A. Ackerman and J.R. Hostetler, Anat. Rec., 166(1970)27
Proliferation and cell traffic L.E. Harris *et al.*, Nature, 201 (1964)884 - B. Von Gaudecker, Z. Zellforsch. 72(1966) 281

Atrophy and regeneration U. Van Haelst, Z. Zellforsch., 80 (1967)153 - P. Gad and S.L. Clark, Jr., Amer. J. Anat., 122(1968)573

Effects of hydrocortisone W.K. Cowan and G.D. Sorenson, Lab. Invest., 13(1964)353

Spleen

General E. Von Herrath, *Bau und Funktion der normalen Milz,* De Gruyter, Berlin, 1958 - W. Stoeckenius, Verhandl. deut. Ges. Pathol. 42(1959)351 - B. Galindo and T. Imaeda, Anat. Rec., 143(1962)399

Function (phagocytic) W.H. Crosby, Blood, 14(1959)399 - L. Weiss, Amer. J. Anat., 111(1962)175 - G. Montaldo *et al.,* Arch. Ital. Anat. Istol. Pat., 38(1964)8 - L. Ceresa-Castellani and G. Lanzavecchia, J. de Microscopie, 5 (1966)65 - R. Pictet *et al.,* Z. Zellforsch., 96(1969)372 - R. Pictet *et al.,* Z. Zellforsch., 96(1969)400

Development L. Zamboni and B. Westin, J. Ultrastruct. Res., 11(1964)469 - E.A. Holyoke *et al.,* J. Ultrastruct. Res., 15(1966)87

Lymph nodes

General Y. Mori and K. Lennert, *Electron Microscopic Atlas of Lymph Node Cytology and Pathology*, Springer, Berlin, 1969

Structure O. Fresen and H.J. Wellensiek, Verhandl. deut. Ges. Pathol., 42(1959)353 - S.S. Han, Anat. Rec., 136(1960) 206 - G.D. Sorenson, Amer. J. Anat., 107(1960)73 - S.S. Han, Amer. J. Anat., 109(1961)183 - S.L. Clark, Jr., Amer. J. Anat., 110(1962)217 - P. Schulze, Morph. Jb., 111(1967)301 - D.A. Zdanov and V.A. Shaklamov, Arkh. Anat. Gistol. Embriol., 55(7)(1968)25 - Y. Ishii and M. Mori, Jap. J. Electr. Micr., 18(2)(1969)128

Function (phagocytic) J.Lindner and U.W. Gusek, Frankf. Z. Path., 70(1960)367

Erythrocytes

General D.C. Pease, J. Hemat., 11(1956)501 - M.C. Bessis and J. Breton-Gorius, Blood, 19(1962)635 - C.W. Bishop and D.M. Surgenor (Eds.), *The Red Blood Cell; A Comprehensive Treatise,* Academic Press, New York, 1964

Structure H.W. Beams and R.G. Kessel, Amer. J. Anat., 118 (1966)471 - J.A. Grasso, Anat. Rec., 156(1966)397 - G. Kent *et al.,* Amer. J. Path., 48(1966)838 - J. Stoubesand *et al.,* Z. Zellforsch., 69(1966)344 - T.W. Tillaek and V.T. Marchesi, J. Cell Biol., 45(1970)649

Cytochemistry D.N. Misra *et al.,* Exper. Cell Res., 34(1964) 325 - V.T. Marchesi and G.E. Palade, J. Cell Biol., 35 (1967)385 - Y. Marikovsky and D. Danon, J. Cell Biol., 43(1969)1

Development L. Ceresa-Castellani and V.G. Leone, Anat. Rec., 165(1969)453 - R.A. Rifkind *et al.,* J. Cell Biol., 40(1969)343 - S.S. Sekhon and H.W. Beams, Amer. J. Anat., 125(1969)353 - G.D. Sorenson, Anat. Rec., 133 (1959)338 - G.A. Ackerman *et al.,* Lab. Invest., 10(1961) 787 - G.D. Sorensen, Lab. Invest., 10(1961)178 - M.C. Bessis and J. Breton-Gorius, Blood, 19(1962)635 - J.A. Grasso *et al.,* J. Cell Biol., 14(1962)235 - O.P. Jones, Anat. Rec., 142(1962)311 - O.P. Jones, J. Ultrastruct. Res., 7(1962)308 - J.R. Warner *et al.,* Science, 138(1962) 1399 - R.A. Rifkind *et al.,* J. Cell Biol., 22(1964)599 - L. Zamboni, J. Ultrastruct. Res., 12(1965)525 - R.H. Edmonds, Anat. Rec., 154(1966)785 - I. Berman, J. Ultrastruct. Res., 17(1967)291 - C.F. Simpson and J.M. Kling, J. Cell Biol., 35(1967)237 - E. Skutelsy and D. Danon, J. Cell Biol., 33(1967)625 - F.R. Campbell, Anat. Rec., 160(1968)539

Dedifferentiation D.B. Harrington, Anat. Rec., 172(1972) 325

Effects of erythropoetin D. Orlic *et al.,* J. Ultrastruct. Res., 13(1965)516

Platelets

General H. Schulz, *Electron Microscopy of Blood Platelets and Thrombosis*, Springer, Berlin, 1968

Structure J.F.D. Ferreira, Int. Rev. Cytol., 17(1964)99 - A.J. Marcus and D. Zucker-Franklin, Blood, 23(1964)389 - E.B. Sandborn *et al.,* Blood, 27(1966)247 - D. Shepro *et al.,* Anat. Rec., 156(1966)203 - O. Behnke, Anat. Rec., 158(1967)121 - O. Behnke, J. Cell Biol., 34(1967)697 - O. Behnke and T. Zelander, J. Ultrastruct. Res., 19(1967) 147 - J.E. French, Brit. J. Haemat., 13(1967)595 - A. Hattori, Jap. J. Electr. Micr., 16(3)(1967)239 - M.D. Silver and J.E. McKinstry, Z. Zellforsch., 81(1967)12 - H.A. Gardner *et al.,* Anat. Rec., 163(1969)509 - J.G. White, Amer. J. Path., 56(2)(1969)267

Cytochemistry A.J. Marcus and D. Zucker-Franklin, J. Clin. Invest., 43(1964)1241 - D. Zucker-Franklin *et al.,* Science, 157(1967)945 - O. Behnke, J. Ultrastruct. Res., 24(1968)51 - M.D. Silver and H.A. Gardner, J. Ultrastruct. Res., 23(1968)366 - J.G. White, Amer. J. Path., 53(5)(1968)791 - S.R. Saba *et al.,* Amer. J. Path., 55(2) (1969)225 - I. Kuruma and T. Okada, Z. Zellforsch., 108 (1970)268 - D. Zucker-Franklin, J. Cell Biol., 47(1970) 293

Function of phagocytosis J.F.D. Ferreira, Z. Zellforsch., 55 (1961)89 - H. Schulz and U.J. Wedel, Klin. Wschr., 40 (1962)1114 - H.Z. Movat *et al.,* J. Cell Biol., 27(1965)531 - M. Martin, Z. Zellforsch., 76(1967)108 - J.G. White, Amer. J. Path., 53(4)(1968)567

Function of aggregation and thrombosis initiation E. Kuhnke, Pflügers Arch. Ges. Physiol., 268(1958)87 - H. Schulz and U.E. Hiepler, Klin. Wschr., 37(1959)273 - O.A. Iseri and E.P. Benditt, Fed. Proc., 20(1961)133 - A. Parmeggiani, Thromb. Diath. Haemorrh., 6(1961)517 - P.A. Castaldi *et al.,* Blood, 20(1962)566 - A. Kjaerheim and T. Hovig, Thromb. Diath. Haemorrh., 7(1962)1 - N.F. Rodman *et al.,* Amer. J. Path., 40(1962)271 - J. Wiener and D. Spiro, Exp. Molec. Path., 1(1962)554 - J.E. French and J.C.F. Poole, Proc. Roy. Soc., Ser. B, 157 (1963)170 - T. Hovig, J. Ultrastruct. Res., 8(1963)195 - J.C.F. Poole *et al.,* J. Clin. Path., 16(1963)523 - N.F. Rodman, Jr. *et al.,* Fed. Proc., 22(1963)1356 - N.F. Rodman, Jr. *et al.,* J. Cell Biol., 16(1963)225 - K.M. Brinkhous *et al.,* Lab. Invest., 14(1965)335 - J.E. French, Ann. Roy. Coll. Surg. Engl. 36(1965)191 - S.A. Johnson *et al.,* Thromb. Diath. Haemorrh., 13(1965)65 - J. Marr *et al.,* Nature, 205(1965)259 - T.P. Ashford and D.G. Freiman, Amer. J. Path., 48(1966)42a - A. Nolte and U.K. Breddin, Thromb. Diath. Haemorrh., 15(1966)93 - J.G. White and W. Krivit, Blood, 27(1966)167 - W.E. Stehbens and T.J. Biscoe, Amer. J. Path., 50(1967)219 - R.H. Edmonds, J. Ultrastruct. Res., 24(1968)295 - T. Hovig *et al.,* J. Lab. Clin. Med., 71(1968)29 - E.J.H. Nathaniel and A.B. Chandler, J. Ultrastruct. Res., 22 (1968)348 - K. Shirasawa and A.B. Chandler, Amer. J. Path., 57(1969)127

Origin and development J.P. Thiery and M. Bessis, Rev. Hemat., 11(1956)162 - E.P. Cronkite *et al.,* Studies on the origin, production and destruction of platelets. In: S.A. Johnson, R. Monto, J. Rebuck, and R.C. Horn (Eds.), *Blood Platelets*, Little, Brown, Boston, 1961, p. 595 - O. Behnke, J. Ultrastruct. Res., 24(1968)412 - H. Schulz and K. Schiller, Z. Zellforsch., 87(1968)389 - D. Graf Keyserlingk and M. Albrecht, Z. Zellforsch., 89 (1968)320

Effects of enzymes T. Hovig, Thromb. Diath. Haemorrh., 13 (1965)84

Effects of colchicine and Vinca alkaloids J.G. White, Amer. J. Path., 53(2)(1968)281 - J.G. White, Amer. J. Path., 54(3) (1969)467

Effects of thrombin H.J. Schmid *et al.*, J. Clin. Invest., 41 (1962)543 - P. Vassalli *et al.*, J. Ultratruct. Res., 11(1964) 374

Effects of plasma clotting and fibrinogen G.J. Steward, J. Appl. Phys. 36(1965)2607 - N.F. Rodman, Jr. *et al.*, Lab. Invest., 15(1966)641

Fibrinogen and fibrin

Structure C.E. Hall and H.S. Slayter, J. Biophys. Biochem. Cytol., 5(1959)11 - E. Kuhnke, Naturwissenschaften, 49 (1962)60 - C.E. Hall, Lab. Invest., 12(1963)998 - B. Kisch, Exper. Med. Surg., 22(1964)237 - G. Koppel, Z. Zellforsch., 77(1967)443 - N. Moe and L. Jorgensen, Acta Path. Microbiol. Scand., 72(1968)519

Megacaryocytes

Structure S.S. Han and B.L. Baker, Anat. Rec., 149(1964) 251 - E. Yamada, Acta Anat., 29(1967)267 - O. Behnke, J. Ultrastruct. Res., 24(1969)412

5. MUSCLE

Skeletal Muscle

General

Structure D.C. Pease and R.F. Baker, Amer. J. Anat., 84 (1949)175 - A.J. Hodge *et al.*, J. Exp. Med., 99(1954)201 - A.J. Hodge, J. Biophys. Biochem. Cytol., 1(1955)361 - A.J. Hodge, J. Biophys. Biochem. Cytol., 2(1956)131 - H.E. Huxley, Endeavour, 15(1956)177 - J.D. Robertson, J. Biophys. Biochem. Cytol., 2(1956)369 - H.S. Bennett. In: G.H. Bourne (Ed.), *The Structure and Function of Muscle, Vol. 1 (Structure)*, Academic Press, New York, 1960, p. 137 - H.E. Huxley. In: D. Nachmansohn (Ed.), *Molecular Biology*, Academic Press, New York, 1960, p. 1 - V.L. Van Breemen, Amer. J. Path., 37(1960)215 - A. Mauro and W.R. Adams, J. Biophys. Biochem. Cytol., 10 (1961)177 - E. Veratti, J. Biophys. Biochem. Cytol., 10 (1961)1 (Suppl.) - E.L. Howes *et al.*, Amer, J. Path., 45 (1964)599 - Y. Uehara and K. Hama, Jap. J. Electr. Micr., 14(1965)34 - H. David *et al.*, Z. Zellforsch., 70(1966)334 - G.F. Gauthier and H.A. Padykula, J. Cell Biol., 28(1966) 333 - R. Mayr *et al.*, Z. Zellforsch., 75(1966)434 - G. Pilar and A. Hess, Anat. Rec., 154(1966)243 - S.A. Shafiq *et al.*, Anat. Rec., 156(1966)283 - T.I. Tikhomirova and N.M. Shestopalova, Arkh. Anat. Gistol. Embriol., 51 (1966)22 - D.E. Ashhurst, J. Cell Science, 2(1967)435 - W.G. Forssmann and A. Matter, Morph. Jb., 111(1967) 319 - H.G. Heumann and E. Zebe, Z. Zellforsch., 78 (1967)131 - P.W. Brandt *et al.*, J. Cell Biol., 38(1968)115 - P.R. Garant, J. Cell Biol., 36(1968)648 - V.P. Guilev *et al.*, Arkh. Anat. Gistol. Embriol., 54(1968)41 - G.G. Knappeis and F. Carlsen, J. Cell Biol., 38(1968)202 - E. Lindner, Z. Zellforsch., 88(1968)370 - H. Schmalbruch, Z. Zellforsch., 85(1968)343 - G.F. Gauthier, Z. Zellforsch., 95(1969)462 - W.S. Bertaud *et al.*, J. Cell Sci., 6 (1970)537

Cytochemistry (enzymes, contractile proteins and ions) R.J. Barrnett and G.E. Palade, J. Biophys. Biochem. Cytol., 6(1959)163 - D.J. Goldstein, Anat. Rec., 134(1959)217 - S. Ebashi and F. Lipmann, J. Cell Biol., 14(1962)389 - A. Margreth *et al.*, Exp. Cell Res., 32(1963)484 - L.L. Constantin *et al.*, Science, 147(1965)158 - S. Winegrad, J. Gen. Physiol., 48(1965)997 - H.D. Fahimi and M.J. Karnovsky, J. Cell Biol., 29(1966)113 - F.A. Pepe, J. Cell Biol., 28(1966)505 - A. Corsi *et al.*, J. Ultrastruct. Res., 19(1967)260 - G.B. Gordon *et al.*, Lab. Invest., 16(1967) 422 - J. Lundin and B. Hellstrom, Z. Zellforsch., 85 (1968)264 - J.E. Rash *et al.*, J. Ultrastruct. Res., 24 (1968)181 - S.H. Fujime and T. Ooi, J. de Microscopie, 8(1969)535 - H. Ishikawa *et al.*, J. Cell Biol., 43(1969) 312 - M.H. Stromer *et al.*, J. Cell Biol., 40(1969)167

Function H. Huxley and J. Hanson, Nature, 173(1954)971 - G.G. Knappeis and F. Carlsen, J. Biophys. Biochem. Cytol., 2(1956)201 - F.S. Sjöstrand and E. Andersson, Exp. Cell Res., 11(1956)493 - D. Spiro, J. Biophys. Biochem. Cytol., 2(1956)157 (Suppl.) - A.F. Huxley and R.E. Taylor, J. Physiol., 144(1958)426 - F. Carlsen *et al.*, J. Biophys. Biochem. Cytol., 11(1961)95 - H. Hoffmeister, Z. Zellforsch., 54(1961)402 - H.E. Huxley, Circulation, 24(1961)328 - R.C. Strohman *et al.*, Exp. Cell Res., 35(1964)617 - W.H. Freygang, Fed. Proc., 24 (1965)1135 - H.E. Huxley, Sci. Amer., 213(1965)18 - M.J. Cohen and A. Hess, Amer. J. Anat., 121(1967)285 - M. Jagendorf-Elfvin, J. Ultrastruct. Res., 17(1967)379 - F.S. Sjöstrand and M. Jagendorf-Elfvin, J. Ultrastruct. Res., 17(1967)348 - A.A. Belousov, Arkh. Anat. Gistol. Embriol., 56(1969)41 - A. Coimbra, Amer. J. Anat., 124 (1969)361 - M. Hagopian, J. Cell Biol., 47(1970)790 - S. Schiaffino *et al.*, J. Cell Biol., 47(1970)107

Development E.D. Hay, Z. Zellforsch., 59(1963)6 - C.H. Waddington *et al.*, Exp. Cell Res., 30(1963)599 - R.J. Przybylski and J.M. Blumberg, Lab. Invest., 15(1966)836 - J.A. Heuson-Stiennon and P. Drochmans, J. de Microscopie, 6(1967)639 - H. Ishikawa *et al.*, J. Cell Biol., 38 (1968)538 - J. Auber, J. de Microscopie, 8(1969)367 - A.M. Kelly and S.I. Zacks, J. Cell Biol., 42(1969)135 - R.H. Warren and K.R. Porter, Amer. J. Anat., 124(1969)1 - R.E. Waterman, Amer. J. Anat., 125(1969)457

Regeneration D. Allbrook, J. Anat., 96(1962)137 - O. Hojiro, Jap. J. Electr. Micr., 12(1963)228 - E.H. Betz *et al.*, Intern. Rev. Cytol., 19(1966)203 - M. Reznick, Lab. Invest., 20(1969)353 - T.L. Lentz, Amer. J. Anat., 124 (1969)447

Proliferation and mitosis H.F. Macconnachie *et al.*, Amer. J. Anat., 114(1964)245 - S.A. Shafiq *et al.*, J. Anat., 103 (1968)135 - G. Goldspink, J. Cell Sci., 6(1970)593 - E.C.B. Hall-Craggs and C.A. Lawrence, Z. Zellforsch., 109(1970)481 - F.P. Moss and C.P. Leblond, J. Cell Biol., 44(1970)459

Regression R. Weber, J. Cell Biol., 22(1964)481

Effects of inorganic cations P.M. Lundin and U. Schelin, Z. Zellforsch., 63(1964)692 - H. Schmalbruch, Z. Zellforsch., 62(1964)246

Effects of free fatty acid mobilization A.B. Maunsback and C. Wirsen, J. Ultrastruct. Res., 16(1966)35

Effects of hormones (thyroid, glucocorticoids, male sex hormones) O. Lindberg, Naturwissenschaften, 52(1965)379 - J.H. Venable, Amer. J. Anat., 119(1966)271 - L.W. Tice and A.G. Engel, Amer. J. Path., 50(1967)311 - Z. Gori *et al.,* Exp. Molec. Path., 6(1967)172 - Z. Gori *et al.,* Exp. Molec. Path., 10(1969)199

Effects of denervation G.R. Schrodt and S.M. Walker, Amer. J. Path., 49(1966)33 - E. Nickel and P.G. Waser, Z. Zellforsch., 88(1968)278

Satellite cells

A. Mauro, J. Biophys. Biochem. Cytol., 9(1961)493 - H. Ishakawa, Z. Anat. Entw. Gesch., 125(1966)43 - J.C.T. Church, J. Anat., 105(1969)419 - E.D. Hay and C.M. Doyle, Anat. Rec., 175(1973)339 - E. Schultz, Anat. Rec., 175 (1973)438

Myotendon junctions

D. Gelber *et al.,* Z. Zellforsch., 52(1960)396 - H.G. Schwarzacher, Acta Anat., 40(1960)59 - K. Schippel and D. Reissig, Z. Mikr.-Anat. Forsch., 75(1966)210 - D. Reissig and K. Schippel, Z. Mikr.-Anat. Forsch., 76(1967)1 - K. Schippel and D. Reissig, Z. Mikr.-Anat., 78(1968)235

Sarcoplasmic reticulum

Structure H.S. Bennett, J. Biophys. Biochem. Cytol., 2 (1956)171 (Suppl.) - K.R. Porter, J. Biophys. Biochem. Cytol., 2(1956)163 (Suppl.) - K.R. Porter and G.E. Palade, J. Biophys. Biochem. Cytol., 3(1957)269 - D.W. Fawcett and J.P. Revel, J. Biophys. Biochem. Cytol., 10 (1961)89 (Suppl.) - K.R. Porter, J. Biophys. Biochem. Cytol., 10(1961)211 (Suppl.) - D.S. Smith, J. Biophys. Biochem. Cytol., 10(1961)61 (Suppl.) - J.P. Revel, J. Cell Biol., 12(1962)571 - C. Franzini-Armstrong, J. Cell Biool., 19(1963)637 - U. Muscatello *et al.,* J. Biophys. Biochem. Cytol., 10(1961)201 (Suppl.) - N. Ikemoto *et al.,* J. Ultrastruct. Res., 23(1968)216

Function G.A. Edwards *et al.,* J. Biophys. Biochem. Cytol., 2(1956)143 (Suppl). - H. Ruska *et al.,* Experientia, 14 (1958)117 - W. Hasselbach, Fed. Proc., 23(1964)909 - J. Rosenbluth, J. Cell Biol., 42(1969)534

Development S. Schiaffino and A. Margreth, J. Cell Biol., 41(1969)855

"T"-system

Structure C. Franzini-Armstrong and K.R. Porter, J. Cell Biol., 22(1964)675 - H.E. Huxley, Nature, 202(1964) 1067 - L.D. Peachey, J. Cell Biol., 25(1965)209 - S.M. Walker and G.R. Schrodt, Anat. Rec., 155(1966)1

Cytochemistry J.A. Zadunaisky, J. Cell Biol., 31(1966)C11

Development E.B. Ezerman and H. Ishikawa, J. Cell Biol., 35(1967)405 - H. Ishikawa, J. Cell Biol., 38(1968)51

Myofilaments

Structure M. Krauss and W.R. Van Antwerp, Exp. Cell Res., 11(1956)637 - H.E. Huxley, J. Biophys. Biochem. Cytol., 3(1957)631 - E.B. Sandborn *et al.,* J. de Microscopie, 6(1967)169 - C.R. Zobel *et al.,* J. Ultrastruct. Res., 18 (1967)637 - W.W. Franke, Z. Zellforsch., 111(1970)143

Function F.S. Sjöstrand and E. Andersson-Cedergren, J. Ultrastruct. Res., 1(1957)74 - V.P. Gilev, J. Cell Biol., 12(1962)135 - F.S. Sjöstrand, Nature, 201(1964)45

Development and regeneration H. Firket, Z. Zellforsch., 78 (1967)313 - D.A. Fischman, J. Cell Biol., 32(1967)557 - H.M. Price *et al.,* Lab. Invest., 13(1964)1279 - D.E. Kelly, Anat. Rec., 163(1969)403

"Z"-band

Structure G.G. Knappeis and F. Carlsen, J. Cell Biol., 13 (1962)323 - C. Franzini-Armstrong and K.R. Porter, Z. Zellforsch., 61(1964)661 - D.E. Kelly, J. Cell Biol., 31 (1966)131A - D.E. Kelly, J. Cell Biol., 34(1967)827 - M.H. Stromer *et al.,* J. Cell Biol., 35(1967)C23 - D.N. Landon, J. Cell Sci., 6(1970)257

Development D.E. Kelly, Anat. Rec., 163(1969)403

Mitochondria

Structure

A.F. Howatson, J. Biophys. Biochem. Cytol., 2(1956)363 (Suppl.) - C.R. Leeson and T.S. Leeson, J. Anat., 105 (1969)363

Function A.G.M. Mattisson and A. Birch-Anderson, J. Ultrastruct. Res., 6(1962)205

Effects of cold G. Schwalbach and U.B. Agostini, Z. Zellforsch., 62(1964)113

Effects of hibernation J.E. Moreland, Anat. Rec., 142(1962) 155

Effects of thyroid hormone and thyroidectomy R.G. Gustafson and J.R. Tata, J. Ultrastruct. Res., 9(1963)396 - R.G. Gustafson *et al.,* J. Cell Biol., 26D(1964)555

Cardiac Muscle

General

Structure H.J. Weinstein, Exp. Cell Res., 7(1954)130 - R. Poche and E. Lindner, Z. Zellforsch., 43(1955)104 - D.H. Moore and H. Ruska, J. Biophys. Biochem. Cytol., 3 (1957)261 - E. Lindner, Z. Zellforsch., 45(1957)702 - J.R. Smith *et al.,* Exp. Cell Res., 20(1960)228 - W. Thoenes and H. Ruska, Z. Zellforsch., 51(1960)560 - C.G. Battig and F.N. Low, Amer. J. Anat., 108(1961)199 - H. Hift *et al.,* Circulation, 24(1961)955 (Abstract) - R.J. Stenger and D. Spiro, J. Biophys. Biochem. Cytol., 9 (1961)325 - G.D. Bloom, Z. Zellforsch., 57(1962)213 - E. Page, J. Ultrastruct. Res., 17(1967)63 - F. Denoit and E. Coraboeuf, J. de Microscopie, 7(1968)245 - D.W. Fawcett, J. Cell Biol., 36(1968)266 - D.W. Fawcett and N.S. McNutt, J. Cell Biol., 42(1969)1 - J.R. Sommer and E.A. Johnson, Z. Zellforsch., 98(1969)437 - Sz. Viragh and C.E. Challice, J.Ultrastruct. Res., 28(1969)321

Histochemistry J.R. Sommer and M.S. Spach, Amer. J. Path., 44(1964)491 - E. Essner *et al.,* J. Cell Biol., 25(1965)201 - J.A. Carney and A.L. Brown, J. Cell Biol., 28(1966)375 - V.J. Ferrans *et al.,* Amer. J. Anat., 125(1969)47 - J.A. Higgins and R.J. Barrnett, J. Cell Sci., 6(1970)29

Function (excitation and contraction) E.A. Johnson and J.R. Sommer, J. Cell Biol., 33(1967)103 - N.A. Stanley and E.S. Benson, J. Cell Biol., 38(1968)99 - P. Anversa *et al.,* Z. Zellforsch., 94(1969)181

Function (lipid synthesis and storage) O. Stein and Y. Stein, J. Cell Biol., 36(1968)63

Development and proliferation R.G. Hibbs, Amer. J. Anat., 99(1956)17 - E. Lindner, Verhandl. Anat. Ges., 22(1957)

305 - G.A. Edwards and C.E. Challice, Exp. Cell Res., 15(1958)247 - H. Meyer and L.T. Queiroga, J. Biophys. Biochem. Cytol., 5(1959)169 - E. Lindner, Anat. Rec., 136(1960)234 (Abstract) - S. Wainrach and J.R. Sotelo, Zellforsch., 55(1961)622 - C.Y. Huang, J. Ultrastruct. Res. 20(1967)211 - P.P. Rumiantzev, Arkh. Anat. Gistol. Embriol., 52(3)(1967)67 - F.J. Manasek, J. Cell Biol., 37 (1968)191 - U. Muscatello *et al.*, J. Ultrastruct. Res., 23 (1968)44 - R.B. Weinstein and E.D. Hay, J. Cell Biol., 47(1970)310

Regeneration O. Klinge, Z. Zellforsch., 80(1967)488

Ageing G.E. Burch *et al.*, Arch. Path., 89(2)(1970)128

Effects of temperature H.M. Albert, Circulation, 24(1961) 875 - L. Merkow and J. Leighton, J. Cell Biol., 28(1966) 127 - L. Merkow and J. Leighton, Amer. J. Path., 50 (1967)975

Effects of unsaturated fatty acid deficiency L. Vitali-Mazza *et al.*, Virchows Arch. Path. Anat., 342(1967)38

Effects of digoxin M.M. Arcasoy and E.A. Smuckler, Lab. Invest., 20(2)(1969)190

Effects of inorganic ions A.R. Muir, J. Anat., 101 (2)(1967)239 - M.J. Legato *et al.*, J. Cell Biol., 37(1968)1 - J.W. Emberson and A.R. Muir, J. Anat., 104(1969)411

Effects of chloroquine R.J. Hendy *et al.*, J. Ultrastruct. Res., 29(1969)485

Effects of cytochalasin B H.G. Sachs, Anat., Rec., 175(1973) 433 - K. Strahs and J.W. Sanger, Anat. Rec., 175(1973) 452

Atrial myocardium

D.w. Fawcett and C.C. Selby, J. Biophys. Biochem. Cytol., 4(1958)63 - J.C. Sosa-Lucero *et al.*, Lab. Invest., 21 (1)(1969)19 - R.G. Hibbs and V.J. Ferrans, Amer. J. Anat., 124(1969)251 - N.S.McNutt and D.W. Fawcett, J. Cell Biol., 42(1969)46

Purkinje cells and conductive system

E. Page, J. Ultrastruct. Res., 17(1966)72 - J.R. Sommer and E.A. Johnson, J. Cell Biol., 36(1968)497 - E. Page *et al.*, J. Ultrastruct. Res., 28(1969)288 - A. Martinez-Palomo *et al.*, J. Cell Biol , 47(1970)1

Intercalated discs

V.L. Van Breemen, Anat. Rec., 117(1953)49 - F.S. Sjöstrand and E. Andersson, Experientia, 10(1954)369 - A.R. Muir, J. Biophys. Biochem. Cytol., 3(1957)193 - F.S. Sjöstrand *et al.*, J. Ultrastruct. Res., 1(1958)271 - C.E. Challice and G.A. Edwards Experientia, 16(1960)70 - P.M. Grimley and G.A. Edwards, J. Biophys. Biochem. Cytol., 8(1960)305 - F.S. Sjöstrand and E. Andersson-Cedergren. In: H.G. Bourne (Ed.), *The Structure and Function of Muscle, Vol. I (Structure)*, Academic Press, New York, 1960, p. 421 - J.P. Revel and M.J. Karnovsky, J. Cell Biol., 33(1967)C7 - D.A. Meddoff and E. Page, J. Ultrastruct. Res., 24(1968)508 - D.G. Rayns *et al.*, J. Cell Biol., 42(1969)322

Sarcoplasmic reticulum and "T"-system

F.O. Simpson and S.J. Oertelis, Nature, 189(1961)758 - F.O. Simpson and S.J. Oertelis, J. Cell Biol., 12(1962)91 - D.A. Nelson and E.S. Benson, J. Cell Biol., 16(1963)297 - W.G. Forssman and L. Girardier, Z. Zellforsch., 72(1966)249 - M.J. Legato and G.A. Langor, J. Cell Biol., 41(1969)401 - M.B. Edge and S.M. Walker, Anat. Rec., 166(1970)51

Mitochondria

A. Policard *et al.*, Z. Zellforsch., 50(1959)818 - E.A. Munn and P.V. Blair, Z. Zellforsch., 80(1967)205

Smooth Muscle

General

Structure J.S. Mark, Anat. Rec., 125(1956)473 - J. Hanson and J. Lowy, Nature, 180(1957)906 - H. Gansler, Z. Zellforsch., 52(1960)60 - H. Gansler, Z. Zellforsch., 55(1961) 724 - J. Hanson and J. Lowy, Proc. Roy. Soc. London, Ser. B., 154(1961)173 - J.W. Harman *et al.*, Exp. Molec. Path., 1(1962)204 - I. Yamamoto, Jap. J. Electr. Micr., 11(3)(1962)212 - G.F. Elliott, Proc. Roy. Soc. London, Ser. B, 160(1964)467 - D.S. Smith *et al.*, J. Cell Sci., 1(1966)49 - G.V. Hehn, Z. Zellforsch., 78(1967)511 - B.J. Panner and C.R. Honig, J. Cell Biol., 35(1967)303 - D.C.Pease, J. Ultrastruct. Res., 23(1968)280 - R.V. Rice *et al.*, J. Cell Biol., 47(1970)183 - P. Weiss, Z. Mikr.-Anat. Forsch., 78(1968)305

Cytochemistry C. Biava and M. West, Amer. J. Path., 47 (1965)287 - N. Carasso and P. Favard, J. de Microscopie, 5(1966)759 - B.P. Lane, J. Cell Biol., 34(1967)713 - F.L. Archer and V.C.Y. Kao, Lab. Invest., 18(6)(1968)669 - R.E. Kelly and R.V. Rice, J. Cell Biol., 37(1968)105 - R.M. Bois, Anat. Rec., 172(1972)273 and 175(1973)274

Function L.D. Peachey and K.R. Porter, Science, 129(1959) 721 - G. Burnstock and C.L. Prosser, Amer. J. Physiol., 199(1960)553 - C.L. Prosser *et al.*, Amer. J. Physiol., 199 (1960)545 - F.W. Schlote, Z. Zellforsch., 52(1960)362 - B.P. Lane and J.A.G. Phodin, J. Ultrastruct. Res., 10 (1964)470 - B.P. Lane, J. Cell Biol., 27(1965)199

Development I. Yamamoto, Jap. J. Electr. Micr., 10(3)(1961) 145 - T.S.L. Cobb and T. Bennett, Z. Zellforsch., 100 (1969)516 - A. Yamauchi and G. Burnstock, J. Anat., 104(1969)1

Regeneration and proliferation I.J. Nad, Arkh. Anat. Gistol. Embriol., 51(12)(1966)21 - J.L.S. Cobb and T. Bennett, Z. Zellforsch., 108(1970)177 - B. Dalley, Anat. Rec., 175 (1973)301

Ageing O. Stein *et al.*, Lab. Invest., 21(5)(1967)386 - J.F. May and W.J. Paule, Anat. Rec., 175(1973)386

Effects of inhibition of cholesterol synthesis I-Li Chen and R.D. Yates, Amer. J. Anat., 121(1967)705

Effects of estrogen and progesterone H. Gansler, Virchows Arch. Path. Anat., 329(1956)235 - R. Ross and S.J. Klebanoff, J. Cell Biol., 32(1967)155 - H.H.R. Friederici and R.J. De Cloux, J. Ultrastruct. Res., 22(1968)402 - W.J. Bo *et al.*, Anat. Rec., 163(1969)121

Effects of pregnancy C.F. Shoenberg, J. Biophys. Biochem. Cytol., 4(1958)609 - Y. Kameya, Jap. J. Electr. Micr., 12(2)(1963)100

Intercellular junctions

R.A. Bergman, Bull. Johns Hopkins Hosp., 102(1958)195 - J.C. Thaemert, J. Biophys. Biochem. Cytol., 6(1959)67 - M.M. Dewey and L. Barr, Science, 137(1962)670 - T. Oosaki and S. Ishii, J. Ultrastruct. Res., 10(1964)567 - J.L.S. Cobb and T. Bennett, J. Cell Biol., 41(1969)287

6. NERVOUS TISSUE

Nervous System

General
J.Z. Young, Endeavour, 15(1956)5 - C.A. Baud, J. Anat. Soc. India, 6(1957)59 - H. Fernandez-Moran and R. Brown, Exp. Cell Res., (1958)5 (Suppl.) - W. Hild, Das Neuron. In: W. Mollendorff and W. Bargmann (Eds.), *Handbuch der mikroskopischen Anatomie des Menschen, Vol. 4, Part 1,* Springer, Berlin, 1959, pp. 1–184 - A. Peters, S. Palay and H. de F. Webster, *The Fine Structure of the Nervous System*, Harper and Row, New York, Evanston, London, 1970

Technical
S.A. Luse, J. Ultrastruct. Res., 4(1960)108 - U. Karlsson and R.L. Schultz, J. Ultrastruct. Res., 14(1966)47 - S.E. Kornguth *et al.,* Exp. Cell Res., 45(1967)656

Neuron

Mitochondria
Structure J.F. Hartmann, J. Biophys. Biochem. Cytol., 2(1956)375 (Suppl.) - D. Duncan and W. Hild, Z. Zellforsch., 51(1960)123 - G. Hudson and J.F. Hartmann, Z. Zellforsch., 54(1961)147 - R.D. Yates and J.C. Yates, Z. Zellforsch., 92(1968)388
Development (formation of new mitochondria) E. Pannese, J. Ultrastruct. Res., 15(1966)57 - E. Pannese, Z. Zellforsch., 72(1966)295

Golgi
Structure R. Honjin, Fol. Anat. Japon., 29(1956)117 - S.K. Malhotra and G.A. Meek, J. Microscop. Sci., 101 (1960)389
Effects of an inhibitor of Na^+ and K^+ transport W.O. Whetsell and R.P. Bunge, J. Cell Biol., 42(1969)490

Subsurface cisterns
J. Rosenbluth, J. Cell Biol., 13(1962)405 - K.A. Siegesmund, Anat. Rec., 162(1968)187

Neurotubules
Structure E. Tani and T. Ametani, J. Cell Biol., 46(1970)159
Effects of spindle inhibitors H. Wisniewski *et al.,* J. Cell Biol., 38(1968)224 - C.B. Basbaum, Anat. Rec., 172(1972)266 - A.H. Bunt, Anat. Rec., 175(1973)281

Neurofilaments
D. Eichner, Z. Zellforsch., 43(1956)501 - E. Pannese, J. Cell Biol., 13(1962) 457

Axons
Structure S.L. Palay *et al.,* J. Cell Biol., 38(1968)193 - S.G. Waxman, Z. Zellforsch., 86(4)(1968)571
Acetylcholinesterase A.J. Darin *et al.,* J. Ultrastruct. Res., 28(1969)27 - M.L. Rennels and E. Nelson, Anat. Rec., 175(1973)423
Function B. Kisch, Exp. Med. Surg., 16(1958)221 - G. Bennett *et al.,* Anat. Rec., 175(1973)270
Effects of pericaryon removal J.R. McClung, Anat. Rec., 172 (1972)359

Coated vesicles
Origin T. Kanaseki and K. Kadota, J. Cell Biol., 42(1969)202
Pinocytosis M.P. Del Carro, Anat. Rec., 172(1972)299

Inclusions (cytoplasmic and nuclear)
A. Ghosh *et al.,* Anat. Rec., 143(1962)195 - R.L. Chandler and R. Willis, J. Cell Sci., 1(1966)283 - Y.J. Le Beux, Anat. Rec., 175(1973)369

Monoamine containing neurons
Cytochemistry K. Fuxe *et al.,* Anat. Rec., 155(1966)33 - T. Hokfelt, Z. Zellforsch., 91(1968)1
Depletion by oxypertine I.J. Bak *et al.,* Z. Zellforsch., 101 (1969)448

5-Hydroxytryptamine containing neurons
H. Braak and H.G. Baumgarten, Z. Zellforsch., 81(1967)416

Adrenergic neurons
Cytochemistry of catecholamines T. Hokfelt, Z. Zellforsch., 79(1967)110 - T.L.B. Spriggs *et al.,* J. de Microscopie, 6(1967)425
Uptake of norepinephrine N.J. Lenn, Amer. J. Anat., 120 (1967)377
Effects of benzoquinolizine (RO4–1284) A. Halaris *et al.,* Z. Zellforsch., 76(1967)100

Cholinergic neurons
Cytochemistry of cholinesterase P.R. Lewis and C.C.D. Shute, J. Cell Sci., 1(1966)381

Solids
R.W. Merriam and W.E. Koch, J. Biophys. Biochem. Cytol., 7(1960)151

Uptake and synthesis of protein
B. Droz, J. de Microscopie, 6(1967)201 - E. Holtzman and E.R. Peterson, J. Cell Biol., 40(1969)863

Growth of plasma membrane M.B. Bunge, Anat. Rec., 175 (1973)280 - K. Pfenninger, J. Cell Biol., 55(1972)203a

Regeneration J.B. Gelderd, Anat. Rec., 172(1972)314 - E.R. Peterson and S.M. Crain, Anat. Rec., 175(1973)411

Embryonic neurons R.P. Skoff, Anat. Rec., 175(1973)444

Ageing (lipofuscin accumulation)
T. Samorajski *et al.,* Anat. Rec., 160(1968)555

Cilia formation after pargyline
M. Milhaud and G.D. Pappas, J. Cell Biol., 37(1968)599

Effects of reserpine
D.L. Griffith, Anat. Rec., 175 (1973) 334

Effects of irradiation
T. Samorajski *et al.,* Anat. Rec., 168(1970)203

Synapses
General E.G. Gray. In: J.D. Boyd, F.R. Johnson and J.D. Lever (Eds.), *Electron Microscopy in Anatomy*, Williams and Wilkins, Baltimore, 1961, pp. 54–73 - V.P. Whittaker and E.G. Gray, Brit. Med. Bull., 18(1962)223
Structure S.L. Palay, J. Biophys. Biochem. Cytol., 2(1956) 193 (Suppl.) - E. De Robertis, Exp. Cell Res., Suppl. 5 (1958)347 - S.L. Palay, Exp. Cell Res., Suppl. 5(1958) 275 - E.G. Gray, J. Anat., 93(1959)420 - E.G. Gray, Nature, 183(1959)1592 - E. De Robertis *et al.,* J. Biophys. Biochem. Cytol., 9(1961)229 - J.D. Robertson *et al.,* J.

Cell Biol., 19(1963)159 - M.V.L. Bennett *et al.*, Science, 141(1963)262 - B.T. Charlton and E.G. Gray, J. Cell Sci., 1(1966)67 - M. Milhaud and G.D. Pappas, J. Cell Biol., 30(1966)437 - E.J.H. Nathaniel and D.R. Nathaniel, J. Ultrastruct. Res., 14(1966)540 - N.I. Artiukhina, Arkh. Anat. Gistol. Embriol., 52(3)(1967)38 - M.W. Brightman and T.S. Reese, J. Cell Biol., 40(1969)648 - G. Jaim-Etcheverry and L.M. Zieher, J. Cell Biol., 42(1969)855 - D.G. Jones, Z. Zellforsch., 95(1969)263 - B. Ehinger *et al.*, Z. Zellforsch., 107(1970)508 - A.M. Mouren-Mathieu, Anat. Rec., 172(1972)371 - F. Gonzalez-Aguilar, Anat. Rec., 175(1973)331 - K. Pfenninger, Synaptic morphology and cytochemistry (A Review). In: *Progr. Histoch. & Cytochem. Vol. 5,* Fischer, Stuttgart, Portland, 1973

Cytochemistry A.J. De Lorenzo, Bull. Johns Hopkins Hosp., 108(1961)258 - E. De Robertis *et al.*, J. Neurochem., 10(1963)225 - E. De Robertis, Science, 156(1967)907 - F.E. Bloom and G.K. Aghajanian, J. Ultrastruct. Res., 22 (1968)361 - H.Hirano *et al.*, Exp. Cell Res., 51(1968)259 - E.L. Rodriquez Echandia and C. Gonzalez, Anat. Rec., 172(1972)393

Function E.J. Furshpan, Science, 144(1964)878 - J. Eccles, Sci. Amer., 212(1965)56 - K. Uchizono, Jap. J. Electr. Micr., 17(1)(1968)55 - J. Heuser and T. Reese, Anat. Rec., 172(1972)329 - A.H. Dickinson and T.S. Reese, Anat. Rec., 175(1973)306 - K. Pfenninger and C.M. Rovainen, Anat. Rec., 175(1973)412

Development and origin of synaptic vesicles D.G. Jones and E. Revell, Z. Zellforsch., 111(1970)179 - D.G. Jones and E. Revell, Z. Zellforsch., 111(1970)195 - L. Vollrath, Z. Zellforsch., 99(1969)146

Formation of new synapses
G. Raisman and P. Field, Anat. Rec., 175(1973)419 - R. Rees *et al.*, Anat. Rec., 175(1973)421

Effects of axotomy M. Cuenod *et al.*, J. Cell Sci., 6(1970)605

Displacement by microglial cells during regeneration K. Blinzinger and G. Kreutzberg, Z. Zellforsch., 85(1968)145

Effects of ischemia due to hemorrhage V. Williams and R.G. Grossman, Anat. Rec., 166(1970)131

Neurosecretion (general)
A.A. Voitkevitch and I.I. Dedov, Arkh. Anat. Gistol. Embriol., 53(8)(1967)18

Neurosecretion in the vascular organ of the lamina terminalis
A. Weindl *et al.*, Z. Zellforsch., 85(1968)552 - P. Röhlich and T. Wenger, Z. Zellforsch., 102(1969)483

Neurosecretion in the subfornical organ
V.U. Rohr, Z. Zellforsch., 75(1966)11

Neurosecretion in the hypothalamo–hypophyseal system

Structure Y.I. Senchik and A.L. Polenov, Arkh. Anat. Gistol. Embriol., 52(3)(1967)45 - D. Zambrano and E. De Robertis, Z. Zellforsch., 81(1967)264 - D. Zambrano and E. De Robertis, Z. Zellforsch., 90(1968)230 - I.G. Akmayev, Z. Zellforsch., 96(1969)609 - W. Bargmann and Br. Von Gaudecker, Z. Zellforsch., 96(1969)495

Secretory cycle D. Zambrano and E. De Robertis, Z. Zellforsch., 73(1966)414

Effects of ageing Ch. Pilgrim, Z. Zellforsch., 109(1970)573

Effects of darkness and light N. Oztan, Z. Zellforsch., 75 (1966)66

Effects of suppression of adrenocortical steroid synthesis G. Garweg *et al.*, Z. Zellforsch., 101(1969)510

Effects of androgen inhibitors T.H. Schiebler and D.W. Meinhardt, Z. Zellforsch., 100(1969)581

Effects of salt loading J.I. Senchik and A.L. Polenov, Z. Zellforsch., 100(1969)118

Effects of inhibition of protein synthesis by puromycin D. Zambrano and E. De Robertis, Z. Zellforsch., 76(1967) 458

Neurosecretion in the arcuate nucleus
J.C. King *et al.*, Anat. Rec., 175(1973)358

Neurosecretion in the median eminence
E.M. Rodriguez, Z. Zellforsch., 93(1969)182 - J.H. Gross, Anat. Rec., 172(1972)320 - K.M. Knigge and A.J. Silverman, Anat. Rec., 172(1972)347 - S.A. Joseph, Anat. Rec., 175 (1973)351

Intraventricular neurosecretion and infundibular recess
T.F. Leveque *et al.*, Z. Zellforsch., 69(1966)381 - H. Leonhardt, Z. Zellforsch., 79(1967)172 - W. Wittkowski, Z. Zellforsch., 92(1968)207

Myelin

Peripheral nerves and Schwann cells

Structure G. Causey and H. Hoffman, J. Anat., 90(1956)1 - J.D. Robertson, J. Physiol., 135(1956)56 - H. Fernandez-Moran and J.B. Finean, J. Biophys. Biochem. Cytol., 3 (1957)725 - J.D. Robertson, J. Physiol., 137(1957)8 - H. Engstrom and J. Wersall, Exp. Cell Res., 14(1958)414 - J.B. Finean and J.D. Robertson, Brit. Med. Bull., 14 (1958)267 - J.D. Robertson, J. Biophys. Biochem. Cytol., 4(1958)39 - J.D. Robertson, Z. Zellforsch., 50(1959)553 - F.O. Schmitt, Rev. Modern Phys., 31(1959)455 - J.S. O'Brien, Science, 147(1965)1099 - A. Bischoff and H. Moor, Z. Zellforsch., 81(1967)571 - L.M. Napolitano and T.J. Scallen, Anat. Rec., 163(1969)1 - J.P. Revel and D.W. Hamilton, Anat. Rec., 163(1969)7 - V. Mizuhira and H. Ozawa, Jap. J. Electr. Micr., 16(2)(1967)169 - L.M. Napolitano and T.J. Scallen, Anat. Rec., 163(1969)1 - J.P. Revel and D.W. Hamilton, Anat. Rec., 163(1969)7 - S.M. Hall and P.L. Williams, J. Cell Sci., 6(1970)767

Cytochemistry L. Napolitano *et al.*, J. Cell Biol., 34(1967) 817 - N. Krishnan and M. Singer, Anat. Rec., 175(1973) 364

Function (including incorporation of choline, transport of histidine) M. Singer and M.M. Salpeter, J. Morph., 120 (1966)281 - W.J. Hendelman and R.P. Bunge, J. Cell Biol., 40(1969)190 - N. Krishan and M. Singer, Anat. Rec., 172(1972)350

Development B.B. Geren and F.O. Schmitt. In: D. Rudnick (Ed.), *Symposium on Cellular Mechanisms in Differentiation and Growth*, Princeton University Press, Princeton, 1956, pp. 213–220 - B.G. Uzman, J. Biophys. Biochem. Cytol., 2(1956)219 (Suppl.) - B.G. Uzman and G. Nogueira-Graf, J. Biophys. Biochem. Cytol., 3(1957)589 - V.L. Boroviaguin, Arkh. Anat. Gistol. Embriol., 52(3) (1967)19 - M.A. Matthews, Anat. Rec., 161(1968)337 - R.L. Friede and T. Samoroski, Anat. Rec., 165(1969)89

Effects of inhibitors of cholesterol synthesis on myelinisation
F.A. Rawlins and B.G. Uzman, J. Cell Biol., 46(1970)505

Effects of axotomy (Wallerian degeneration) R. Honjin and A. Takahashi, Jap. J. Electr. Micr., 11(3)(1962)139

Technical (effects of fixation, dehydration and embedding on structure) J.B. Finean, J. Biophys. Biochem. Cytol., 8

(1960)13 - J.B. Finean, J. Biophys. Biochem. Cytol., 8 (1960)31 - R.M. Condie *et al.*, J. Biophys. Biochem. Cytol., 9(1961)429

Central nervous system

Structure E. Horstmann, Z. Zellforsch., 45(1956)18 - A. Peters, J. Biophys. Biochem. Cytol., 11(1961)733 - U. Karlsson, J. Ultrastruct. Res., 15(1966)451 - F.I. Khattab, Anat. Rec., 156(1966)91 - A. Bischoff and H. Moor, Z. Zellforsch., 81(1967)303 - A. Hirano and H.M. Dembitzer, J. Cell Biol., 34(1967)555 - W.F. Blakemore, J. Ultrastruct. Res., 29(1969)496 - A. Hirano and H.M Dembitzer, J. Ultrastruct. Res., 28(1969)141

Development and origin S.A. Luse, J. Biophys. Biochem. Cytol., 2(1956)777 - E. De Robertis *et al.*, J. Biophys. Biochem. Cytol., 4(1958)651- A. Peters, J. Biophys. Biochem. Cytol., 8(1960)431 - M.G. Bunge *et al.*, J. Cell Biol., 12(1962)448

Regeneration M.B. Bunge *et al.*, J. Biophys. Biochem. Cytol., 10(1961)67

Glia

General

Structure S.A. Luse, Anat. Rec., 124(1956)329 (Abstract) - A. Bairati *et al.*, Z. Mikr.-Anat. Forsch., 63(1958)423 - E. De Robertis *et al.* In: D.B. Tower and J.P. Schade (Eds.), *Structure and Function of the Cerebral Cortex*, Elsevier, Amsterdam, 1960, pp. 69–80 - E. De Robertis and H.M. Gerschenfeld, In: C.C. Pfeiffer and J.R. Smythies (Eds.), *International Review of Neurobiology,* Academic Press, New York, 1961, p. 1 - A.L. Mikeladze, Arkh. Anat. Gistol. Embriol., 52(3)(1967)29 - C.H. Phelps, Anat. Rec., 175(1973)412 - V. Williams, Anat. Rec., 175(1973) 470

Origin J. Paterson *et al.*, Anat. Rec., 172(1972)380

Effects of thiamine deficiency G.H. Collins, Amer. J. Path., 50(1967)791

Astrocytes

Structure J. Wolff, Acta Neuropath., Suppl. 4(1968)33–39 - C.S. Raine and H. Wisniewski, Anat. Rec., 167(1970)303

Cytochemistry (glycogen) A. Oksche, Z. Zellforsch., 54 (1961)307 - J. Koizumi *et al.*, Jap. J. Electr. Micr., 19(4) (1970)355

Function (pinocytosis) M.P. Del Carro, Anat. Rec., 172 (1972)299

Development J.E. Vaughn and A. Peters, Amer. J. Anat., 121(1967)131

Oligodendroglia

Structure S.A. Luse, Anat. Rec., 138(1960)481 - L. Kruger and D.S. Maxwell, Amer. J. Anat., 118(1966)411

Function (production of central myelin) A. Hirano, J. Cell Biol., 38(1968)637

Function (reaction to chromatolytic neurons) J.S. Dixon, Anat. Rec., 163(1969)101

Ependyma, Subependyma and Choroid Plexus

Structure

M. Murakami, Jap. J. Electr. Micr., 10(2)(1961)77 - M. Murakami, Jap. J. Electr. Micr., 11(1)(1962)22 - W. Bargmann and E. Katritsis, Z. Zellforsch., 75(1966)366 - P.F. Doolin and W.J. Birge, J. Cell Biol., 29(1966)333 - H. Leonhardt, Z. Zellforsch., 74(1966)1 - A. Hirano and H.M. Zimmerman, Anat. Rec., 158(1967)293 - T.C. Anano Kumar, Z. Zellforsch., 90(1968)28 - H. Leonhardt, Z. Zellforsch., 88(1968) 297 - R.C. Santolaya and E.L. Rogriguez Echandia, Z. Zellforsch., 92(1968)43 - P.F. Doolin and W.J. Birge, Anat. Rec., 165(1969)515 - A. Weindl *et al.*, Z. Zellforsch., 100 (1969)300 - H. Leonhardt, Z. Zellforsch., 105(1970)595 - G.P. Kozlowski, Anat. Rec., 175(1973)363

Cytochemistry (glycogen, ATPase) G. Yasuzumi and I. Tsubo, Jap. J. Electr. Micr., 14(4)(1965)350 - A. Oksche *et al.*, Z. Zellforsch., 94(1969)232

Function, including neurosecretion and phagocytosis G. Sterba and G. Bruckner, Z. Zellforsch., 81(1967)457 - W. Wittkowski, Z. Zellforsch., 86(1968)111 - S.J. Carpenter *et al.*, Z. Zellforsch., 110(1970)471

Development W.F. Blakemore, J. Anat., 104(1969)423

Ageing A. Oksche and M. Vaupel-von Harnack, Z. Zellforsch., 93(1969)1

Intraventricular Axons

H. Leonhardt and H. Prien, Z. Zellforsch., 92(1968)394 - H. Leonhardt and A. Backhus-Roth, Z. Zellforsch., 97(1969)369 - W. Noack and J.R. Wolff, Z. Zellforsch., 111(1970)572 - I. Vigh-Teichmann *et al.*, Z. Zellforsch., 108(1970)17

Brain

Extracellular space and ground substance

Structure K. Niessing and W. Vogell, Z. Naturforsch., 12b (1957)641 - K. Niessing and W. Vogell, Z. Zellforsch., 52(1960)216 - W. Bondareff, Z. Zellforsch., 72(1966)487 - R.M. Torack, J. Ultrastruct. Res., 14(1966)590 - A. Van Harreveld and S.K. Malhotra, J. Cell Sci., 1(1966)223 - W. Bondareff, Z. Zellforsch., 81(1967)366 - P.V. Johnston and B.I. Roots, J. Cell Sci., 2(1967)377 - A. Van Harreveld and S.K. Malhotra, J. Anat., 101(2)(1967)197 - R.G. Frederickson and F.N. Low, Amer. J. Anat., 125 (1969)123 - F. Gonzalez-Aguilar, J. Ultrastruct. Res., 29 (1969)76 - A. Van Harreveld and J. Steiner, Anat. Rec., 166(1970)117 - A. Van Harreveld and J. Steiner, J. Cell Sci., 6(1970)793

Histochemistry A. Hess, J. Anat., 92(1958)298 - H. Amon, Z. Zellforsch., 88(1968)39

Development J.J. Pysh, Amer. J. Anat., 124(1969)411 - S.M. Sumi, J. Ultrastruct. Res., 29(1969)398

Cerebral cortex (general)

Structure E.G. Gray, J. Biophys. Biochem. Cytol., 6(1959) 121 - J.S. King, Anat. Rec., 161(1968)111 - V.S. Petrov, Arkh. Anat. Gistol. Embriol., 54(3)(1968)77 - T.V. Davydova and G.D. Smirnov, Arkh. Anat. Gistol. Embriol., 56(7)(1969)3 - A. Peters and I.R. Kaiserman-Agramof, Z. Zellforsch., 100(1969)487

Development H. Ramsey, Anat. Rec., 139(1961)333 (Abstract) - K. Meller *et al.*, Z. Zellforsch., 72(1966)525 - S. Duckett, Anat. Rec., 161(1968)231 - I.I. Glezer, Arkh. Anat. Gistol. Embriol., 56(4)(1969)77 - R. Johnson and M. Armstrong-James, Z. Zellforsch., 110(1970)540

Olfactory cortex

Effects of puromycin P. Gambetti *et al.*, J. Cell Biol., 36 (1968)379

Effects of axotomy L.E. Westrum, Z. Zellforsch., 98(1969) 157

Motor cortex

Structure K. Meller *et al.*, Z. Zellforsch., 92(1968)217

Development K. Meller *et al.*, Z. Zellforsch., 86(1968)171 - K. Meller *et al.*, Z. Zellforsch., 99(1969)443

Visual cortex

Phagocytosis of ferritin L. Selwood, Z. Zellforsch., 107 (1970)6

Hippocampus

Structure H.J. Nafstad and T.W. Blackstad, Z. Zellforsch., 73(1966)234 - Y. Ibata and N. Otsuka, Z. Zellforsch., 91(1968)547

Cytochemistry (cholinesterase) C.C.D. Shute and P.R. Lewis, Z. Zellforsch., 69(1966)334

Effects of methoxypyridoxin, dithizon, reserpin and iproniazid W. Niklowitz, Z. Zellforsch., 70(1966)220 - N. Otsuka and Y. Ibata, Jap. J. Electr. Micr., 16(4)(1967)340 - W.L. Niklowitz, Z. Zellforsch., 101(1969)192

Mammillary bodies

A.L. Mikeladze and I.L. Lazriyev, Arkh. Anat. Gistol. Embriol. 56(1)(1969)28

Median eminence and arcuate nucleus

Structure U.K. Rinne, Z. Zellforsch., 74(1966)98 - G.J. Etcheverry and A. Pellegrino de Iraldi, Anat. Rec., 160 (1968)239 - H. Leonhardt, Z. Zellforsch., 103(1970)420

Effects of castration, estrous cycle and hypothalamic deafferentiation D. Zambrano and E. De Robertis, Z. Zellforsch., 87(1968)409 - D. Zambrano, Z. Zellforsch., 93(1969)560 - D.E. Scott and K.M Knigge, Z. Zellforsch., 105(1970)1

Infundibulum

M. Mazzuca, J. de Microscopie, 7(1968)135 - R.M. Bergland and R.M. Torack, Z. Zellforsch., 99(1969)1

Corpus callosum

R.L. Schultz *et al.*, Amer. J. Anat., 100(1957)369 - K. Fleischhauer and H. Wartenberg, Z. Zellforsch., 83(1967)568

Corpus striatum and globus pallidus

Structure S. Mori, Z. Zellforsch., 70(1966)461

Effects of psychotropic drugs J. Koizumi and H. Shiraishi, Jap. J. Electr. Micr., 19(2)(1970)182

Thalamus, ventrobasal and posterior

M.M. Herman and H.J. Ralston, Anat. Rec., 167(1970)183

Lateral geniculate body

Structure U. Karlsson, J. Ultrastruct. Res., 16(1966)429 - U. Karlsson, J. Ultrastruct. Res., 16(1966)482 - A. Peters and S.L. Palay, J. Anat., 100(3)(1966)451 - P.F. Doolin *et al.*, Amer. J. Anat., 121(1967)601 - P.F. Doolin *et al.*, Anat. Rec., 159(1967)219 - R.W. Guillery, Amer. J. Anat., 120(1967)583 - U. Karlsson, J. Ultrastruct. Res., 17(1967)137 - J.A. Campos-Ortega *et al.*, Z. Zellforsch., 87(1968)82 - J.P. Saavedra *et al.*, Z. Zellforsch., 89(1968) 462 - R.W. Guillery, Z. Zellforsch., 96(1969)1 - R.W. Guillery and M. Colonnier, Z. Zellforsch., 103(1970)90

Development U. Karlsson, J. Ultrastruct. Res., 17(1967)158

Effects of eye enucleation and of blinding U.J. McMahan, Z. Zellforsch., 76(1967)116 - J.P. Saavedra *et al.*, Z. Zellforsch., 93(1969)164

Hypothalamo–hypophyseal system

H. Braak, Z. Zellforsch., 83(1967)398 - A. Bjorklund *et al.*, Z. Zellforsch., 89(1968)590 - N. Stosic *et al.*, Z. Zellforsch., 102(1969)554

Supraoptic and paraventricular nuclei

Structure A.M. Suburio and A. Pellegrino de Iraldi, J. Anat., 105(1969)439

Effects of dehydration H.F. Reinhardt *et al.*, Z. Zellforsch., 102(1969)172

Effects of castration D. Zambrano and E. De Robertis, Z. Zellforsch., 86(1968)487

Amygdala

E. Hall, Z. Zellforsch., 92(1968)169

Subfornical organ

K. Akert *et al.*, Z. Zellforsch., 81(1967)537 - H. Rudert *et al.*, Z. Zellforsch., 88(1968)145

Subcommissural organ

Structure R.M. Barlow *et al.*, Z. Zellforsch., 77(1967)299 - N.X. Papacharalampous *et al.*, Z. Zellforsch., 90(1968) 202

Development H.S. Lin and I.L. Chen, Z. Zellforsch., 96 (1969)186

Brain Stem

Red Nucleus

J.S. King, Z. Zellforsch., 106(1970)309

Substantia nigra and locus coeruleus

Structure K. Hirosawa, Z. Zellforsch., 88(1968)187

Uptake of labeled norepinephrine L. Descarries and B. Droz, J. Cell Biol., 44(1970)385

Area postrema

E. Lindner and H. Leonhardt, Z. Zellforsch., 86(1968)453

Reticular substance

R.C. Santolaya and E.M. Rodriguez, Z. Zellforsch., 79(1967) 537

Vestibular nuclei

Effects of thiamine deficiency I. Tellez and R.D. Terry, Amer. J. Path., 52(4)(1968)777

Trapezoid body and ventral cochlear nuclei

N.J. Lenn and T.S. Reese, Amer. J. Anat., 118(1966)375

Cerebellum

Structure

C.H. Good, Anat. Rec., 139(1961)231 (Abstract) - L.L. Ross *et al.*, J. Cell Biol., 14(1962)19 - S. Gobel, J. Ultrastruct. Res., 15(1966)310 - R. Morales and D. Duncan, J. Ultrastruct. Res., 15(1966)480 - R. Morales and D. Duncan, Z. Zellforsch., 83(1967)49 - M.P. Del Cerro and R.S. Snider, Anat. Rec., 165(1969)127 - K.U. Petersen, Z. Zellforsch.,

100(1969)616 - K. Takahashi, Jap. J. Electr. Micr., 18(4) (1969)312 - D. Duncan *et al.*, Anat. Rec., 168(1970)1 - S.U. Kim, Z. Zellforsch., 107(1970)454 - K. Takahashi and R.L. Wood, Z. Zellforsch., 110(1970)311

Cytochemistry (sodium) K.A. Siegesmund, J. Anat., 105(1969) 403

Development L.N. Diyatchkova and I. Hamori, Arkh. Anat. Gistol. Embriol., 52(2)(1967)30 - K. Dvorak and J. Bueck, Z. Zellforsch., 111(1970)51

Cranial Nerves

Olfactory

Structure B. Berger, Arch. d'Anat. Micr., 58(1969)41

Development J. Ochi, Z. Zellforsch., 76(1967)339

Optic

Structure H.R. Maturana, J. Biophys. Biochem. Cytol., 7 (1960)107 - A. Peters and J.E. Vaughn, J. Cell Biol., 32 (1967)113

Development J.E. Vaughn, Z. Zellforsch., 94(1969)293

Effects of axotomy (Wallerian degeneration) L. Kruger and D.S. Maxwell, Amer. J. Anat., 125(1969)247

Ciliary ganglion

A.J. de Lorenzo, J. Biophys. Biochem. Cytol., 7(1960)31 - K. Takahashi, Z. Zellforsch., 83(1967)70

Trigeminal nerve root and ganglion

A. Pineda *et al.*, Amer. J. Anat., 121(1967)461 - J.H. Hardin *et al.*, Anat. Rec., 164(1969)403 - D.S. Maxwell *et al.*, Anat. Rec., 164(1969)113

Acoustic and vestibular

J. Rosenbluth and S.L. Palay, J. Biophys. Biochem. Cytol., 9(1961)853 - J. Rosenbluth, J. Cell Biol., 12(1962)329 - E.L. Rodriguez Echandia, Z. Zellforsch., 85(1968)183

Spinal Cord

Structure

F. Valverde, Z. Zellforsch., 71(1966)297 - A. Rapoport and J. Stempak, Anat. Rec., 161(1968)361 - K. Kohno, Z. Zellforsch., 94(1969)565 - V.A. Maisky and L.A. Savoskina, Arkh. Anat. Gistol. Embriol., 57(7)(1969)26

Development and tissue cultures H.J. Gamble, J. Anat., 104 (1969)435 - K. Meller *et al.*, Z. Zellforsch., 101(1969)135

Regeneration of axons P. Lampert and M. Cressman, Lab. Invest., 13(1964)825

Spinal nerve roots

W.W. Schlaepfer, Z. Zellforsch., 88(1968)441

Spinal ganglia

Structure G.M. Wyburn, J. Anat., 92(1958)528 - E. Pannese, Z. Zellforsch., 52(1960)567 - J. Rosenbluth and S.L. Palay, Anat. Rec., 136(1960)268 (Abstract) - K.H. Andres, Z. Zellforsch., 55(1961)1 - M.B. Bunge *et al.*, J. Cell Biol., 32(1967)439 - W. Brzin *et al.*, J. Cell Biol., 31(1966)215 - A. Novikoff *et al.*, J. Cell Biol., 29(1966) 525 - T.L. Lentz, Anat. Rec., 158(1967)453

Development V.M. Tennyson and M. Brzin, J. Cell Biol., 46 (1970)64

Regeneration E. Pannese, Z. Zellforsch., 60(1963)711

Effects of axotomy (retrograde degeneration) K.H. Andres, Z. Zellforsch., 55(1961)49

Spinal nerves

Structure W. Thornburg and E. De Robertis, J. Biophys. Biochem. Cytol., 2(1956)475 - J.D. Robertson, J. Biophys. Biochem. Cytol., 3(1957)1043 - F.O. Schmitt, J. Cell Comp. Physiol., 49(1957)165 (Suppl. 1) - F.O. Schmitt, Exp. Cell Res., Suppl. 5(1958)33 - B.G. Uzman and G.M. Villegas, J. Biophys. Biochem. Cytol., 7(1960)761 - T. Samorajski and R.L. Friede, Anat. Rec., 161(1968)281 - R.L. Friede and T. Samorajski, Anat. Rec., 167(1970)379

Development A. Peters and A.R. Muir, Quart. J. Exp. Physiol., 44(1959)117 - H.J. Gamble, J. Anat., 100(3) (1966)487 - E.T. Hedley-Whyte *et al.*, Lab. Invest., 21(6) (1969)536 - G. Allt, J. Anat., 105(1969)283

Regeneration A. Pellegrino de Iraldi and E. De Robertis, Z. Zellforsch., 87(1968)330 - C. Estable *et al.*, Z. Zellforsch., 46(1957)387 - S. Ohmi, Z. Zellforsch., 56(1962)625 - S. Blumcke and H.R. Niedorf, Virchows Arch. Path. Anat., 340(1965)93

Effects of anisotonic solutions J.D. Robertson, J. Biophys. Biochem. Cytol., 4(1958)349 - L.G. Elfvin, J. Ultrastruct. Res., 7(1962)1

Effects of axotomy H.D. Webster, J. Cell Biol., 12(1962)361

Neuromuscular Junctions

Skeletal muscle

Structure E. Andersson-Cedergren, J. Ultrastruct. Res.,Suppl. 1(1959)1 - J.E. Gruner, Compt. Rend. Soc. Biol. Pan's, 155(1961)1841 - M.V. During, Z. Zellforsch., 81(1967)74 - H. Hirano, Z. Zellforsch., 79(1967)198 - E. Nickel *et al.*, Z. Zellforsch., 78(1967)261 - H.A. Padykula and G.F. Gauthier, J. Cell Biol., 46(1970)27 - H. Teräväinen, Z. Zellforsch., 96(1969)206 - J. Rosenbluth, Anat. Rec., 175(1973)428

Histochemistry R. Davis and G.B. Koelle, J. Cell Biol., 34 (1967)157 - M.M. Salpeter, J. Cell Biol., 32(1967)379 - A.W. Rogers *et al.*, J. Cell Biol., 41(1969)665 - M.M. Salpeter, J. Cell Biol., 42(1969)122

Development and tissue cultures H. Teräväinen, Z. Zellforsch., 87(1968)249 - D.W. James and R.L. Tresman, Z. Zellforsch., 100(1969)126 - A.M. Kelly and S.I. Zacks, J. Cell Biol., 42(1969)154

Effects of acetylcholinesterase inhibitors H.J. Preusser, Z. Zellforsch., 80(1967)436

Effects of axotomy H. Teräväinen and K. Huikuri, Z. Zellforsch., 102(1969)466

Autonomic

Ganglia

Structure G. Causey and H. Hoffman, J. Anat., 90(1956)502 - A.A. Barton and G. Causey, J. Anat., 92(1958)399 - G.M. Wyburn, Scot. Med. J., 3(1958)385 - J.S. Dixon, Anat. Rec., 156(1966)239 W.G. Forssmann and C. Rouiller, Z. Zellforsch., 70(1966)364 - T.N. Radostina and I.F. Ivanov, Arkh. Anat. Gistol. Embriol., 50(5)(1966)66 - I.F. Ivanov and T.N. Radostina, Arkh. Anat. Gistol. Embriol., 53(8)(1967)50 - J. Pick, Z. Zellforsch., 82(1967) 118 - K. Becker, Z. Zellforsch., 88(1968)318 - L.M. Diyatchkova and V.P. Badmindra, Arkh. Anat. Gistol. Embriol., 54(3)(1968)30 - L.G. Elfvin, J. Ultrastruct.

Res., 22(1968)37 - G. Siegrist *et al.*, J. Ultrastruct. Res., 25(1968)381 - G.L. Colborn and N.J. Adamo, Anat. Rec., 164(1969)185 - M.J.T. Fitzgerald and R.W. Alexander, J. Anat., 105(1969)27 - M.R. Matthews and G. Raisman, J. Anat., 105(1969)255 - C.O. Sangiacomo, Z. Zellforsch., 95(1969)290 - M.A. Grillo, J. Cell Biol., 45(1970)100 - H. Watanabe, Amer. J. Anat., 130(1971)305 - V.M. Tennyson, Anat. Rec., 175(1973)456

Cytochemistry (sulfated protein inclusions) R. Seite, Z. Zellforsch., 101(1969)621

Effects of axotomy E. Holtzman *et al.*, J. Cell Biol., 33 (1967)419 - J. Hamori *et al.*, Z. Zellforsch., 90(1968)37 - A.R. Lieberman, J. Anat., 104(1969)49 - A.R. Lieberman, J. Anat., 104(1969)309 - J.S. Dixon, Anat. Rec., 168(1970)179

Effects of ascorbic acid deficiency D.F. Sulkin *et al.*, Lab. Invest., 19(1)(1968)55

Effects of glucose deprivation P. Nicolescu *et al.*, J. Cell Biol., 29(1966)267

Paraganglia

P. Böck, Z. Zellforsch., 110(1970)243 - I. Li Chen and R.D. Yates, Z. Zellforsch., 108(1970)309

Nerve fibers and terminals (general)

Structure A. Hess, Proc. Roy. Soc., 144(1956)496 - L.G. Elfvin, J. Ultrastruct. Res., 1(1958)428 - L.G. Elfvin, J. Ultrastruct. Res., 5(1961)51 - L.G. Elfvin, J. Ultrastruct. Res., 5(1961)374 - L.G. Elfvin, J. Ultrastruct. Res., 5 (1961)388 - K.C. Richardson, Anat. Rec., 164(1969)359

Uptake of labeled norepinephrine G.S. Budd and M.M. Salpeter, J. Cell Biol., 41(1969)21

Effects of axotomy J.J. Mire *et al.*, J. Cell Biol., 45(1970)9

Afferent visceral fibers

Effects of axotomy G. Ungváry and C. Léránth, Z. Zellforsch., 110(1970)185

Autonomic innervation of heart

Structure S. Viragh and A. Porte, Z. Zellforsch., 55(1961) 282 - J.C. Thaemert, J. Cell Biol., 29(1966)156 - R. Hadek and P.J. Talso, J. Ultrastruct. Res., 17(1967)257 - J.C. Thaemert, Anat. Rec., 163(1969)575 - T. Chiba and A. Yamauchi, Z. Zellforsch., 108(1970)324 - S. Hayashi *et al.*, Jap. J. Electr. Micr., 19(2)(1970)176 - E. Nilsson and B. Sporrong, Z. Zellforsch., 111(1970)404

Histochemistry H. Hirano and K. Ogawa, Jap. J. Electr. Micr., 16(4)(1967)313

Autonomic innervation of vessels

Structure S. Sato, Amer. J. Anat., 118(1966)873 - F.O. Simpson and C.E. Devine, J. Anat., 100(1)(1966)127 - M. Dragiyev, Arkh. Anat. Gistol. Embriol., 53(9)(1967)67 - E. Hagen and W. Wittkowski, Z. Zellforsch., 95(1969)429

Development W. Calvo and J. Forteza-Vila, Amer. J. Anat., 126(1969)355

Effects of axotomy J.D. Lever *et al.*, J. Anat., 103(1) (1968)15 - T. Iwayama, Z. Zellforsch., 109(1970)465

Autonomic innervation of visceral (non-vascular) smooth muscle

Structure R. Caesar *et al.*, J. Biophys. Biochem. Cytol., 3 (1957)867 - K.C. Richardson, Amer. J. Anat., 103(1958) 99 - T. Yamamoto, Acta Neuroveget. Vienna, 21 (1960)406 - H. Gansler, Acta Neuroveget. Vienna, 22 (1961)192 - J.C. Thaemert, J. Cell Biol., 28(1966)37 - C.E. Devine and F.O. Simpson, Amer. J. Anat., 121 (1967)153 - N.C.R. Merrillees, J. Cell Biol., 37(1968)794 - A.M. Novi, Anat. Rec., 160(1968)123 - D.C. Rogers, Z. Zellforsch., 89(1968)80 - I. Kushiya, Jap. J. Electr. Micr., 17(2)(1968)127 - A. Yamauchi and G. Burnstock, J. Anat., 104(1969)17 - H.G. Baumgarten *et al.*, Z. Zellforsch., 106(1970)376 - J.A. Gosling and J.S. Dixon, Z. Zellforsch., 108(1970)127

Histochemistry P.M. Robinson and C. Bell, J. Cell Biol., 33 (1967)93 - H.G. Baumgarten *et al.*, Z. Zellforsch., 90 (1968)81 - P.M. Robinson, J. Cell Biol., 41(1969)462

Uptake of labeled catecholamines J. Taxi and B. Droz, Arkh. Anat. Gistol. Embriol., 55(7)(1968)35

Effects of axotomy C.D. Roth and K.C. Richardson, Amer. J. Anat., 124(1969)341

Autonomic innervation of glands

See subsequent chapters on the various visceral systems

Meninges (Dura, Arachnoid, Pia)

Structure H. Thomas, Z. Mikr.-Anat. Forsch., 75(1966)270 - K.H. Andres, Z. Zellforsch., 79(1967)272 - K.H. Andres, Z. Zellforsch., 82(1967)92 - M. Rascol and J. Izard, J. de Microscopie, 8(1969)1017

Nerve Sheaths (Endoneurium, Perineurium, Epineurium)

Structure P. Röhlich and A. Knoop, Z. Zellforsch., 53 (1961)299 - W.E. Burkel, Anat. Rec., 158(1967)177 - J.S. McCabe and F.N. Low, Anat. Rec., 164(1969)15 - A. Saito and S.I. Zacks, Anat. Rec., 164(1969)379 - D. Kerjaschki and L. Stockinger, Z. Zellforsch., 110(1970) 386 - F.R. Haller and F.N. Low, Amer. J. Anat., 131 (1971)1 - M.D. Ross and W. Burkel, Amer. J. Anat., 130 (1971)73

Transport of large and small molecules across nerve sheaths J.D. Waggener *et al.*, J. Neuropath. Exp. Neurol., 24 (1965)430 - H. Klemm, Z. Zellforsch., 108(1970)431

Regeneration after Wallerian degeneration R.D. Terry and J.C. Harkin, Exp. Cell Res., 13(1957)193

Connective Tissue of Ganglia

A.R. Lieberman, Z. Zellforsch., 89(1968)95

7. CIRCULATORY SYSTEM

General

D.W. Fawcett, The fine structure of capillaries, arterioles and small arteries. In: S.R.M. Reynolds and B.W. Zweifach (Eds.), *The Microcirculation*, University of Illinois Press, Urbana, 1959, pp. 1–27

Capillaries and Endothelium

General

Structure W. Bargmann, Deut. Med. Wochschr., 83(1958) 1704 - A. Policard and A. Collet, Rev. Franc. Etud. Clin. Biol., 3(1958)205 - H.S. Bennett *et al.*, Amer. J. Physiol., 196(1959)381 - H.W. Florey *et al.*, J. Pathol. Bacteriol.,

77(1959)625 - K. Hama, Anat. Rec., 139(1961)437 - J.A.G. Rhodin, J. Ultrastruct. Res., 6(1962)171 - J. Wolff, Z. Zellforsch., 73(1966)143 - J. Wolff and H.J. Merker, Z. Zellforsch., 73(1966)174 - J.N.H. Anh *et al.*, Z. Mikr.-Anat. Forsch., 77(1967)432 - A. Cecio, Z. Zellforsch., 83(1967)40 - V.A. Shakhlamov, Arkh. Anat. Gistol. Embriol., 52(1)(1967)24 - H.H.R. Friederici, J. Ultrastruct. Res., 23(1968)444 - G.E. Palade and R.R. Bruns, J. Cell Biol., 37(1968)633 - A.A. Voitkevitch and I.I. Dedov, Arkh. Anat. Gistol. Embriol., 55(12)(1968)25 - G.J. Dohrman and P.B. Herdson, Exp. Molec. Path., 11 (2)(1969)163 - R.M. Ludatscher and W.E. Stehbens, Z. Zellforsch., 97(1969)169 - K.F. Steinsiepe and E.R. Weibel, Z. Zellforsch., 108(1970)105

Cytochemistry (acid polysaccharides, ATPase) J.H. Luft, Fed. Proc., 25(1966)1771 - W.G. Campbell, Jr., Lab. Invest., 18(3)(1968)304

Function (permeability) G.D. Pappas and V.M. Tennyson, J. Cell Biol., 15(1962)227 - M.J. Karnofsky, J. Cell Biol., 35(1967)213 - A.A. Veitkevitch and I.I. Dedov, Arkh. Anat. Gistol. Embriol., 57(12)(1969)3 - J.H. Luft. In: B.W. Zweifach *et al.* (Eds.), The Inflammatory Process p. 121, Academic Press, New York, 1965 - A.L. Shabo and M.W. Brightman, Anat. Rec., 172(1972)404 - P.P. De Bruyn and S. Michelson, Anat. Rec., 175(1973)303 - A.F. Payer, Anat. Rec., 175(1973)408

Function (leucocyte emigration inflammation) V.T. Marchesi, Quart, J. Exp. Physiol. 46(1961)115

Function (contraction) R.S. De Santo and P.L. Dudley, J. Ultrastruct. Res., 28(1969)259

Development F. Gonzalez-Crussi, Amer. J. Anat., 130(1971) 441

Ageing R. Morales *et al.*, Texas Repts. Biol. Med., 18 (1960)247

Effects of histamine and serotonin G. Majno and G.E. Palade, J. Biophys. Biochem. Cytol., 11(1961)571 - G. Majno *et al.*, J. Cell Biol., 42(1969)647

Effects of adrenaline P.H. Burri and E.R. Weibel, Z. Zellforsch., 88(1968)426

Effects of Vit. E deficiency V.W. Fischer and J.S. Nelson, Anat. Rec., 175(1973)319

Effects of X-rays M.M. Sholley, Anat. Rec., 175(1973)441

Effects of thrombosis L. Cossel, Beitr. Path. Anat., 135 (1967)377

Capillaries of bone marrow

L. Weiss, Bull. Johns Hopkins Hosp., 108(1961)171 - L. Zamboni and D. C. Pease, J. Ultrastruct. Res., 5(1961)65

Capillaries of thymus

L. Weiss, Anat. Rec., 145(1963)413 - B. Kramarsky *et al.*, J. Cell Biol., 35(1967)464

Capillaries (sinusoids) of spleen

L. Weiss, J. Biophys. Biochem. Cytol., 3(1957)599 - L. Weiss, Anat. Rec., 139(1961)286 - L. Weiss, Amer. J. Anat., 111 (1962)131 - R.D. Moore *et al.*, Exp. Molec. Path., 3(1964)31 - G. Simon and R. Pictet, Acta Anat., 57(1964)163 - C.E. Thomas, Amer. J. Anat., 120(1967)527

Capillaries of lymphnodes

A. Policard *et al.*, Z. Zellforsch., 56(1962)203

Capillaries of muscle

Structure F. Hammersen, Z. Zellforsch., 69(1966)296 - R.R. Bruns and G.E. Palade, J. Cell Biol., 37(1968)244 - E. Nickel and E. Grieshaber, Z. Zellforsch., 95(1969)445

Function (transport of ferritin) R.R. Bruns and G.E. Palade, J. Cell Biol., 37(1968)277

Capillaries of heart

G.E. Palade, Circulation, 24(1961)368

Capillaries of nervous system

Structure E.A. Maynard *et al.*, Amer. J. Anat., 100(1957)409 - H. Hager, Acta Neuropath. Berlin, 1(1961)9 - E. Nelson *et al.*, Neurology (Minneap.), 11(1961)285 - J.M. Rivera-Pomar, Z. Zellforsch., 75(1966)542 - A. Schwink and R. Wetzstein, Z. Zellforsch., 73(1966)56 - H. Leonhardt, Z. Zellforsch., 76(1967)511 - E. Sluga and F. Seitelberger, Z. Zellforsch., 78(1967)303 - W. Wittkowski, Z. Zellforsch., 81(1967)344 - W. Lierse, Acta Neuropath., Berlin, Suppl. 4(1968)40 - G. Gabbiani and G. Majno, Z. Zellforsch., 97(1969)111

Histochemistry (nucleoside phosphatase) R.M. Torack and R.J. Barnett, J. Neuropath. Exp. Neurol., 23(1964)46

Function (blood–brain barrier to peroxidase) T.S. Reese and M.J. Karnovsky, J. Cell Biol., 34(1967)207 - T.S. Bodenheimer and M.W. Brightman, Amer. J. Anat., 122(1968) 249

Development S. Donahue and G.D. Pappas, Amer. J. Anat., 108(1961)331 - N.N. Bogolepov, Arkh. Anat. Gistol. Embriol., 52(6)(1967)83

Capillaries of other organs

See subsequent chapters

Arterioles

R.G. Hibbs *et al.*, Amer. Heart. J., 56(1958)662 - A. Policard *et al.*, Bull. Microsc. Appl., 2(1960)17 - G.P. Epling, Anat. Rec., 155(1966)513 - J.A.G. Rhodin, J. Ultrastruct. Res., 18 (1967)181 - P. Röhlich and I. Olah, J. Ultrastruct. Res., 18 (1967)667 - E. Westergaard and M.W. Brightman, Anat. Rec., 175(1973)469

Muscular Arteries

D.H. Moore and H. Ruska, J. Biophys. Biochem. Cytol., 3 (1957)457 - F. Parker, Amer. J. Anat., 103(1958)247 - H.W. Florey, Proc. Roy. Soc. Med., 53(1960)13 - D.C. Pease and S. Molinari, J. Ultrastruct. Res., 3(1960)447 - H.A. Hackensellner and H. David, Frankf. Z. Path., 71(1961)194 - J. Lang and A. Nordwig, Z. Zellforsch., 73(1966)313 - W.E. Burkel, Anat. Rec., 167(1970)329 - N. Cauna, Anat. Rec., 168(1970) 9 - F. Hammersen, Z. Zellforsch., 109(1970)380

Structural role of calcium in endothelial junctions P. Constantinides, Anat. Rec., 172(1972)295

Function (possible endothelial secretion) R.S. Piezzi, Anat. Rec., 165(1969)229

Permeability of endothelium J.E. French, Int. Rev. Exp. Path. 5(1966)253 - I. Hüttner *et al.*, Am. J. Path., 61 (1970)395 - I. Hüttner *et al.*, Am. J. Path., 66(1972)46a - P. Constantinides, Proc. 4th Europ. Congr. Pathol., Budapest 1973, In Acta Morph. Acad. Sci. Hung. Suppl. XIV (1973)

Ageing M. Grunnet, Arch., Path., 88(3)(1969)314

Regeneration after injury P. Constantinides, Arch. Path., 85 (1968)280

Endothelial effects of high-fat diet A.D. Ashburn *et al.*, Anat.

Rec., 165(1969)379

Endothelial effects of oral fatty acids and of ketoacids P. Constantinides, Anat. Rec., 175(1973)296

Endothelial effects of pH, osmolarity and cyanide P. Constantinides and M. Robinson, Arch. Path., 88(1969)99

Endothelial effects of vasoactive amines P. Constantinides and M. Robinson, Arch. Path. 88(1969)106 - P.C. Phelps and J.H. Luft, Amer. J. Anat., 125(1969)399 - P. Constantinides. In: *The Artery and the Process of Arteriosclerosis, Vol. 16A,* p. 185, Plenum Press, New York 1971 - P. Constantinides, Fed. Proc., 32(1973)855

Endothelial effects of enzymes and surfactants P. Constantinides and M. Robinson, Arch. Path., 88(1969)113 - F. Parl and W.H. Gutstein, Fed. Proc., 32(1973)855

Elastic Arteries

Structure R.C. Buck, J. Biophys. Biochem. Cytol., 4(1958) 187 - M.K. Keech, J. Biophys. Biochem. Cytol., 7(1960) 533 - D.C. Pease and W.J. Paule, J. Ultrastruct. Res., 3 (1960)469 E.S. Sachs and W.T. Daems, Z. Zellforsch., 73(1966)553 - P.M. Rees, J. Anat., 103(1)(1968)35

Histochemistry of elastic laminae S.Y. Yu and S.E. Lai, Jap. J. Electr. Micr., 19(4)(1970)362

Development H.E. Karrer, J. Ultrastruct. Res., 4(1960)420 - K. Takagi and O. Kawase, Jap. J. Electr. Micr., 16(4) (1967)330 - J. Bartman, J. de Microscopie, 7(1968)355

Ageing H.E. Karrer, J. Ultrastruct. Res., 5(1961)1 - D.N. McMartin *et al.,* Arch. Path., 89(2)(1970)164

Effects of copper deficiency J. Waisman *et al.,* Amer. J. Path., 54(1)(1969)107 - J. Waisman *et al.,* Lab. Invest., 21(6)(1969)548

Carotid Body

Structure L.L. Ross, J. Biophys. Biochem. Cytol., 6(1959) 253 - W.E. Stehbens and M.D. Silver, J. Cell Biol., 26 (1965)669 - T.J. Biscoe and W.E. Stehbens, J. Cell Biol., 30(1966)563 - R. Hoglund, Z. Zellforsch., 76(1967)568 - F. Al-Lami and R.G. Murray, J. Ultrastruct. Res., 24 (1968)465 - E. Morita *et al.,* J. Ultrastruct. Res., 28 (1969)399 - P. Böch *et al.,* Z. Zellforsch., 105(1970)543 - E. Morita *et al.,* Anat. Rec., 167(1970)309

Function (uptake of labelled amine precursors) I. Li Chen and R D. Yates, J. Cell Biol., 42(1969)794

Cytochemistry (biogenic amines) G. Battaglia, Z. Zellforsch., 99(1969)529

Effects of reserpine D. Duncan and R. Yates, Anat. Rec., 157(1967)667 - I. Li Chen *et al.,* J. Cell Biol., 42(1969) 804

Effects of CO_2, anoxia and sinus nerve stimulation S. Blumcke *et al.,* Z. Zellforsch., 81(1967)557 - F. Al-Lami and R.G. Murray, Anat. Rec., 160(1968)697 - R.D. Yates *et al.,* J. Cell Biol., 46(1970)544

Venules

Structure J.A.G. Rhodin, J. Ultrastruct. Res., 25(1968)452 - M. Takada, Anat, Rec., 166(1970)605 - C. Ropke *et al.,* Anat. Rec., 172(1972)393

Passage of lymphocytes through endothelial junctions E.J. Wenk *et al.,* Anat. Rec., 175(1973)468

Effects of ferritin and thorotrast on endothelial junctions R.P. Becker, Anat. Rec., 172(1971)267

Veins

R.M. Ludatscher, J. Anat., 103(2)(1968)345 - C.H. Tsao *et al.,* Anat. Rec., 166(1970)529 - A.W. El Bermani, Anat. Rec., 172(1972)306

Lymphatic Capillaries

R. Moe, Anat. Rec., 136(1960)245 (Abstract) - E.E. Fraley and L. Weiss, Amer. J. Anat., 109(1961)85 - L.V. Leak and J.F. Burke, Amer. J. Anat., 118(1966)785 - L.V. Leak, J. Morph., 125(1968)419 - L.V. Leak and J.F. Burke, J. Cell Biol., 36(1968)129 - H.J. Oehmke, Z. Zellforsch., 90(1968) 320 - R.H. Borst *et al.,* Z. Zellforsch., 101(1969)338 - G.L. Todd, Anat. Rec., 172(1972)419 and 175(1973)457

Lymphatic Ducts

W. Kuhnel, Z. Zellforsch., 70(1966)519 - R. Schipp, J. Ultrastruct. Res., 19(1967)250

Endocardium and Heart Valves

Structure W. Kuhnel, Z. Zellforsch., 69(1966)452 - W. Kuhnel, Z. Zellforsch., 72(1966)462 - R. Kolb *et al.,* Z. Mikr.-Anat. Forsch., 76(1967)184 - Y. Mitomo, Amer. J. Anat., 125(1969)147

Effects of high-fat diet W.R. Lockwood *et al.,* Amer. J. Anat., 126(1969)185

Myocardium

See Ch. 5, Muscle

Pericardium

Structure T. Kluge and T. Hovig, Acta Path. Microbiol. Scand., 71(1967)529

Function - Uptake of thorium dioxide T. Kluge, Acta Path. Microbiol. Scand., 72(1968)64

8. RESPIRATORY SYSTEM

General

H. Schulz, *Die submikroskopische Anatomie und Pathologie der Lunge,* Springer, Berlin, 1959

Nasal, tracheal and bronchial epithelium

Structure J. Rhodin and T. Dalhamn, Exp. Cell Res., 9(1955) 371 - J. Rhodin and T. Dalhamn, Z. Zellforsch., 44(1956) 345 - J. Rhodin, Ann. Otol. Rhinol. Laryngol., 68(1959) 964 - J.M. Frasca *et al.,* Exp. Molec. Path., 4(1965)340 - J.M. Frasca *et al.,* Exp. Molec. Path., 6(1967)261 - J.M. Frasca *et al.,* Exp. Molec. Path., 7(1967)92 - J.M. Frasca *et al.,* Exp. Molec. Path., 9(1968)363

Structure (sensory innervation) N. Cauna *et al.,* Amer. J. Anat., 124(1969)187

Structure ("chemoreceptor" cells in respiratory epithelium) L. Luciano *et al.,* Z. Zellforsch., 85(1968)350

Structure (secretomotor innervation) S. Blümcke *et al.,* Z. Zellforsch., 100(1969)474

Cytochemistry (ATPase) H.R. Cress *et al.,* Exp. Molec. Path.,

6(1967)314

Function (transmission of stimuli) J. Graf and L. Stockinger, Z. Zellforsch., 72(1966)184

Development T.S. Leeson, Anat. Anz., 110(1961)214- R.E. Dirksen and T.T. Crocker, J. de Microscopie, 5(1966)629

Bronchiolar epithelium

Structure A. Policard *et al.*, Compt. Rend. Acad. Sci., Paris, 241(1955)148 - H.E. Karrer, J. Biophys. Biochem. Cytol., 2(1956)115 (Suppl.) - H.E. Karrer, J. Ultrastruct. Res., 2(1958)96 - A. Policard *et al.*, Presse Méd., 26(1960)999 - P. Petrik and A. Collet, Z. Zellforsch., 103(1970)232

Bronchiole innervation

K.S. Hung *et al.*, Anat. Rec., 175(1973)348

Alveolar epithelium, general and type I cells

Structure B. Kisch, Exp. Med. Surg., 13(1955)101 - R. Giese-king, Beitr. Pathol. Anat. Allgem. Pathol., 116(1956)177 - K. Itagi, Acta tuberc. Japon., 6(1956)91 - H.E. Karrer, J. Biophys, Biochem. Cytol., 2(1956)287 (Suppl.) - F.N. Low and M.M. Sampaio, Anat. Rec., 127(1957)51 - J. Driessens *et al.*, Compt. Rend. Soc. Biol. Paris, 153(1959) 626 - A. Policard *et al.*, Z. Zellforsch., 50(1959)561 - W. Bargmann and A. Knoop, Z. Zellforsch., 54(1961)541 - O.K. Reiss, J. Cell Biol., 30(1966)45 - D.H. Bowden *et al.*, Arch. Path., 86(1968)667 - B. Meyrick and L. Reid, J. Ultrastruct. Res., 23(1968)71 - L. Luciano, Z. Zellforsch., 95(1969)198 - K.S. Hung *et al.*, Anat. Rec., 172(1972)333

Cytochemistry T. Caulet *et al.*, Z. Zellforsch., 91(1968)478 - C. Kuhn, Amer. J. Path., 53(5)(1968)809 - A.E. Vatter *et al.*, J. Cell Biol., 38(1968)80

Development G.L. Woodside and A.J. Dalton, J. Ultrastruct. Res., 2(1958)28 - C.N. Sun, J. Ultrastruct. Res., 15(1966) 380 - Y. Kikkawa *et al.*, Amer. J. Path., 52(1)(1968)177

Effects of carbon dioxide and oxygen H. Schulz, Naturwissenschaften, 43(1956)205 - B. Cedergren *et al.*, Acta Paediat., 48(1959)477

Effects of uracil mustard R.H. Curry *et al.*, J. Ultrastruct. Res., 28(1969)335

Effects of temperature H. Hayek *et al.*, Wien. Z. Inn. Med. Grenzgeb., 38(1957)165

Effects of hibernation H. Schulz, Z. Zellforsch., 46(1957)583

Effects of vagotomy V.E. Goldenberg *et al.*, Lab. Invest., 16(1967)693

Alveolar epithelium type II cells

Structure M. Campiche, J. Ultrastruct. Res., 3(1960)302 - Y. Kikkawa and R. Spitzer, Anat. Rec., 163(1969)525 - R.E. Brooks, Z. Zellforsch., 106(1970)484

Cytochemistry (acid phosphatase) B. Corrin *et al.*, J. Anat., 104(1969)65

Function (phospholipid synthesis) S. Buckingham *et al.*, Amer. J. Path., 48(1966)1027 - G. Chevalier and A.J. Collet, Anat. Rec., 172(1972)289

Development J.U. Balis and P.E. Conen, Lab. Invest., 13 (1964)1215 - Y. Kikkawa *et al.*, Amer. J. Path., 47(1965) 877 - Y. Kikkawa and R. Spitzer, Anat. Rec., 163(1969) 525

Surfactant layer on alveolar epithelium

Structure W.H. Chase, Exp. Cell Res., 18(1959)15 - P. Petrik and B. Riedel, Z. Zellforsch., 88(1968)204 - J. Groniowski and W. Biczyslkowa, Lab. Invest., 20(5)(1969)430

Development P. Petrik and B. Riedel, Lab. Invest., 18(1) (1968)54

Technical (methods of preservation) G.B. Dermer, J. Ultrastruct. Res., 27(1969)88 - Y. Kikkawa, Anat. Rec., 167 (1970)389

Lamellated materials in alveolar space

T.S. Leeson and C.R. Leeson, J. Cell Biol., 28(1966)577 - E.R. Weibel *et al.*, Z. Zellforsch., 69(1966)418 - G.A. Harrison and J. Weibel, J. Ultrastruct. Res., 24(1968)334

Alveolar septum and capillaries

Structure A. Policard and A. Collet, J. Physiol., 48(1956)687 - W. Bargmann and A. Knoop, Z. Zellforsch., 44(1956) 263 - H.E. Karrer, J. Biophys. Biochem. Cytol., 2(1956) 241 - A. Policard *et al.*, Acta Anat., 30(1957)624 - M. De Groodt *et al.*, Nature, 181(1958)1066 - J. Groniowski and W. Djaczenko, Z. Zellforsch., 53(1961)639 - A. Policard *et al.*, Z. Zellforsch., 57(1962)37

Function (permeability to peroxidase) E.E. Schneeberger-Keeley and M.J. Karnovsky, J. Cell Biol., 37(1968)781

Connective tissue of alveolar septum

Structure A. Policard *et al.*, Bull. Micr. Appl., 9(1959)93 - E.A. Laitinen, Acta Path. Microbiol. Scand., 49(1960)136 - F.N. Low, Anat. Rec., 139(1961)105

Alveolar phagocytes

Structure H.E. Karrer, J. Biophys. Biochem. Cytol., 4(1958) 693

Function M.M. Sampaio, Anat. Rec., 124(1956)501 - R. Gieseking, Ergebn. Pathol., 38(1958)92 - H.E. Karrer, J. Biophys. Biochem. Cytol., 7(1960)357 - R.D. Moore and M.D. Schoenberg, Amer. J. Path., 45(1964)991 - A.J. Collet, Anat. Rec., 167(1970)277

Effects of smoking S.A. Pratt *et al.*, Anat. Rec., 163(1969) 497

Mesothelium of pleura

P.M. Andrews and M.A. Bonneville, Anat. Rec., 172(1972) 262

9. ALIMENTARY SYSTEM

Oral Mucosa and Gingiva

Structure R.F. Sognnaes and J.T. Albright, Anat. Rec., 126 (1956)225 - E. Fasske and H. Themann, Z. Zellforsch., 49 (1959)447 - J.T. Albright, Ann. N.Y. Acad. Sci., 85(1960) 351 - M.A. Listgarten, Amer. J. Anat., 119(1966)147 - M. Kumegawa *et al.*, J. Cell Biol., 34 (1967)897 - F.R. Susi *et al.*, J. Cell Biol., 34(1967)686 - A. Weinstock and J.T. Albright, J. Ultrastruct. Res., 17(1967)245 - R.M. Frank and G. Cimasoni, Z. Zellforsch., 109(1970)356

Development G.R. Smiley and A.D. Dixon, Anat. Rec., 161 (1968)293

Tongue

Fungiform papillae

L.J. Stensaas, Amer. J. Anat., 131(1971)443

von Ebner's glands

A.R. Hand, J. Cell Biol., 44(1970)340

Tooth

Enamel organ and ameloblasts

Structure H. Warshawsky, Anat. Rec., 161(1968)211 - P.D. Frazier, J. Ultrastruct. Res., 22(1968)1 - E. Kallenbach, Anat. Rec., 172(1972)340

Function E.J. Reith, J. Ultrastruct. Res., 17(1967)503 - W.K. Elwood and M.H. Bernstein, Amer. J. Anat., 122(1968)73 - A. Weinstock and R.W. Young, Anat. Rec., 172(1972) 424 - M. Weinstock, Anat. Rec., 172(1972)424

Development E. Kallenbach, J. Ultrastruct. Res., 14(1966) 518 - P.R. Garant and J. Nalbandian, J. Ultrastruct. Res., 23(1968)427 - E. Kallenbach, J. Ultrastruct. Res., 22 (1968)90 - H. Jessen, J. Ultrastruct. Res., 22(1968)120 - A. Boyde, Z. Zellforsch., 93(1969)583 - M.E. Matthiessen and F.A. von Bülow, Z. Zellforsch., 101(1969)232 - P.R. Garant, Anat Rec., 166(1970)167 - A.E. Zaki *et al.*, Anat. Rec. 168(1970)79

Enamel organ capillaries

P.R. Garant and R. Gillespie, Anat. Rec., 163(1969)71

Odontoblasts and dentin

Structure A. Boyde, Z. Zellforsch., 94(1969)479 - R.M. Frank, Z. Zellforsch., 95(1969)310

Development H.C. Slavkin *et al.*, Anat. Rec., 165(1969)237 - M.E. Mathiessen and F.A. von Bülow, Z. Zellforsch., 105 (1970)569 - A.R. Ten Cate *et al.*, Anat. Rec., 168(1970) 491

Cementum

K.S. Lester, J. Ultrastruct. Res., 27(1969)63 - R.S. Jande and L.F. Belanger, Anat. Rec., 167(1970)439

Peridental ligament

G. Bevelander and H. Nakahara, Anat. Rec., 162(1968)313 - G. Zampichi, J. de Microscopie, 7(1968)1081

Pulp nerves

A. Pischinger and L. Stockinger, Z. Zellforsch., 89(1968)44

Resorptive cells

J.A. Yaeger and E. Kraucunas, Anat. Rec., 164(1969)1

Salivary Glands

General

Structure B.L. Scott and D.C. Pease, Amer. J. Anat., 104 (1959)115 - B. Tandler, Virchows Arch. Path. Anat., 341 (1966)317 - A.L. Kierszenbaum, J. Ultrastruct. Res., 29 (1969)459 - B. Tandler, Z. Zellforsch., 94(1969)555 - A.R. Hand, Anat. Rec., 168(1970)565

Cytochemistry (nucleoside diphosphatase and thiamine pyrophosphatase) A.R. Hand, Amer. J. Anat., 130(1971)141

Myoepithelial

F. Haguenau, Compt. Rend. Acad. Sci., 249(1959)182

Parotid gland

Structure H. Ferner and H. Gansler, Z. Zellforsch., 55(1961) 148 - H.F. Parks, Amer. J. Anat., 108(1961)303 - H.F. Parks, J. Cell Biol., 14(1962)221 - M.R. Robinovitch *et al.*, Exp. Cell Res., 42(1966)634

Cytochemistry (peroxidase) V. Herzog and F. Miller, Z. Zellforsch., 107(1970)403

Function H.F. Parks, J. Ultrastruct. Res., 6(1962)449 - A. Amsterdam *et al.*, J. Cell Biol., 41(1969)753

Effects of actinomycin D S.S. Han, Amer. J. Anat., 120 (1967)161

Effects of isoproterenol J.V. Simson, Z. Zellforsch., 101 (1969)175 - R.S. Bressler *et al.*, Anat. Rec., 172(1972) 276 - J.A. Simson and S.S. Spicer, Anat. Rec., 175(1973 442

Effects of liquid metrecal diet W.H. Wilborn and C.A. Schneyer, Z. Zellforsch., 103(1970)1

Submaxillary (submandibular) gland

Structure B. Tandler, Amer. J. Anat., 111(1962)287 - A. Tamarin, J. Ultrastruct. Res., 16(1966)320 - M. Sato *et al.*, Jap. J. Electr. Micr., 15(1)(1966)1 - M. Kumegawa *et al.*, J. Cell Biol., 33(1967)720 - A.C. Luzzatto *et al.*, J. Ultrastruct. Res., 22(1968)185

Structure (secretomotor innervation) M. Kagayama, Amer, J. Anat., 131(1971)185 - E.O. Butcher, Anat. Rec., 172 (1972)282

Function K. Kurosumi *et al.*, Z. Zellforsch., 55(1961)297

Development C.R. Leeson and F. Jacoby, J. Anat., 93(1959) 287 - M. Dvorak, Z. Zellforsch., 99(1969)346 - S.K. Kim *et al.*, Anat. Rec., 168(1970)463 - T. Yohro, Z. Zellforsch., 110(1970)173

Regeneration C.T. Hanks and A.P. Chaudry, Amer. J. Anat., 130(1971)195

Effects of isoproterenol and isoprenaline M. Takahama and T. Barka, J. Ultrastruct. Res., 17(1967)452 - T. Kanda *et al.*, Exp. Molec. Path., 9(1968)189 - J.M. Radley, Z. Zellforsch., 97(1969)196

Effects of sex and castration F. Caramia, J. Ultrastruct. Res., 16(1966)505 - F. Caramia, J. Ultrastruct. Res., 16(1966) 524

Esophageal Epithelium

Structure P.F. Parakkal, Amer. J. Anat., 121(1967)175

Histochemistry (phospholipids) I. Olah and P. Rohlich, Z. Zellforsch., 73(1966)205

Keratinising Stomach Epithelium

N. Pipan, Z. Zellforsch., 86(1968)546

Stomach

General and surface epithelium

Structure H. Helander and R. Ekholm, J. Ultrastruct. Res., 3(1959)74 - G. Causey, Proc. Roy. Soc. Med., 53(1960) 171 - H.F. Helander, J. Ultrastruct. Res., Suppl. 4(1962) 1 - S. Ito and R.J. Winchester, J. Cell Biol., 16(1963)541 - F.R. Johnson and B.A. Young, J. Anat., 102(3)(1968)541 - W. Rubin *et al.*, Lab. Invest., 19(6)(1968)598 - R.J. Stephens and C.J.Pfeiffer, J. Ultrastruct. Res., 22(1968) 45 - R.M. Lanker, J. Cell Biol., 41(1969)657

Function T.Moussa and F.I. Khattab, J. Morph., 101(1957) 191

Effects of endocrines (hypophysectomy and cortisone) R.E. Corpron, Amer. J. Anat., 118(1966)53 - R. Laumonier *et al.*, Ann. Anat. Path., 11(3)(1966)265

Parietal (oxyntic) cells

Structure C.E. Challice *et al.*, Exp. Cell Res., 13(1957)488 - A.W. Sedar, Anat. Rec., 127(1957)482 (Abstract) - A.D. Hally, J. Anat., 93(1959)217 - A.D. Hally, J. Anat., 94 (1960)425 - A.M. Lawn, J. Biophys. Biochem. Cytol., 7 (1960)161 - J.D. Vial and H. Orrego, J. Biophys. Biochem. Cytol., 7(1960)367 - W. Gusek, Z. Zellforsch., 55

(1961)790 - S. Ito, J. Biophys. Biochem. Cytol., 11(1961) 333 - A.W. Sedar, J. Biophys. Biochem. Cytol., 10(1961) 47 - V.L. Van Breemen and D.E. McChesney, Anat. Rec., 139(1961)324 (Abstract) - C.W. Philpott and D.E. Copeland, J. Cell Biol., 18(1963)389 - C.W. Philpott, J. Cell Biol., 35(1967)104A - W.B. Winborn and D.E. Bockman, Anat. Rec., 159(1967)387 - C.B. Lillibridge, J.Ultrastruct. Res., 23(1968)243 - S. Ito, Anat. Rec., 172(1972)334 - T.S. Leeson, Anat. Rec., 172(1972)353

Cytochemistry (enzymes) W. Rubin, J. Cell Biol., 42(1969) 332

Function A.D. Hally, Nature, 183(1959)408 - A.W. Sedar and M.H. Friedman, Fed. Proc., 18(1959)141 (Abstract) - A.W. Sedar and M.H.F. Friedman, J. Biophys. Biochem. Cytol., 11(1961)349 - A.W. Sedar, Fed. Proc., 24(1965) 1360

Development and origin A.F. Hayward, J. Anat., 101(1) (1967)69 - W.B. Winborn and D.E. Bockman, Lab. Invest., 19(3)(1968)256 - G.E. Wise and D.M. Prescott, Anat. Rec., 175(1973)472

Effects of pilocarpine A.D. Hally, In: J.D. Boyd, F.R. Johnson and J.D. Lever (Eds.), *Electron Microscopy in Anatomy*, Williams and Wilkins, Baltimore, pp. 225–234

Chief (zymogenic) cells

Structure C.B. Lillibridge, J. Biophys. Biochem. Cytol., 10 (1961)145

Proliferation and renewal C.P. Leblond and B. Messier, Anat. Rec., 132(1958)247

Function K. Kurosumi, Int. Rev. Cytol., 11(1961)1

Argentaffine cells

H.F. Helander, J. Ultrastruct. Res., 5(1961)257 - M.R. Dollinger and B. Gardner, Surg. Gyn. Obst., 122(1966)1335 - K.L. Melmon, Gastroenterol., 55(1968)545

Endocrine cells

E. Solcia *et al.*, Z. Zellforsch., 81(1967)474 - W.G. Forssmann and L. Orci, Z. Zellforsch., 101(1969)419 - M.H. Greider *et al.*, Gastroenterol., 63(1972)572

New cell types

J.B. Hammond and L. Ladeur, Anat. Rec., 161(1968)393 - K. Kataoka, Z. Zellforsch., 100(1969)93

Intestine

Absorptive epithelium

Structure S.L. Golden, Dokl. Akad. Nauk U S S R, 106(1956) 721 - R.E. Hartman *et al.*, J. Biophys. Biochem. Cytol., 5(1959)171 - L. Zamboni, Anat. Rec., 139(1961)290 (Abstract) - A.L. Brown, J. Cell Biol., 12(1962)623 - L.S. Gottlieb *et al.*, Amer. J. Path., 41(1962)747 - R. Laguens and M. Briones, Lab. Invest., 14(1965)1616 - T. Oda and S. Seki, Jap. J. Electr. Micr., 14(3)(1965)210 - J.C. Hampton and B. Rosario, Anat. Rec., 156(1966)369 - W.G. Forssmann and M. Baumann, Morph. Jb., 111(1967)250 - T.M. Mukherjee and A.W. Williams, J. Cell Biol., 34(1967) 447 - D.K. Jasper and J.R. Bronk, J. Cell Biol., 38(1968) 277 - C.A.R. Boyd and D.S. Parsons, J. Cell Biol., 41 (1969)646 - S.A. Pratt and L. Napolitano, Anat. Rec., 165(1969)197 - A. Takeuchi *et al.*, Anat. Rec., 164(1969) 79 - W.J. Krause, Anat. Rec., 167(1970)473

Cytochemistry (iron, calcium, enzymes) R.S. Hartman *et al.*, J. Appl. Phys. 31(1960)1841 (Abstract) - J.D. Lever. In: J.D. Boyd, F.R. Johnson and J.D. Lever (Eds.), *Electron Microscopy in Anatomy*, Williams and Wilkins, Baltimore, 1961, pp. 278–286 - P.F. Millington *et al.*, J. Cell Science, 1(1966)415 - J. Hugon and M. Borgers, J. Cell Biol.. 33 (1967)212 - M. Corriveau and J.S. Hugon, Anat. Rec., 175(1973)297

Function (fat absorption) S.L. Palay and L.J. Karlin, Anat. Rec., 124(1956)343 (Abstract) - S.L. Palay and L.J. Karlin, J. Biophys. Biochem. Cytol., 5(1959)373 - S.L. Palay, J. Biophys. Biochem. Cytol., 7(1960)391 - W.A. Thomas and R.M. O'Neal, Arch. Path., 69(1960)121 - J.C. Hampton, Anat. Rec., 139(1961)306 (Abstract) - M. Bergener, Z. Zellforsch., 57(1962)428 - D. Lacy and A.B. Taylor, Amer. J. Anat., 110(1962)155 - R.A. Jersild, Jr., J. Cell Biol., 31(1966)413 - R.A. Jersild, Jr., Amer. J. Anat., 118(1966)135 - R.R. Cardell *et al.*, J. Cell Biol., 34(1967)123 - G.B. Dermer, J. Ultrastruct. Res., 20 (1967)51 - G.B. Dermer, J. Ultrastruct. Res., 20(1967) 311 - F.S. Sjöstrand and B. Borgstrom, J. Ultrastruct. Res., 20(1967)140 - L. Napolitano and J. Howard, Anat. Rec., 160(1968)25 - R.A. Jersild and R.T. Clayton, Amer. J. Anat., 131(1971)481 - P.B. Berendsen, Anat. Rec., 172 (1972)269

Function (absorption of protein, general) S.L. Clark, Jr., J. Biophys. Biochem. Cytol., 5(1959)41 - W. Schmidt, Z. Zellforsch., 54(1961)803 - J.P. Kraehenbuhl *et al.*, Z. Zellforsch., 76(1967)170 - D.E. Bockman and W.B. Winborn, Anat. Rec., 155(1966)603 - R. Cornell and H.A. Padykula, Amer. J. Anat., 125(1969)291

Function (absorption of antibodies) J.P. Kraehenbuhl and M.A. Campiche, J. Cell Biol., 42(1969)345 - R. Rodewald, J. Cell Biol., 45(1970)635

Function (absorption of carbohydrate (galactose)) C.E. Stirling and W.B. Kinter, J. Cell Biol., 35(1967)585

Function (absorption of vitamin B_{12}*)* H. Weisberg *et al.*, Lab. Invest., 19(5)(1968)516

Function (absorption of particulate materials and methoxychlor) E. Sanders and C.T. Ashworth, Exp. Cell Res., 22 (1961)137 H. Imai and F. Coulston, Exp. Molec. Path., 8(1968)135

Function (formation of cell coat (glycocalyx)) G. Bennett, J. Cell Biol., 45(1970)668 - G. Bennett and C.P. Leblond, J. Cell Biol., 46(1970)409

Development J. Shaw Dunn, J. Anat., 101(1967)57 - T.E. Staley *et al.*, Anat. Rec., 161(1968)497 - H. Cheng, Anat. Rec., 172(1972)288

Proliferation and renewal J.C. Hampton and H. Quastler, J. Biophys. Biochem. Cytol., 10(1961)140 - W.D. Troughton and J.S. Trier, J. Cell Biol., 41(1969)251

Exfoliation mechanism H. David, Virchows Arch. Path. Anat., 342(1967)19

Effects of water, ions and osmolarity C. Ruska, Z. Zellforsch., 52(1960)748 - C. Ruska, Z. Zellforsch., 56(1962) 498 - P.F. Millington and J.B. Finean, J. Cell Biol., 14 (1962)125

Effects of calcium removal M.M. Cassidy and C.S. Tidball, J. Cell Biol., 32(1967)685

Effects of sodium fluoride E. Malmquist and H. Löw, J. Ultrastruct. Res., 29(1969)276

Effects of fasting S.L. Palay and L.J. Karlin, J. Biophys. Biochem. Cytol., 5(1959)363

Effects of essential fatty acid deficiency R.L. Snipes, Lab. Invest., 18(2)(1968)179

Effects of surfactants and lipid solvents C. Ruska, Z. Zellforsch., 53(1961)867 - C. Ruska, Z. Zellforsch., 56(1962) 762

Effects of actinomycin D R.K.A. Wesley and T.E. Jensen, J.

Ultrastruct. Res., 27(1969)306
Possible effects of neurosecretion E. Thomsen, Z. Zellforsch., 75(1966)281

Mucous (Goblet) cells
Structure J.J. Taylor, Anat. Rec., 133(1959)434 (Abstract) - H.W. Florey, Quart. J. Exp. Physiol., 45(1960)329 - K.C. Kanwar, Experientia, 17(1961)228 - K.H. Hollmann, Ann. N.Y. Acad. Sci., 106(1963)545 - J.A. Freeman, Anat. Rec., 154(1966)121 - D.G. Silva, J. Ultrastruct. Res., 18(1967)127
Cytochemistry (acid mucosubstances, peroxidase) M.G. Wetzel *et al.*, J. Cell Biol., 30(1966)299 - J.D. Berlin, J. Cell Biol., 32(1967)760 - M.A. Venkatachalam *et al.*, J. Cell Biol., 46(1970)168
Function (uptake of glucose and galactose) M. Neutra and C.P. Leblond, J. Cell Biol., 30(1966)119 - M. Neutra and C.P. Leblond, J. Cell Biol., 30(1966)137
Function (site of sulfation) N. Lane *et al.*, J. Cell Biol., 21 (1964)339

Paneth cells
A.D. Hally, J. Anat., 92(1958)268 - J. Pitha, Z. Zellforsch., 90(1968)563 - H. Cheng. Anat. Rec., 175(1973)289 - S.L. Erlandsen and T. Taylor, Anat. Rec., 175(1973)315

Argentaffine cells
M.N. Ferreira, Amer. J. Anat., 131(1971)315

Brunner's glands
Structure H. Moe, J. Ultrastruct. Res., 4(1960)58 - C.R. Leeson and T.S. Leeson, Anat. Rec., 156(1966)253 - C.R. Leeson and T.S. Leeson, Anat. Rec. 159(1967)409 - T.S. Leeson and C.R. Leeson, J. Anat., 103(2)(1968)263
Function (protein synthesis) H.P. Rohr *et al.*, Z. Zellforsch., 80(1967)183
Function (polysaccharide synthesis) J. Schmalbeck and H. Rohr, Z. Zellforsch., 80(1967)329

Lamina propria
H.W. Deane, Anat. Rec., 149(1964)453 - W.J. Krause and C.R. Leeson, J. Anat., 104(1969)467

Capillaries of lamina propria
Structure E. Horstmann, Z. Zellforsch., 72(1966)364
Function (transport of peroxidase) J.C. Hampton and B. Rosario, Anat. Rec., 159(1967)159

Nerves and ganglia
Structure R. Honjin *et al.*, Jap. J. Electr. Micr., 14(1)(1965) 43 - G. Gabella, J. de Microscopie, 6(1967)863 - J. Pick, Anat. Rec., 159(1967)131 - D.G. Silva *et al.*, Anat. Rec., 162(1968)157
Function (uptake of norepinephrine) C.E. Devine and F.O. Simpson, J. Cell Biol., 38(1968)184

Perianal glands
C. Kuhn, Z. Zellforsch., 90(1968)554

Liver

General
K. Tanikawa, *Ultrastructural Aspects of the Liver and its Disorders*, Springer and Igaku Shoin, Berlin, Heidelberg, New York, and Tokyo, 1968

Hepatocyte (general)
Structure N.D. Chapman *et al.*, J. Exp. Med., 113(1961)981 - H. David, Z. Zellforsch., 55(1961)220 - C. Bruni and K.R. Porter, Amer. J. Path., 46(1965)691 - T. Heath and S.L. Wissig, Amer. J. Anat., 119(1966)97 - R.J. Stein *et al.*, Exp. Molec. Path., 5(1966)195 - H.D. Fahimi, Lab. Invest., 16(1967)736 - J.J. Curgy, J. de Microscopie, 7(1968)63 M.N. Berry and D.S. Friend, J. Cell Biol., 43(1969)506 - E.R. Weiber *et al.*, J. Cell Biol., 42(1969)68 - J.P. Chalcroft and S. Bullivant, J. Cell Biol., 47(1970)49 - D.A. Goodenough and J.P. Revel, J. Cell Biol., 45(1970)272
Cytochemistry (ATPase, nucleotidase and acid phosphatase) E. Essner *et al.*, J. Biophys. Biochem. Cytol., 4(1958)711 - A.B. Novikoff and E. Essner, Amer. J. Med., 29(1960) 102 - S.J. Holt and A.M. Hicks, J. Biophys. Biochem. Cytol., 11(1961)47 - H. Ohkita *et al.*, Jap. J. Electr. Micr., 14(4)(1965)345
Cytochemistry (β-glucuronidase) M. Hayashi *et al.*, J. Cell Biol., 36(1968)289
Cytochemistry (ferritin) D.N.S. Kerr and A.R. Muir, J. Ultrastruct. Res., 3(1960)313 - J.C. Hampton, Blood, 15 (1960)480
Cytochemistry (very low density lipoproteins) R.L. Hamilton *et al.*, Lab. Invest., 16(1967)305
Cytochemistry (calcium, strontium) T.S. Leeson and H. Kalant, J. Biophys. Biochem. Cytol., 10(1961)95 - J.W. Greenawalt and E. Carafoli, J. Cell Biol., 29(1966)37
Function (synthesis of proteins, enzymes and membranes) G. Dallner *et al.*, J. Cell Biol., 30(1966)97 - C.A. Ashley and T. Peters, J. Cell Biol., 43(1969)237
Function (synthesis of glycogen) A. Coimbra and C.P. Leblond, J. Cell Biol., 30(1966)151
Function (synthesis of triglycerides, phospholipids and lipoproteins) Y. Suzuki, Jap. J. Electr. Micr., 9(1)(1960)24 - A.L. Jones *et al.*, Proc. Soc. Exp. Biol. Med., 123(1966)4 - O. Stein and Y. Stein, J. Cell Biol., 33(1967)319 - H.F. Parks, Amer. J. Anat., 124(1969)513 - O. Stein and Y. Stein, J. Cell Biol., 40(1969)461 - A. Claude, J. Cell Biol., 47(1970)745
Function (uptake of protein, pinocytosis and phagocytosis) J. Hampton, Acta Anat., 32(1958)262 - G. Roschlau and C. Kemmer, Virchows Arch. Path. Anat., 343(1968)265 - R.C. Graham *et al.*, Lab. Invest., 20(3)(1969)298 - S. Goldfischer *et al.*, J. Cell Biol., 44(1970)513
Function (uptake of chylomicrons) O. Stein *et al.*, J. Cell Biol., 43(1969)410
Function (secretion) M. Dvorak and D. Horky, Z. Zellforsch., 76(1967)486
Development (including embryonic hemopoiesis) G.D. Sorenson, Amer. J. Anat., 106(1960)27 - H.E. Karrer, J. Ultrastruct. Res., 5(1961)116 - A.M. Jezequel *et al.*, Lab. Invest., 14(1965)1894 - M. Dvorak and K. Mazanec, Z. Zellforsch., 80(1967)370 - R.J. Stephens and R.F. Bils, J. Ultrastruct. Res., 18(1967)456 - S. Goldfischer and J. Bernstein, J. Cell Biol., 42(1969)253
Ageing W. Andrew, Amer. J. Anat., 110(1962)1
Effects of electromagnetic fields K.A. Zufarov and V.B. Shneivais, Arkh. Anat. Gistol. Embriol., 57(8)(1969)47
Effects of radiation I.B. Tokin, Arkh. Anat. Gistol. Embriol., 57(8)(1969)23
Effects of light and darkness cycles (circadian rhythms) O. Muller *et al.*, Z. Zellforsch., 69(1966)438
Effects of hibernation I. Toro and Sz. Viragh, Z. Zellforsch., 69(1966)403
Nutritional effects (fasting) N.L. Trotter, J. Cell Biol., 34

(1967)703 - G.F.J.M. Vrensen and Ch.M.A. Kuyper, J. de Microscopie, 8(1969)599 - R. Cardell, Amer. J. Anat., 131(1971)21

Nutritional effects (protein and amino acid deficiency) J.M. Ordy *et al.*, Amer. J. Path., 48(1966)769 - O.S. Kochar, Exp. Cell Res., 49(1968)598 - H. Shinozuka *et al.*, Lab. Invest., 18(1)(1968)72

Nutritional effects (protein and amino acid deficiency) J.M. Smithson, Lab. Invest., 20(2)(1969)207

Nutritional effects (choline deficiency) G. Sugioka *et al.*, Amer. J. Path., 57(2)(1969)431

Nutritional effects (riboflavin deficiency) B. Tandler *et al.*, Amer. J. Path., 52(1)(1968)69 - G. Sugioka *et al.*, Amer. J. Path., 54(1)(1969)1

Nutritional effects (vitamin E deficiency) W. Djaczenko *et al.*, J. de Microscopie, 8(1969)139

Effects of orotic acid E.A. Porta *et al.*, Arch. Path., 86(1968) 217 - S. Rajalakshmi *et al.*, J. Cell Biol., 41(1969)625

Effects of inhibitors (actinomycin D) H. Shinozuka and E. Farber, J. Cell Biol., 41(1969)280 - P.J. Goldblatt *et al.*, Lab. Invest. , 20(3)(1969)283 - E.R. Suter and J.C. Salomon, Exp. Cell Res., 43(1966)248

Effects of inhibitors (fluorouracil) U. Stenram and R. Willen, Z. Zellforsch., 82(1967)270

Effects of inhibitors (cycloheximide) C. Harris *et al.*, J. Ultrastruct. Res., 22(1968)240

Effects of metals (iron) G.S. Pechet. Lab. Invest., 20(1) (1969)119

Effects of metals (copper) W. Wessel *et al.*, Virchows Arch. Path. Anat., 340(1966)206

Effects of organic halogens (carbon tetrachloride) N.J. Unakar, J. de Microscopie, 8(1969)355

Effects of organic halogens (iodoform) D.A. Sell and E.S. Reynolds, J. Cell Biol., 41(1969)736

Effects of carcinogens (dimethylaminoazo benzene) M. Arcasoy *et al.*, Amer. J. Path., 52(4)(1968)841

Effects of alkaloids (retrozsine) B.A. Afzelius and R. Schoental, J. Ultrastruct. Res., 20(1967)328

Effects of dyes (neutral red) M.A. Alousi *et al.*, Exp. Molec. Path., 9(1968)97

Effects of choleretics and cholecystectomy G. Hegewald *et al.*, Morph. Jb., 111(1967)240 - K. Yamada, Anat. Rec., 162(1968)373

Effects of hormones (thyroid) U. Stenram, Z. Zellforsch., 100(1969)402

Effects of hormones (cortisone) R.W. Mahley *et al.*, Lab. Invest., 19(4)(1968)358 - M.W. Rancourt and G. Litwack, Exp. Cell Res., 51(1968)413 - J. Wiener *et al.*, J. Cell Biol., 37(1968)47 - J.P. Dupouy and A. Jost, Arch. d'Anat. Micr., 58(1969)183

Effects of hormones (diabetes and insulin) C.R. Morgan and R.A. Jersild, Anat. Rec., 166(1970)575 and 172(1972) 368

Effects of hormones (glucagon) A.U. Arstila and B.F. Trump, Amer. J. Path., 53(5)(1968)687

Effects of hormones (estrogen and gonadectomy) D.R. Nathaniel and E.J. H. Nathaniel, Amer. J. Anat., 118 (1966)537 - T.J. Nicholls *et al.*, Z. Zellforsch., 90(1968) 19

Regeneration and dedifferentiation F.F. Becker and B.P. Lane, Amer. J. Path., 47(1965)783 - F.F. Becker and B.P. Lane, Amer. J. Path., 49(1966)227 - B.P. Lane and F.F. Becker, Amer. J. Path., 48(1966)183 - R.J. Stenger and D.B. Confer, Exp. Molec. Path., 5(1966)455 - B.P. Lane and F.F. Becker, Amer. J. Path., 50(1967)435

Hepatocyte, polysomes and RER

P. Pfuderer and D.C. Swartzendruber, J. Cell Biol., 30(1966) 193 - H. David and J. Noçon, Z. Zellforsch., 94(1969)56

Hepatocyte, SER

Structure W.R. Richter *et al.*, Z. Zellforsch., 70(1966)180

Effects of phenobarbital (synthesis of new enzyme membranes) S. Orrenius *et al.*, J. Cell Biol., 25(No. 3, part 1)(1965)627 - A.L. Jones and D.W. Fawcett, J. Histochem. Cytochem., 14(1966)215 - S. Orrenius and J.L. Ericsson, J. Cell Biol., 28(1966)181 - S. Orrenius and J.L. Ericsson, J. Cell Biol., 31(1966)243 - E. Loker *et al.*, Anat. Rec., 168(1970)221

Hepatocyte, Golgi apparatus

Function (in glycogen formation) H.E. Karrer, J. Ultrastruct. Res., 4(1960)149

Function (in transport of albumin) H. Glaumann and J.L.E. Ericsson, J. Cell Biol., 47(1970)555

Effects of dietary factors L. Estes and B. Lombardi, Lab. Invest., 21(5)(1969)374 - H.H. Mollenhauer *et al.*, Exp. Molec. Path., 11(2)(1969)113

Hepatocyte, lysosomes

Structure W.T. Daems and T.G. Van Rijssel, J. Ultrastruct. Res., 5(1961)263 - T.P. Ashford and K.R. Porter, J. Cell Biol., 12(1962)198 - T. Amakawa, Jap. J. Electr. Micr., 16(2)(1967)154 - M. Dvorak and H. Konecna, Z. Zellforsch., 99(1969)277

Cytochemistry J.C.H. De Man *et al.*, J. Ultrastruct. Res., 4 (1960)43 - P. Baudhuin *et al.*, J. Cell Biol., 26(1965)219

Function C. De Duve, Sci. Amer., 208(1963)64 - G. Kent *et al.*, Amer. J. Path., 46(1965)803 - W.D. Bradford *et al.*, Amer. J. Path., 56(2)(1969)201

Development A.B. Novikoff *et al.*, Fed. Proc., 23(1964)1010 - I. Bartok *et al.*, Virchows. Arch. Path. Anat., 343(1967) 1 - R.L. Wood, Anat. Rec., 166(1970)635

Effects of glucagon (autophagocytosis) R.L. Deter *et al.*, J. Cell Biol., 35(1967)C11

Hepatocyte, microbodies

Structure L. Biempica, J. Cell Biol., 29(1966)383 - W.T. Daems, J. de Microscopie, 5(1966)295 - H. Tsukada *et al.*, J. Cell Biol., 28(1966)449 - B. Tandler and C.L. Hoppel, Z. Zellforsch., 110(1970)166

Cytochemistry (peroxidase, catalase) H.D. Fahimi, J. Cell Biol., 43(1969)275 - T.K. Shnitka, J. Ultrastruct. Res., 16(1966)598

Development M. Dvorak *et al.*, Arkh. Anat. Gistol. Embriol., 52(3)(1967)86 - H. Tsukado *et al.*, J. Cell Biol., 37(1968) 231

Effects of chlorophenoxyisobutyrate (stimulation) D.J. Svoboda and D.L. Azarnoff, J. Cell Biol., 30(1966)442 - P.G. Legg and R.L. Wood, J. Cell Biol., 45(1970)118

Effects of amino-triazole (inhibition) R.L. Wood and P.G. Legg, J. Cell Biol., 45(1970)576

Effects of male sex hormone D. Svoboda *et al.*, J. Cell Biol., 40(1969)734

Genetic effects (acatalasemia) J. Reddy *et al.*, J. Cell Biol., 42(1969)587

Hepatocytes, mitochondria

Structure W.T. Daems and E. Wisse, J. Ultrastruct. Res., 16 (1966)123 - U. Glas and G.F. Bahr, J. Cell Biol., 29(1966) 507 - J. Stempak, J. Ultrastruct. Res., 18(1967)619

Structure (topographic association with RER, nucleus and desmosomes) W. Bernhard and C. Rouiller, J. Biophys. Biochem. Cytol., 2(1956)73 (Suppl.) - R.J. North and J.K. Pollak, J. Ultrastruct. Res., 5(1961)497 - I. Sternlieb, Z. Zellforsch., 93(1969)249

Origin by division of pre-existing mitochondria B. Tandler *et al.*, J. Cell Biol., 41(1969)477

Cytochemistry (enzymes) C. Schnaitman *et al.*, J. Cell Biol., 32(1967)719 - G.L. Sottocasa *et al.*, J. Cell Biol., 32 (1967)415 - C. Schnaitman and J.W. Greenawalt, J. Cell Biol., 38(1968)158 - A. Mizutani and H. Fujita, Jap. J. Electr. Micr., 18(1)(1969)17

Hepatocyte, cytoplasmic inclusions

"Hyaline" inclusions G. Roschlau and C. Kemmer, Morph. Jb., 111(1967)208

Lipid inclusions C.T. Ashworth *et al.*, J. Cell Biol., 31(1966) 301 - H.F. Parks, Amer. J. Anat., 120(1967)253

Pigments E. Essner and A.B. Novikoff, J. Ultrastruct. Res., 3(1960)374

Hepatocyte, nucleus

Structure A. Monneron and Y. Moule, Exp. Cell Res., 51 (1968)531 - T. Unuma *et al.*, Exp. Cell Res., 52(1968)101

Cytochemistry M. Amano, Exp. Cell Res., 46(1967)169

Function (RNA synthesis) E. Bresnick *et al.*, Exp. Cell Res., 46(1967)396

Inclusions (glycogen and "glycogen bodies") M. Himes and A.W. Pollister, Anat. Rec., 132(1958)453 - F. Caramia *et al.*, J. Ultrastruct. Res., 19(1967)573 - M. Mori *et al.*, Jap. J. Electr. Micr., 19(2)(1970)163

Inclusions (ferritin) G.W. Richter, J. Biophys. Biochem. Cytol., 9(1961)263

Sinusoids, general

Structure F. Wasserman, Z. Zellforsch., 49(1958)13 - P. Nicolescu and C. Rouiller, Z. Zellforsch., 76(1967)313

Development P.M. Carsten, Z. Zellforsch., 54(1961)252 - P.W. Bankston, Anat. Rec., 172(1972)265

Sinusoids, Kupffer cells and RES

Structure F.C. Schmidt, Anat. Rec., 136(1960)274 (Abstract) - R.K. Boler, Anat. Rec., 163(1969)483 - A. Matter *et al.*, J. Ultrastruct. Res., 23(1969)272 - D.M. Mills and D. Zucker-Franklin, Amer. J. Path., 54(2)(1969)147

Function (phagocytosis and pinocytosis) C.T. Ashworth *et al.*, Exp. Molec. Path., Suppl. 1(1963)83 - J. Wiener *et al.*, Amer. J. Path., 45(1964)783 - L. Orci *et al.*, J. de Microscopie, 6(1967)413 - H. Dariush Fahimi, J. Cell Biol., 47(1970)247

Effects of steroids on phagocytosis J. Wiener *et al.*, Amer. J. Path., 50(1967)187

Sinusoids, space of Disse and contents

L. Cossel, Klin. Wochschr., 37(1959)743 - R. Caesar, Z. Zellforsch., 54(1961)793 - W.E. Burkel and F.N. Low, Amer. J. Anat., 118(1966)769

Bile canaliculi

Structure C. Rouiller, Acta. Anat., 26(1956)94 - C.T. Ashworth and E. Sanders, Amer. J. Path., 37(1960)343 - J.M. Davis, Nature, 188(1960)1123 - W.T. Daems, Acta Anat., 46(1961)1 - H. David, Acta Anat., 47(1961)216 - R.L. Wood, Anat. Rec., 139(1961)287 (Abstract) - R.L. Wood, Anat. Rec., 140(1961)207

Bile preductules, ductules and ducts

Structure J.W. Steiner and J.S. Carruthers. Amer. J. Path., 38(1961)639

Origin and proliferation J.W. Grisham and E.A. Porta, Exp. Molec. Path., 3(1964)242

Common bile duct

K. Yamada, J. Anat., 105(1969)511

Gall bladder epithelium

Structure G.B. Chapman *et al.*, Anat. Rec., 154(1966)579 - K. Yamada, Z. Zellforsch., 84(1968)463

Development A.F. Hayward, J. Anat., 100(2)(1966)245

Function (absorption and fluid transport) A.F. Hayward, Z. Zellforsch., 56(1962)197 - G. Kaye *et al.*, J. Cell Biol., 30(1966)237

Pancreas

Acinar cell

Structure G.E. Palade, J. Biophys. Biochem. Cytol., 2(1956) 417 - R. Ekholm and Y. Edlund, J. Ultrastruct. Res., 2(1959)453 - R. Ekholm *et al.*, J. Ultrastruct. Res., 7 (1962)61 - P. Bannasch, J. Ultrastruct. Res., 15(1966)528 - R. Fedou *et al.*, Exp. Cell Res., 42(1966)389

Cytochemistry (enzymes and RNA) P. Siekevitz and G.E. Palade, J. Biophys. Biochem. Cytol., 7(1960)631 - P. Siekevitz and G.E. Palade, J. Cell Biol., 13(1962)217 - M.L. Seligman *et al.*, Exp. Molec. Path., Suppl. 3(1966) 21 - P. Siekevitz and G.E. Palade, J. Cell Biol., 30(1966) 519

Function (enzyme synthesis, transport and secretion) L.C. Junqueira and G.C. Hirsch, Int. Rev. Cytol., 5(1956)323 - L.G. Caro, J. Biophys. Biochem. Cytol., 10(1961)37 - G.E. Palade. In: J.D. Boyd, F.R. Johnson and J.D. Lever, (Eds.), *Electron Microscopy in Anatomy*, Williams and Wilkins, Baltimore, 1961, pp. 176–206 - L.G. Caro and G.E. Palade, J. Cell Biol., 20(1964)473 - J. Jamieson and G.E. Palade, J. Cell Biol., 34(1967)597 - J.D. Jamieson and G.E. Palade, J. Cell Biol., 34(1967)577 - H. Luppa and A. Ermisch., Morph. Jb., 110(1967)245 - S.H. Shapiro and S.S. Lazarus, Exp. Molec. Path., 6(1967)320

Development B.L. Munger, Amer. J. Anat., 103(1958)1 - N. Pipan, Z. Zellforsch., 52(1960)291 - R.J. Przybylski, J. Morph., 123(1967)85 - I. Parsa *et al.*, Amer. J. Path., 57(3)(1969)457

Regeneration P.J. Fitzgerald *et al.*, Amer. J. Path., 52(5) (1968)983

Effects of radiation K.F. Wellmann *et al.*, Lab. Invest., 15 (1966)1007

Effects of protein deficiency B. Weisblum *et al.*, J. Cell Biol., 12(1962)313

Effects of pilocarpine N. Watari and N. Baba, Jap. J. Electr. Micr., 17(4)(1968)327

Effects of inhibitors (ethionine) R. Ekholm *et al.*, J. Ultrastruct. Res., 7(1962)102 - L. Herman and P.J. Fitzgerald, J. Cell Biol., 12(1962)277 - L. Herman and P.J. Fitzgerald, J. Cell Biol., 12(1962)297

Effects of inhibitors (actinomycin D) T.G. Rodriguez, J. Ultrastruct. Res., 19(1967)116

Effects of inhibitors (fluorouracil) B.F. Martin *et al.*, J. Anat., 104(1969)93

Ducts

W. Gusek and J. Kracht, Endokrinologie, 38(1959)316 - R. Ekholm *et al.*, J. Ultrastruct. Res., 7(1962)73

Capillaries
F. Gloor, Acta Anat., 35(1958)63

Nerves
T. Zelander *et al.*, J. Ultrastruct. Res., 7(1962)84 - N. Watari, Z. Zellforsch., 85(1968)291

Peritoneal Mesothelium

Structure A. Vogel, Experientia, 13(1957)54 - K. Hama, J. Biophys. Biochem. Cytol., 7(1960)575 - M.D. Felix, J. Nat. Cancer Inst., 27(1961)713

Cytochemistry R.S. Cotran and C. Nicca, Lab. Invest., 18(4)(1968)407

Function (uptake and transport of protein and particles) M.D. Felix and A.J. Dalton, J. Biophys. Biochem. Cytol., 2(1956)109 (Suppl.) - D.L. Odor, J. Biophys. Biochem. Cytol., 2(1956)105 (Suppl.) - R. Cotran and M.J. Karnovsky, J. Cell Biol., 37(1968)123

Proliferation and regeneration
I. Chow, Anat. Rec., 175(1973)291 - W.B. Watters and R.C. Buck, Anat. Rec., 172(1972)423

Effects of triglycerides M.A. Williams and I. Carr, Exp. Cell Res., 51(1968)196

10. URINARY SYSTEM

Kidney

General

Structure W. Bargmann *et al.*, Z. Zellforsch., 42(1955)386 - D.C. Pease, J. Histochem. Cytochem., 3(1955)295 - D.C. Pease, Anat. Rec., 121(1955)723 - P. Meriel *et al.*, Compt. Rend. Acad. Sci., 246(1958)2600 - J. Rhodin, Amer. J. Med., 24(1958)661 - A. Siadat-Pour, Beitr. Pathol. Anat. Allgem. Pathol., 120(1959)382 - E. Anderson, J. Morph., 106(1960)205 - J.B. Longley *et al.*, J. Biophys. Biochem. Cytol., 7(1960)103 - C. Rouiller, Schweitz. Med. Wochschr., 91(1961)65 - A.B. Maunsbach *et al.*, J. Ultrastruct. Res., 6(1962)511 - J.A.G. Rhodin, Electron microscopy of the kidney. In: D.A.K. Black (Ed.), *Renal Disease*, Blackwell, Oxford, 1962, pp. 117–156 - J.A.G. Rhodin, The structure of the kidney. In: M.B. Strauss and L.G. Welt (Eds.), *Diseases of the Kidney*, Little, Brown, Boston, 1963, pp. 10–55 - R.E. Bulger and B.F. Trump, Amer. J. Anat., 118(1966)685 - A.J. Dalton and F. Haguenau, *Ultrastructure of the Kidney*, Academic Press, New York, London, 1967 - J.L.E. Ericsson *et al.*, Acta Path. Microbiol. Scand., 69(1967)493 - L.D. Griffith *et al.*, Lab. Invest., 16(1967)220 - F.R. Johnson and S.J. Darnton, Z. Zellforsch., 81(1967)390 - C.C. Tisher *et al.*, Lab. Invest., 18(6)(1968)655 - M.E. Beard and A.B. Novikoff, J. Cell Biol., 42(1969)501

Function B. Schmidt-Nielsen *et al.*, Amer. J. Physiol., 200 (1961)1119 - W. Thoenes, Klin. Wochschr., 39(1961)504 - J.B. Caulfield and B.F. Trump, Amer. J. Path., 40(1962) 199 - L.E. Davis and B. Schmidt-Nielsen, J. Morph., 121 (1967)255

Development S.L. Clark, Jr., J. Biophys. Biochem. Cytol., 3(1957)349 - T.S. Leeson, Exp. Cell Res., 12(1957)670 - T.S. Leeson, Amer. J. Anat., 105(1959)165 - T.S. Leeson, J. Anat., 94(1960)100

Effects of unilateral neophrectomy W.A. Anderson, Amer. J. Anat., 121(1967)217

Effects of hyperparathyroidism B. Engfelt *et al.*, Acta Endocrinol., 29(1958)15

Glomerulus, general

Structure in mammals R.T.W. Reid, Austral. J. Exp. Biol. Med. Sci., 32(1954)235 - C.B. Mueller *et al.*, Amer. J. Med., 18(1955)267 - A. Policard *et al.*, Arch. Anat. Micr., 44(1955)1 - J.F. Rinehart, Arch. Path., 59(1955)439 - E. Yamada, J. Biophys. Biochem. Cytol., 1(1955)551 - A. Bergstrand, Lab. Invest., 6(1957)191 - R.K.F. Pak Poy, Austral. J. Exp. Biol. Med. Sci., 35(1957)437 - A. Bergstrand and H. Bucht, Z. Zellforsch., 48(1958)51 - C.B. Mueller, Amer. Heart J., 55(1958)304 - D.B. Jones *et al.*, Amer. J. Path., 41(1962)373 - M.L. Zimny and E. Rigamer, Anat. Rec., 154(1966)87 - F. Jorgensen and M. Weis Bentzon, Lab. Invest., 18(1)(1968)42

Structure in fishes, amphibia, reptiles and birds R.K.F. Pak Poy, Austral. J. Exp. Biol. Med. Sci., 35(1957)583 - R.K.F. Pak Poy and J.S. Robertson, J. Biophys. Biochem. Cytol., 3(1957)183 - R.K.F. Pak Poy, Austral. J. Exp. Biol. Med. Sci., 36(1958)191 - R.K.F. Pak Poy, Austral. J. Exp. Biol. Med. Sci., 37(1959)153

Histochemistry D.B. Jones, Lab. Invest., 21(3)(1969)119

Function (plasma filtration) B.V. Hall, Amer. Heart J., 54 (1957)1 - M.G. Farquhar and G.E. Palade, J. Biophys. Biochem. Cytol., 7(1960)297 - M.G. Farquhar *et al.*, J. Exp. Med., 113(1961)47 - J.A. James and C.T. Ashworth, Amer. J. Path., 38(1961)515

Development S.M. Kurtz, Exp. Cell Res., 14(1958)355 - S.M. Kurtz and J.F.A. McManus, Amer. Heart J., 58(1959)357 - L. Zamboni and C. De Martino, Arch. Path., 86(1968) 279

Glomerulus, capillaries and basement membrane

Structure J. Rhodin, Exp. Cell Res., 8(1955)572 - R.K.F. Pak Poy, Amer. J. Path., 34(1958)885 - V.L. Van Breemen *et al.*, J. Biophys. Biochem. Cytol., 2(1956)283 (Suppl.) - S.M. Kurtz and J.F.A. McManus, J. Utrastruct. Res., 4(1960)81 - S.M. Kurtz, Lab. Invest., 10(1961)1189

Development S.M. Kurtz and J.D. Feldman, J. Ultrastruct. Res., 6(1962)19

Ageing C.T. Ashworth *et al.*, Amer. J. Path., 36(1960)165

Glomerulus, visceral epithelium (podocytes)

Structure H. Latta, J. Ultrastruct. Res., 6(1962)407 - W. Thoenes, Z. Zellforsch., 78(1967)561 - D.C. Pease, J. Ultrastruct. Res., 23(1968)304 - W.A. Webber, Anat. Rec., 175(1973)465

Function (protein absorption) B.W. Dick and S.M. Kurtz, Lab. Invest., 19(4)(1968)412

Development H. Buss, Z. Zellforsch., 111(1970)346

Glomerulus, mesangium

Structure A. Policard *et al.*, Bull. Microsc. Appl., 5(1955)5 - H. Latta *et al.*, J. Ultrastruct. Res., 4(1960)455 - D. Huhn *et al.*, Z. Zellforsch., 56(1962)213 - H. Latta and A.B. Maunsbach, J. Ultrastruct. Res., 6(1962)562 - L. Zamboni and C. De Martino, Z. Zellforsch., 86(1968)364

Function (phagocytosis, possible secretion) M.G. Farquhar and G.E. Palade, J. Cell Biol., 13(1962)55 - F.W. Dunihue and W.G. Boldosser, Lab. Invest., 12(1963)1228

Glomerulus, extracellular materials
E. Yamada, J. Biophys. Biochem. Cytol., 7(1960)407 - H. Latta, J. Ultrastruct. Res., 5(1961)364

Juxtaglomerular (secretory) cells
Structure C. Oberling and P.Y. Hatt, Ann. Anat. Pathol., 5 (1960)441 - C. Oberling and P.Y. Hatt, Compt. Rend. Acad. Sci., 250(1960)929 - O. Bucher and E. Reale, Z. Zellforsch., 54(1961)167 - P.M. Hartroft and L.N. Newmark, Anat. Rec., 139(1961)185 - O. Bucher and E. Reale, Z. Zellforsch., 56(1962)344 - H. Latta and A.B. Maunsbach, J. Ultrastruct. Res., 6(1962)547 - L. Barajas and H. Latta, Lab. Invest., 12(1963)257 - S. Chandra *et al.*, Lab. Invest., 14(1965)1834 - C.G. Biava and M. West, Amer. J. Path., 49(1966)679 - C.G. Biava and M. West, Amer. J. Path., 49(1966)955 - B. Riedel and O. Bucher, Z. Zellforsch., 79(1967)244 - S. Rosen and C.C. Tisher, Lab. Invest., 18(3)(1968)240 - R.E. Bulger and B.F. Trump, Amer. J. Anat., 124(1969)77
Function (secretion) S. Chandra *et al.*, Lab. Invest., 13(1964) 1192 - L. Barajas, J. Ultrastruct. Res., 15(1966)400 - J.C. Lee *et al.*, Lab. Invest., 15(1966)1459
Effects of adrenalectomy L. Barajas and H. Latta, Lab. In vest., 12(1963)1046
Effects of ischemia P.Y. Hatt, Compt. Rend. Acad. Sci., 252 (1961)1851

Proximal tubule
Structure (general) F.S. Sjostrand and J. Rhodin, Exp. Cell Res., 4(1953)426 - J. Rhodin, Int. Rev. Cytol., 7(1958) 485 - B.F. Trump and J.L. Ericsson, Lab. Invest., 14 (1965)1245 - J.L.E. Ericsson, J. de Microscopie, 5(1966) 97 - A.B. Maunsbach, J. Ultrastruct. Res., 15(1966)283 - C.C. Tisher *et al.*, Lab. Invest., 15(1966)1357 - L.V. Leak, J. Ultrastruct. Res., 25(1968)253 - C.C. Tisher *et al.*, Amer. J. Path., 56(3)(1969)469
Structure (brush border (microvilli)) A. Policard *et al.*, Compt. Rend. Acad. Sci., 239(1954)936 - M.M. Sampaio *et al.*, J. Biophys. Biochem. Cytol., 4(1958)335 - L. Thuneberg and J. Rostgaard, Exp. Cell Res., 51(1968)123
Structure (cell membrane and cell coat) H.H.R. Friederici, Lab. Invest., 21(6)(1969)459 - J. Groniowski *et al.*, J. Cell Biol., 40(1969)585
Structure (cytoplasmic organelles) R.K. Boler and R.B. Arhelger, Lab. Invest., 15(1966)302 - Y. Clermont and G. Pereira, Anat. Rec., 156(1966)215 - J.L. Ericsson and B.F. Trump, Lab. Invest., 15(1966)1610 - K. Kurosumi *et al.*, J. Ultrastruct. Res., 16(1966)269 - K.H. Langer, Z. Zellforsch., 90(1968)432 - C.C. Tisher *et al.*, Lab. Invest., 19(1)(1968)1
Structure (cytoplasmic inclusions) W. Thoenes, J. Cell Biol., 12(1962)433 - A.B. Maunsbach, J. Ultrastruct. Res., 14 (1966)167 - R.E. Bulger, J. Ultrastruct. Res., 24(1968) 150
Structure (cell base and basement membrane) H. Ruska *et al.*, J. Biophys. Biochem. Cytol., 3(1957)249 - D. Waugh *et al.*, Amer. J. Anat., 121(1967)775 - W. Thoenes, Z. Zellforsch., 86(1968)351
Cytochemistry (ATPase and phosphatases) E.R.G. Molbert *et al.*, J. Biophys. Biochem. Cytol., 7(1960)387 - J.L. Ericsson and B.F. Trump, Lab. Invest., 13(1964)1427 - A.B. Maunsbach, J. Ultrastruct. Res., 16(1966)197 - M.T. Tellez de Inon and M.H. Burgos, J. de Microscopie, 5(1966)181
Inon and M.H. Burgos, J. de Microscopie, 5(1966)181
Cytochemistry (cytochrome oxidase) M.J. Karnovsky, Exp. Molec. Path., 2(1963)347 - A.M. Seligman *et al.*, J. Cell Biol., 34(1967)787
Cytochemistry (leucin aminopeptidase) H.J. Mohr, Beitr. Z. Path. Anat., 134(1966)52
Cytochemistry (sodium ions) R.E. Bulger, J. Cell Biol., 40 (1969)79 - C.C. Tisher *et al.*, Amer. J. Path., 57(2) (1969)231
Function (transport of ions and water) H. Latta *et al.* In: J.D. Boyd, F.R. Johnson and J.D. Lever (Eds.), *Electron Microscopy in Anatomy*, Williams and Wilkins, Baltimore, pp. 235–240 - A. Nolte, Z. Zellforsch., 72(1966)562
Function (uptake and storage of hemoglobin, ferritin and ionic iron) F. Miller, J. Biophys. Biochem. Cytol., 8 (1960)689 - J.F. Reger *et al.*, J. Ultrastruct. Res., 5(1961) 28 - A.B. Maunsbach, J. Ultrastruct. Res., 16(1966)1 - H.B. Neustein and A.B. Maunsbach, J. Ultrastruct. Res., 16(1966)141 - H.B. Neustein, J. Ultrastruct. Res., 17 (1967)565 - A.B. Maunsbach and H.B. Neustein, J. Ultrastruct. Res., 25(1968)183 - A. Engberg *et al.*, Z. Zellforsch., 98(1969)378
Function (uptake and storage of proteins) W. Straus, J. Cell Biol., 20(1964)497 - R. Marx *et al.*, Virchows Arch. Path. Anat., 341(1966)9 - A.B. Maunsbach, J. Ultrastruct. Res., 15(1966)197
Function (uptake and storage of saccharose) A.B. Yolac, Verhandl. Deut. Ges. Pathol., 43(1959)235 - H.P. Rohr and H.U. Zollinger, Virchows Arch. Path. Anat., 341(1966) 115
Function (uptake and storage of colloidal materials and dyes) J.M. Weiss, J. Exp. Med., 101(1955)213 - W. Schmidt, Z. Zellforsch., 52(1960)598 - B.F. Trump, J. Ultrastruct. Res., 5(1961)291 - J.L. Ericsson *et al.*, Lab. Invest., 14 (1965)1341
Function (uptake of gold by mitochondria) J. Stuve and P. Galle, J. Cell Biol., 44(1970)667
Development Y. Suzuki, Jap. J. Electr. Micr., 6(1958)52
Effects of hibernation H. Amon *et al.*, Z. Zellforsch., 77 (1967)204
Effects of choline-deficiency A.J. Monserrat *et al.*, Arch. Path., 85(1968)419
Effects of alloxan diabetes G. Ditscherlein and I. Marx, Z. Mikr.-Anat. Forsch., 80(1969)484
Effects of phenacetin overloading J. Torhorst *et al.*, Virchows Arch. Path. Anat., 342(1967)70
Effects of calcium-free media R.E. Bulger and B.F. Trump, J. Ultrastruct. Res., 28(1969)301
Effects of hypophysectomy W. Schwarz and J. Wolff, Z. Zellforsch., 71(1966)441

Loop of Henle, general and thin limb
Structure W. Thoenes, Klin. Wochschr., 39(1961)827 - L. Osvaldo and H. Latta, J. Ultrastruct. Res., 15(1966)144 - R.E. Bulger *et al.*, Lab. Invest., 16(1967)124 - S.J. Darnton, Z. Zellforsch., 93(1969)516
Cytochemistry (glutamic oxalacetic transaminase) S.H. Lee, J. Cell Biol., 45(1970)644
Function (electrolyte transport) D.J. Marsh and S. Solomon, Amer. J. Physiol., 208(1965)1119

Loop of Henle, thick limb
T. Suzuki and F.K. Mostofi, J. Cell Biol., 33(1967)605

Distal tubule
Structure W. Thoenes, Z. Zellforsch., 55(1961)486

Cytochemistry (mucosubstances) L.D. Griffith *et al.*, Anat. Rec., 160(1968)643

Collecting tubules

Structure C.E. Myers *et al.*, Lab. Invest., 15(1966)1921 - F. Miller, J. Biophys. Biochem. Cytol., 9(1961)157

Function (synthesis of polysaccharides) S.J. Darnton, Z. Zellforsch., 102(1969)273

Effects of vasopressin on water transport C.E. Ganote *et al.*, J. Cell Biol., 36(1968)355 - J.J. Grantham *et al.*, J. Cell Biol., 41(1969)562

Interstitial cells

Structure L. Osvaldo and H. Latta, J. Ultrastruct. Res., 15 (1966)589 - D.B. Moffat, J. de Microscopie, 6(1967)1073 - H.M. Nissen, Z. Zellforsch., 97(1969)274

Function L. Tobian, Proc. Symposium on *Vascular Reactivity in Hypertension,* Fed. Amer. Soc. Exp. Biol., Atlantic City, April 1973, In press

Development T.S. Leeson, Lab. Invest., 10(1961)466

Blood vessels

D.C. Pease, Anat. Rec., 121(1955)701 - D.B. Moffat, J. Ultrastruct. Res., 19(1967)532

Lymphatics

F. Huth, Beitr. Z. Path. Anat., 136(1968)341

Nerves

L. Barajas, Lab. Invest., 13(1964)916 - J.A. Gosling and J.S. Dixon, Anat. Rec., 165(1969)503 - J. Newstead and I. Munkacsi, Z. Zellforsch., 97(1969)465

Renal Pelvis and Ureter

Transitional epithelium

Structure R.M. Hicks, J. Cell Biol., 30(1966)623 - G. Petry and H. Amon, Z. Zellforsch., 69(1966)587 - B. Monis and D. Zambrano, Z. Zellforsch., 87(1968)101 - B. Monis and D. Zambrano, Z. Zellforsch., 85(1968)165

Function (permeability) R.M. Hicks, J. Cell Biol., 28 (1966)21

Nerves

R.G. Notley, J. Anat., 105(1969)393 - J.S. Dixon and J.A. Gosling, Z. Zellforsch., 103(1970)328

Urinary Bladder Epithelium

Structure R.K.F. Pak Poy and P.J.Bentley, Exp. Cell Res., 20(1960)235 - B.E. Walker, J. Ultrastruct. Res., 3(1960) 345 - J.K. Choi, Anat. Rec., 139(1961)214 (Abstract) - S. Jard *et al.*, J. de Microscopie, 5(1966)31 - L.G. Koss, Lab. Invest., 21(2)(1969)154 - R.M. Hicks and B. Ketterer, J. Cell Biol., 45(1970)542 - F.J. Chlapowski, Anat. Rec., 175(1973)291

Function (water transport) L.D. Peachy and H. Rasmussen, J. Biophys. Biochem. Cytol., 10(1061)529 - N. Carasso *et al.*, J. de Microscopie, 5(1966)519

Effects of vitamin A deficiency R.M. Hicks, J. Ultrastruct. Res., 22(1968)206

11. FEMALE REPRODUCTIVE SYSTEM

Ovary

General

Structure A.D. Chiquoine, Anat. Rec., 139(1961)29 - E.J. Blanchette, J. Cell Biol., 31(1966)501 - B.S. Weakley, J. Anat., 105(1969)129

Structure (nerves) K. Unsicker, Z. Zellforsch., 109(1970)46

Development D.L. Odor and R.J. Blandau, Amer. J. Anat., 125(1969)177 - D.L. Odor and R.J. Blandau, Amer. J. Anat., 124(1969)163 - J.R. Ruby *et al.*, Z. Zellforsch., 105(1970)252 - J.R. Ruby *et al.*, Anat. Rec., 167(1970)1

Effects of silver R. Hadek, J. Ultrastruct. Res., 15(1966)66

Effects of hormonal (gonadotrophic) stimulation K. Nagai *et al.*, Z. Zellforsch., 79(1967)550 - H.J. Merker, Z. Zellforsch., 94(1969)605

Follicle, general

Structure E. Anderson and H.W. Beams, J. Ultrastruct. Res., 3(1960)432 - L.L. Franchi, J. Biophys. Biochem. Cytol., 7(1960)397 - A. Porte and J.P. Zahnd, Compt. Rend. Soc. Biol., 155(1961)1058 - A.T. Hertig and E.C. Adams, J. Cell Biol., 34(1967)647 - A.G.S. Byskov, Z. Zellforsch., 100(1969)285 - J. Priedkalns and A.F. Weber, Z. Zellforsch., 91(1968)554

Function (estrogen production) R. Moricard, Ann. Endocrinol., 19(1958)943

Development H.J. Merker, Z. Zellforsch., 54(1961)677 - B.S. Weakley, J. Anat., 100(3)(1966)503 - B.S. Weakley, J. Anat., 101(3)(1967)435

Effects of an ovulation inhibitor (melengestrol) J. Priedkalns, Z. Zellforsch., 93(1969)56

Oocyte (ovum)

Structure (human oocyte) H. Wartenberg and H.E. Stegner, Z. Zellforsch., 52(1960)450 - H.E. Stegner and H. Wartenberg, Z. Zellforsch., 53(1961)702 - M. Baca and L. Zamboni, J. Ultrastruct. Res., 19(1967)354 - T.G. Baker and L.L. Franchi, J. Cell Sci., 2(1967)213 - A.T. Hertig, Amer. J. Anat., 122(1968)107

Structure (mammalian (non human) oocyte) G. Petry and S. Zuleger, Z. Zellforsch., 47(1958)683 - E. Anderson and H.W. Beams, Anat. Rec., 134(1959)525 (Abstract) - J.R. Sotelo, Z. Zellforsch., 50(1959)749 - J.R. Sotelo and K.R. Porter, J. Biophys. Biochem. Cytol., 5(1959)327 - A.D. Chiquoine, Amer. J. Anat., 106(1960)149 - D.L. Odor, J. Biophys. Biochem. Cytol., 7(1960)567 - E.J. Blanchette, J. Ultrastruct. Res., 5(1961)349 - L. Zamboni and L. Mastroianni, J. Ultrastruct. Res., 14(1966)95 - L. Zamboni and L. Mastroianni, J. Ultrastruct. Res., 14 (1966)118 - D. Szollosi, Anat. Rec., 158(1967)59 - B.S. Weakley, Z. Zellforsch., 83(1967)582 - B.S. Weakley, Z. Zellforsch., 81(1967)91 - R. Honjin, J. Electr. Micr., 17 (3)(1968)193 - C. Krauskopf, Z. Zellforsch., 92(1968)275 - B.S. Weakley, Z. Zellforsch., 96(1969)229 - B.S. Weakley, Z. Zellforsch., 101(1969)394

Structure (amphibian oocyte) J.G. Gall, J. Biophys. Biochem. Cytol., 2(1956)393 (Suppl.) - N.E. Kemp, J. Biophys. Biochem. Cytol., 2(1956)281 - S. Wischnitzer, J. Ultrastruct. Res., 1(1958)201 - C.A. Brown and H. Ris, J. Morph., 104(1959)377 - H. Wartenberg and W. Gusek, Exp. Cell Res., 19(1960)199 - S. Wischnitzer, J. Biophys. Biochem. Cytol., 8(1960)558 - S. Wischnitzer, Z Zellforsch., 57(1962)202 - U. Scheer, J. Cell Biol., 45(1970) 445

Structure (invertebrate oocyte) J.R. Sotelo and O. Trujillo-Cenoz, J. Biophys. Biochem. Cytol., 3(1957)301 - L.E. Franklin, Exp. Cell Res., 43(1966)673 - A.K. Bal *et al.*, J. Ultrastruct. Res., 25(1968)15 - L.I. Rebhun and G. Sander, Amer. J. Anat., 130(1971)35 - R.G. Skalko *et al.*, Anat. Rec., 175(1973)443

Function (formation of yolk) G. Yasuzumi and H. Tanaka, Exp. Cell Res., 12(1957)681 - R.G. Kessel, J. Ultrastruct. Res., 16(1966)305 - J. Dumont and E. Anderson, J. de Microscopie, 6(1967)791 - E. Anderson, J. Morph., 125 (1968)23

Function (uptake of lipoprotein and protein) T.F. Roth and K.R. Porter, J. Cell Biol., 20(1964)313 - S. Schlafke and A.C. Enders, Anat. Rec., 172(1972)400 - R.A. Hastings, Anat. Rec., 175(1973)339

Function (nucleocytoplasmic exchange) R.G. Kessel, J. Ultrastruct. Res., 15(1966)181

Function (formation of inclusion in nuclear envelope) T.G. Baker and L.L. Franchi, Z. Zellforsch., 93(1969)45

Function (polar body formation) D.L. Odor and D.F. Renninger, Anat. Rec., 137(1960)13

Development (cytoplasmic and nuclear maturation) N.E. Kemp, J. Biophys. Biochem. Cytol., 2(1956)187 (Suppl.) - O. Trujillo-Cenoz and J.R. Sotelo, J. Biophys. Biochem. Cytol., 2(1959)347 - E.C. Adams and A.T. Hertig, J. Cell Biol., 21(1964)397 - E. Anderson, J. Cell Biol., 35(1967) 193 - D. Szollosi, Anat. Rec., 159(1967)431 - S. Wischnitzer, J. Morph., 121(1967)29 - A.K. Bal *et al.*, Z. Zellforsch., 100(1969)180 - R.G. Kessel, Z. Zellforsch., 94 (1969)441

Ageing and atretic changes G.H. Vazquez-Nin and J.R. Sotelo, Z. Zellforsch., 80(1967)518 - D. Szollosi, Amer. J. Anat., 130(1971)209

Effects of radiation D.F. Parsons, J. Cell Biol., 14(1962)31

Effects of fertilisation (sperm entry) L.H. Colwin and A.L. Colwin, J. Biophys. Biochem. Cytol., 7(1960)315 - H. Wartenberg and W. Schmidt, Z. Zellforsch., 54(1960)118 - C. Barros and L.E. Franklin, J. Cell Biol., 37(1968)C13 - H.J. Merker and E. Kohler, Z. Zellforsch., 86(1968)603

Granulosa cells

Structure and development G.M. Wyburn *et al.*, Z. Zellforsch., 72(1966)53 - L. Bjersing, Z. Zellforsch., 82(1967)173 - B. Gondos, Anat. Rec., 165(1969)67 - J.D. O'Shea, Anat. Rec., 167(1970)127 - T.M. Crisp *et al.*, Anat. Rec., 172 (1972)296

Function (uptake of protein)
A.F. Payer, Anat. Rec., 172(1972)380

Lutein cells

Structure and development J.D. Lever, Anat. Rec., 124 (1956)111 - A.C. Enders, Anat. Rec., 139(1961)225 (Abstract) - A.C. Enders, J. Cell Biol., 12(1962)101 - E.J. Blanchette, J. Cell Biol., 31(1966)517 - E.G. Rennels, Endocrinol., 79(1966)373 - L. Bjersing, Z. Zellforsch., 82 (1967)187 - T.M. Crisp and H.C. Browning, Amer. J. Anat., 122(1968)169 - S.W. Gillim *et al.*, Amer. J. Anat., 126(1969)409

Involution P. Motta, Z. Zellforsch., 98(1969)233

Effects of menstrual cycle E.C. Adams and A.T. Hertig, J. Cell Biol., 41(1969)696

Effects of pregnancy G. Cohere *et al.*, J. de Microscopie, 6(1967)657 - E.C. Adams and A.T. Hertig, J. Cell Biol., 41(1969)716

Effects of lactation H. Breinl *et al.*, Z. Mikr.-Anat. Forsch., 77(1967)442

Stroma cells and capillaries

Structure O. Nilsson, J. Ultrastruct. Res., 1(1957)170 - Y. Toji, Jap. J. Electr. Micr., 5(1957)43 - U. Borell *et al.*, Acta Obstet. Gynecol. Scand., 38(1959)203 - N. Björkman and B. Fredricsson, Z. Zellforsch., 51(1960)589 - Y. Le Beux, J. de Microscopie, 7(1968)445 - H.C. Fertuck and J.D. Newstead, Z. Zellforsch., 103(1970)447

Histochemistry B. Fredricsson, Acta Anat., 37(1959)3 (Suppl.)

Function (secretion) N. Björkman and B. Fredricsson, Z. Zellforsch., 55(1961)500

Development D.L. Odor, Anat. Rec., 139(1961)331 (Abstract) - H.E. Stegner, Z. Zellforsch., 55(1961)247

Effects of hormones and estrous cycle U. Borell *et al.*, Acta Obstet. Gynecol. Scand., 35(1956)35 - O. Nilsson, Exp. Cell Res., 14(1958)341

Uterus

Endometrium, general

Structure after implantation of ovum J.F. Larsen, Amer. J. Anat., 109(1961)319 - A.C. Enders and S. Schlafke, Amer. J. Anat., 120(1967)185 - D.M. Potts, J. Anat., 103 (1)(1968)77 - R. Abraham *et al.*, Exp. Molec. Path., 13 (1970)329 - G. Sevcenko and Z. Vacek, Arkh. Anat. Gistol. Embriol., 53(10)(1967)72

Effects of estrogen H. Nemetschek-Gansler, Virchows Arch. Path. Anat., 343(1968)197

Effects of estrous and menstrual cycle H.A. Krone and K. Rickers, Beitr. Z. Path. Anat., 135(1967)390 - K. Rickers and H.A. Krone, Beitr. Z. Path. Anat., 136(1967)180 - H.J. Merker *et al.*, Z. Zellforsch., 86(1968)139 - Y. Kojima and U. Selander, Z. Zellforsch., 104(1970)69

Endometrium, surface epithelium of body of uterus

Structure (in body of uterus) J.F. Larsen, J. Cell Biol., 14 (1962)49

Involution post partum in rodents E. Anton *et al.*, Anat. Rec., 164(1969)231

Effects of hormones O. Nilsson, Exp. Cell Res., 14(1958)434 - O. Nilsson, J. Ultrastruct. Res., 2(1959)373 - L.E. Maraspin, Anat. Rec., 175(1973)383

Effects of estrous cycle Y. Kojima and U. Selander, Z. Zellforsch., 104(1970)557

Endometrium, glands of body of uterus (human)

Effects of menstrual cycle (general) U. Borell *et al.*, Acta Obstet. Gynecol. Scand., 38(1959)364 - W. Wessel, Z. Zellforsch., 51(1960)633 - A. Sengel and P. Stoebner, Z. Zellforsch., 109(1970)260

Effects of follicular phase of cycle O. Nilsson, J. Ultrastruct. Res., 6(1962)413

Effects of luteal phase of cycle O. Nilsson, J. Ultrastruct. Res., 6(1962)422

Endometrial stroma

Structure (granular cells of primates, possibly relaxin-secreting) R.R. Cardell *et al.*, Amer. J. Anat., 124(1969)307

Structure (ciliated stromal cells) S. Tachi *et al.*, J. Anat., 104(1969)295

Effects of menstrual cycle (in man) A. Sengel and P. Stoebner, Z. Zellforsch., 109(1970)245

Effects of pregnancy (in rodents) C.A. Finn and A.M. Lawn, J. Ultrastruct. Res., 20(1967)321

Endometrial epithelium of cervix

Structure H.E. Karrer, J. Biophys. Biochem. Cytol., 7(1960)

181 - C. Grubb *et al.*, J. Ultrastruct. Res., 22(1969)458 - M. Hackemann *et al.*, J. Ultrastruct. Res., 22(1968)443 - D.L. Odor, Anat. Rec., 175(1973)401

Myometrium
Structure and innervation D.G. Silva, Anat. Rec., 158 (1967)21
Effects of castration and estrogen R.A. Bergman, J. Cell Biol., 36(1968)639

Mesometrium, "metrial gland" of rodents
Structure and possible relaxin secretion L.H. Larkin and C.J. Flickinger, Amer. J. Anat., 126(1969)337

Involution post partum
Collagen resorption W. Schwarz and F.H. Guldner, Z. Zellforsch., 83(1967)416
Phagocytosis of debris D. Brandes and E. Anton, J. Cell Biol., 41(1969)450

Avian Uterus

Endometrium, protein and polysaccharide glands
Function (secretion) K.V. Trainis, Arkh. Anat. Gistol. Embriol., 55(10)(1968)17

Endometrium, calcium (shell) glands
Structure W. Hohman and H. Schraer, J. Cell Biol., 30(1966) 317
Effects of calcium-deficient diet T.J. Nevalainen, Anat. Rec., 164(1969)127

Vagina

Epithelium
Function (formation of keratin) A. Cuadros and R.A. Cooper, Z. Zellforsch., 84(1968)429
Effects of sex hormones and estrous cycle (in rodents) R.A. Cooper *et al.*, Z. Zellforsch., 77(1967)377 - H.E. Stegner and M. Iwata, Z. Mikr.-Anat. Forsch., 76(1967)491 - E.M. Eddy and B.E. Walker, Anat. Rec., 164(1969)205

Placenta

General and comparative morphology
E.W. Dempsey, Histophysiological considerations. In: C.A. Villee (Ed.), *The Placenta and Fetal Membranes,* Williams and Wilkins, New York, 1960, pp. 29–35 - Z. Vacek and G. Sevcenko, Arkh. Anat. Gistol. Embriol., 53(7)(1967)56

Human placenta - villus, general
Structure C. Sawasaki *et al.*, Endocrinol. Jap., 4(1957)1 - R. Vokaer. In: J. Snoeck (Ed.), *Le Placenta Humaine,* Masson, Paris, 1958, pp. 149 - M. Hashimoto *et al.*, J. Jap. Obstet. Gynecol. Soc., 7(1960)44 - M. Hashimoto *et al.*, J. Jap. Obstet. Gynecol. Soc., 7(1960)122 - J. Terzakis and J.A.G. Rhodin, Anat. Rec., 139(1961)279 (Abstract) - J. Rhodin and J. Terzakis, J. Ultrastruct. Res., 6(1962) 88 - C.A. Ashley, Arch. Path., 80(1965)377 - A.C. Enders, Amer. J. Anat., 122(1968)419 - M. Knoth, J. Ultrastruct. Res., 25(1968)423 - T.H. Shiebler and P. Kaufmann, Z. Zellforsch., 102(1969)242
Histochemistry (ATPase) Y. Okudaira *et al.*, Jap. J. Electr. Micr., 17(4)(1968)42

Human placenta - syncytiotrophoblast
Structure W. Bargmann and A. Knoop, Z. Zellforsch., 50 (1959)472 - G.B. Pierce and A.R. Midgley, Amer. J. Path., 43(1963)153 - J.D. Boyd *et al.*, J. Anat., 102(3)(1968) 553 - J.D. Boyd *et al.*, Z. Zellforsch., 88(1968)57
Development (origin from cytotrophoblast) J.D. Boyd and W.J. Hamilton, J. Anat., 100(3)(1966)535 - Y. Hashimoto and K. Hayakawa, Jap. J. Electr. Micr., 17(1)(1968)47

Human placenta - Hofbauer cells
A.C. Enders and B.F. King, Anat. Rec., 167(1970)231

Human placenta - chorionic plate
R. Bartolini *et al.*, Z. Mikr.-Anat. Forsch., 80(1969)358

Primate placenta - villus
Structure and development G.B. Pierce *et al.*, Lab. Invest., 13(1964)451 - W.P. Luckett, Anat. Rec., 167(1970)141

Dog placenta - villus including capillaries
Function (endothelial niacropinocytosis) J.W. Anderson, Anat. Rec., 165(1969)15

Sheep and coat placenta - villus
A.M. Lawn *et al.*, J. Anat., 105(1969)557

Bovine placenta - villus
Structure N.H. Björkman, Anat. Rec., 163(1968)17 - N. Björkman, Z. Zellforsch., 90(1968)535 - N.H. Björkman, J. Ultrastruct. Res., 24(1968)249
Function (trophoblastic phagocytosis) N.H. Björkman, Anat. Rec., 163(1969)17

Rodent and marsupial placenta - villus
Structure I. Toro, Jr. and P. Rohlich, Anat. Rec., 155(1966) 385 - A.C. Enders and W.A. Wimsatt, Amer. J. Anat., 122(1968)453 - D.A. Ollerich, J. Cell Biol., 37(1968)188 - A.A. Sinha, Anat. Rec., 160(1968)187 - E.C. Carlson and D.A. Ollerich, J. Ultrastruct. Res., 28(1969)150 - A.C. Enders and R.K. Enders, Anat. Rec., 165(1969)431 - W.P. Jollie, Anat. Rec., 165(1969)1 - B.E. King and F.D. Tibbitts, Anat. Rec., 163(1969)543
Function (attachment to and phagocytosis and lysis of endometrium) A.C. Enders and S. Schlafke, Amer. J. Anat., 125(1969)1
Function (uptake and transport of protein (ferritin, peroxidase)) T.W. Tillack, Lab, Invest., 15(1966)896 - B.F. King and A.C. Enders, Amer. J. Anat., 130(1971)409
Function (uptake and storage of thorotrast) S.J. Carpenter and V.H. Ferm, Amer. J. Anat., 125(1969)429

Rodent paraplacentar chorion
J.F. Larsen and J. Davies, Anat. Rec., 143(1962)27

Amniotic Epithelium

Human
H. Bautzmann and W. Schmidt, Z. Zellforsch., 51(1960)571 - G.L. Bourne and D. Lacy, Nature, 186(1960)952 - A.D. Hoyes, J. Anat., 105(1969)149

Rodent
E.K. Bakhtin, Arkh. Anat. Gistol. Embriol., 52(3)(1967)61

Yolk Sac

Human
Structure H. Hesseldahl and J.F. Larsen, Amer. J. Anat., 126 (1969)315
Function (hemopoiesis) A.D. Hoyes, Z. Zellforsch., 99(1969) 469

Rodent

Structure P.G. Calarco and F.H. Moyer, J. Morph., 119 (1966)341 - D.G. Porter, Anat. Rec., 154(1966)847 - W.P. Jollie, Amer. J. Anat., 122(1968)513 - R.J. Stephens and N. Easterbrook, Amer. J. Anat., 124(1969)47

Function (transport of materials) R.O. Lambson, Amer. J. Anat., 118(1966)21

Effects of detergents P.W. Schultz *et al.,* Amer. J. Anat., 119(1966)199

Blastomeres (First Embryonic Cells)

Structure C.N. Hebard and R.C. Herold, Exp. Cell Res., 46 (1967)553 - S. Schlafke and A.C. Enders, J. Anat., 102(1) (1967)13 - C. Krauskopf, Z. Zellforsch., 92(1968)296 - V.D. Vacquier, Exp. Cell Res., 52(1968)571

12. MALE REPRODUCTIVE SYSTEM

Testis

General

Structure D.W. Fawcett and S. Ito, J. Biophys. Biochem. Cytol., 4(1958)135 - B.V. Kingsley Smith and D. Lacy, Nature, 184(1959)249 - K. Kubota *et al.,* Anat. Rec., 136(1960)226 (Abstract) - H.H. Mollenhauer and W. Zebrun, J. Biophys. Biochem. Cytol., 8(1960)761 - W. Zebrun and H.H. Mollenhauer, J. Biophys. Biochem. Cytol., 7(1960)311 - L. Nicander, Z. Zellforsch., 83 (1967)375 - M.H. Ross, Amer. J. Anat., 121(1967)523

Development L.J. Pelliniemi and M. Niemi, Z. Zellforsch., 99(1969)507

Effects of estrogen P. Baust *et al.,* Z. Zellforsch., 69(1966) 686

Spermatogonia

Structure (including sex chromosomes) L.L. Tres and A.J. Solari, Z. Zellforsch., 91(1968)75 - L. Nicander and L. Plöen, Z. Zellforsch., 99(1969)221 - R. Sugihara and G. Yasuzumi, Z. Zellforsch., 107(1970)466

Spermatocytes

Structure (including synaptinemal complex, sex chromosomes and sex vesicle) T. Nagano, Anat. Rec., 141(1961) 73 - B.R. Nebel and E.M. Hackett, Z. Zellforsch., 55 (1961)556 - E.H.R. Ford and D.H.M. Woollam, J. Anat., 100(4)(1966)787 - A.J. Solari and L.L. Tres, Exp. Cell Res., 47(1967)86 - A.J. Solari and L.L. Tres, J. Cell Biol., 45(1970)43 - Y. Clermont and R. Pelletier, Anat. Rec., 172(1972)292

Spermatids

Structure M.H. Burgos and D.W. Fawcett, J. Biophys. Biochem. Cytol., 2(1956)223 - Y. Clermont, Exp. Cell Res., 11(1956)214 - Y. Clermont, J. Biophys. Biochem. Cytol., 2(1956)119 (Suppl.) - T. Nagano, J. Cell Biol., 14(1962) 193 - P.J. Gardner, Anat. Rec., 155(1966)235 - J.R. McIntosh and K.R. Porter, J. Cell Biol., 35(1967)153 - L.E. Franklin, Anat. Rec., 161(1968)149 - R. Hadek, J. Ultrastruct. Res., 27(1969)396 - H. Pedersen, Z. Zellforsch., 98(1969)148

Development J.R. Sotelo and O. Trujillo-Cenoz, Z. Zellforsch., 51(1960)243

Function of "chromatoid body" G. Yasusumi *et al.,* Z. Zellforsch., 110(1970)231 - E.M. Eddy, Anat. Rec., 172 (1972)304

Spermatozoa

Structure D.W. Fawcett, Int. Rev. Cytol., 7(1958)195 - B.I. Afzelius, J. Biophys. Biochem. Cytol., 5(1959)269 - G. Bloom and L. Nicander, Z. Zellforsch., 55(1961)833 - A.L. Colwin and L.H. Colwin, J. Biophys. Biochem. Cytol., 10(1961)211 - A. Telkka *et al.,* Anat. Rec., 141(1961)231 - L. Nicander and A. Bane, Z. Zellforsch., 57(1962)390 - P.R. Burton, J. Morph., 120(1966)397 - S.K. Makielski, J. Morph., 118(1966)11 - L. Nicander and A. Bane, Z. Zellforsch., 72(1966)496 - S.E. Dietert, J. Morph., 120(1966)317 - J.M. Bedford, Amer. J. Anat., 121(1967)443 - L.G. Elfvin, J. Ultrastruct. Res., 24 (1968)259 - T. Nagano, Z. Zellforsch., 97(1969)491 - H. Pedersen, Z. Zellforsch., 94(1969)542 - T. Fujita *et al.,* Z. Zellforsch., 105(1970)483 - D.M. Woolley, J. Cell Sci., 6(1970)865

Cytochemistry (sulfhydryl groups and lysosomal enzymes) L. Nelson, J. Ultrastruct. Res., 4(1960)182 - H.M. Dott and J.T. Dingle, Exp. Cell Res., 52(1968)523

Differentiation M. Gordon and K.G. Bensch, J. Ultrastruct. Res., 24(1968)33 - D. Fawcett and D.M. Phillips, Anat. Rec., 165(1969)153

Regression E.C. Roosen-Runge and J. Leik, Amer. J. Anat., 122(1968)275

Function (penetration into ovum) A.L. Colwin and L.H. Colwin, J. Biophys. Biochem. Cytol., 7(1960)321 - L.H. Colwin and A.L. Colwin, J. Biophys. Biochem. Cytol., 10(1961)231 - A.L. Colwin and L.H. Colwin, J. Biophys. Biochem. Cytol., 10(1961)255 - D.G. Szollosi and H. Ris, J. Biophys. Biochem. Cytol., 10(1961)275 - H.J. Merker and D. Neubert, Z. Zellforsch., 95(1969)594

Spermatogenesis

G. Yasuzumi, J. Biophys. Biochem. Cytol., 2(1956)445 - J.S. Kaye, J. Morph., 102(1958)347 - J.S. Kaye, J. Morph., 103 (1958)311 - E. Horstmann, Z. Zellforsch., 54(1961)68 - J. Andre, J. Ultrastruct. Res., Suppl. 3(1962)1–185 - D.M. De Kretser, Z. Zellforsch., 98(1969)477 - F.R. Susi *et al.,* Amer. J. Anat., 130(1971)251 - Y. Clermont and A. Girard, Anat. Rec., 175(1973)294 - L. Hermo, Anat. Rec., 175(1973)343

Sertoli cell

Structure T. Nagano, Z. Zellforsch., 73(1966)89 - M.H. Burgos and R. Vitale-Calpe, J. Ultrastruct. Res., 19(1967) 221 - C. Flickinger and D.W. Fawcett, Anat. Rec., 158 (1967)207 - T. Nagano, Z. Zellforsch., 89(1968)39

Development C.J. Flickinger, Z. Zellforsch., 78(1967)92 - V.H. Black and A.K. Christensen, Amer. J. Anat., 124 (1969)211

Function (phagocytosis) I. Carr *et al.,* J. Anat., 102(3) (1968)501 - V.H. Black, Amer. J. Anat., 131(1971)415

Function (hormone production) D. Cameron *et al.,* Anat. Rec., 172(1972)284

Leydig cell

Structure D.W. Fawcett and M.H. Burgos, Amer. J. Anat., 107(1960)245 - A.K. Christensen, J. Cell Biol., 26(1965) 911 - A.K. Christensen and D.W. Fawcett, Amer. J. Anat., 118(1966)551 - M. Murakami, Z. Zellforsch., 72(1966) 139 - W.D. Belt and L.F. Cavazos, Anat. Rec., 158(1967) 333 - D.M. De Kretser, Z. Zellforsch., 80(1967)594 - A.A. Sinha and U.S. Seal, Anat. Rec., 164(1969)35

Cytochemistry S. Murota *et al.*, Steroids, 5(1965)409 - A.L. Frank and A.K. Christensen, J. Cell Biol., 36(1968)1 - G.A. Bubenik *et al.*, Anat. Rec., 175(1973)280

Development I. Ichihara, Z. Zellforsch., 108(1970)475 - J. Russo and J.C. De Rosas, Amer. J. Anat., 130(1971)461

Ageing G. Yasusumi *et al.*, Exp. Cell Res., 45(1967)261

Effects of gonadotrophin D.M. De Kretser, Z. Zellforsch., 83(1967)344 - L. Merkow *et al.*, Amer. J. Path., 53(6)(1968)989 - L. Merkow *et al.*, Amer. J. Path., 57(3)(1969)581

Rete

A.J. Ladman and W.C. Young, J. Biophys, Biochem. Cytol., 4(1958)219 - M. Dym, Anat. Rec., 172(1972)304

Ductuli efferentes

N.M. Montorzi and M.H. Burgos, Z. Zellforsch., 83(1967)58 - A. Hoffer, Anat. Rec., 172(1972)331

Epididymis

Structure E. Horstmann, Z. Zellforsch., 57(1962)692 - E. Horstmann *et al.*, Z. Zellforsch., 69(1966)69 - A.M. Dupuy-Coin and S.R. Kalifat, J. de Microscopie, 7(1968) 1031 - M. Luthman, Z. Zellforsch., 91(1968)475 - C.J. Flickinger, Anat. Rec., 163(1969)39

Function (relating to hormones) D.W. Hamilton, Anat. Rec., 172(1972)324 - M.A. Bonneville and R.M. Wilkins, Anat. Rec., 175(1973)275

Development C.J. Flickinger, Z. Zellforsch., 96(1969)344 - C.J. Flickinger, J. Ultrastruct. Res., 27(1969)344

Effects of castration R.L. Van De Velde and S. Van De Velde, Anat. Rec., 161(1968)427

Vas Deferens

D.S. Friend and M.G. Farquhar, J. Cell Biol., 35(1967)357

Seminal Vesicle

Structure H.W. Deane and K.R. Porter, Z. Zellforsch., 52 (1960)697 - A. Riva, J. Anat., 102(1)(1967)71

Development C.J. Flickinger, Z. Zellforsch., 109(1970)1

Ageing V.F. Allisoñ and G.W. Cearley, Anat. Rec., 172(1972) 262

Effects of castration P.G. Toner and A.H. Baillie, J. Anat., 100(1)(1966)173

Prostate

Structure (epithelium) D. Brandes, Lab. Invest., 12(1963)290 - P. Mao and A. Angrist, Lab. Invest., 15(1966)1768

Structure (corpora amylacea) A.J. Marx *et al.*, Arch. Path., 80(1965)487 - G.R. Schrodt and M. Murray, Arch. Path., 82(1966)518

Cytochemistry P. Mao *et al.*, Lab. Invest., 15(1966)422

Ageing J.C. Harkin, Lab. Invest., 10(1961)696

Effects of castration D. Brandes *et al.*, Lab. Invest., 11(1962) 339

Coagulating Gland of Rodents

C. Rowlatt, J. Ultrastruct. Res., 22(1968)393

Bulbo-Urethral Gland (of Cowper)

Structure S. Grzycki and M. Latalski, Z. Mikr.-Anat. Forsch., 80(1969)191 - K.H. Wrobel, Z. Zellforsch., 101(1969)607

13. ENDOCRINES

Anterior Pituitary

General

Structure M.G. Farquhar and J.F. Rinehart, Endocrinol., 54 (1954)516 - R.R. Peterson, Anat. Rec., 127(1957)346 - M. Yamada *et al.*, Jap. J. Electr. Micr., 9(1)(1960)43 - M. Sano, J. Cell Biol., 15(1962)85 - H.D. Purves, Cytology of the adenohypophysis. In: G.W. Harris and B.T. Donovan (Eds.), *The Pituitary Gland, Vol. 1*, University of California Press, Berkeley, 1966, p. 147 - A. Dekker, Anat. Rec., 158(1967)351 - A. Costoff and W.H. McShan, J. Cell Biol., 43(1969)564 - J.T. Tesar *et al.*, J. Cell Biol., 40(1969)225 - S.I. Mikami, Z. Zellforsch., 105(1970)457 - B.A. Young and R.J. Harrison, Z. Zellforsch., 103(1970) 475

Function (secretory process and products) B.G. Barnes, Endocrinol., 71(1962)618 - W.C. Hymer and W.H. McShan, J. Cell Biol., 17(1963)67 - R.E. Smith, J. Cell Biol., 19 (1963)66A - M. Herlant, Internat. Rev. Cytol., 17(1964) 299 - H. Salazar and R.R. Peterson, Amer. J. Anat., 115 (1964)199 - R.E. Smith and M.G. Farquhar, J. Cell Biol., 31(1966)319

Function (uptake of labeled aminoacids) A. Tixier-Vidal and R. Picart, J. Cell Biol., 35(1967)501

Effects of light and darkness A. Tixier-Vidal *et al.*, Arch. d'Anat. Microsc., 55(1966)539

Effects of hibernation Y. Kobayashi and L. Herman, 6th Intern. Congr. for Electron Microscopy, Kyoto, 2(1966) 537

Effects of gamma radiation A.A. Voitkevitch *et al.*, Arkh. Anat. Gistol. Embriol., 54(6)(1968)19

Effects of vitamin E deficiency I. Ichihara, J. Anat., 104 (1969)455

Effects of pinealectomy and re-implantation F. Clementi *et al.*, 6th Intern. Congr. for Electron Microscopy, Kyoto, 2(1966)539

Luteotrophic (lactotrophic) cells

Structure A. Dekker, Anat. Rec., 162(1968)123

Effects of estrogen V. Pantic and O. Genbacev, Z. Zellforsch., 95(1969)280

Somatotrophic cells

A. Leznoff *et al.*, Proc Soc. Exp. Biol. Med., 104(1960)232 - P.W. Coates *et al.*, Anat. Rec., 172(1972)293

Gonadotrophic cells

Structure M.W. Hartley *et al.*, J. Biophys. Biochem. Cytol., 7(1960)209 - F. Yoshimura and K. Harumiya, Endocrin. Jap., 12(2)(1965)119 - K. Kurosumi and Y. Oota, Z. Zellforsch., 85(1968)34 - M. Herlant, Z. Zellforsch., 101 (1969)212

Function (pinocytosis) E.B. Cramer and C.A. Ely, Anat. Rec., 175(1973)298

Effects of LH-releasing hormone M. Shiino *et al.*, Anat. Rec., 172(1972)405

Effects of estrogen W.C. Hymer *et al.*, Endocrinol., 69(1961) 81 - P.M. Lundin and U. Schelin, Acta. Path. Scand., 54 (1962)66 - P.R. Potvliege, Anat. Rec., 160(1968)595
Effects of castration J.F. Foncin and J. Le Beau, J. de Microscopie, 5(1966)523
Effects of lactation (in pigeons) A. Tixier-Vidal and I. Assenmacher, Z. Zellforsch., 69(1966)489

Corticotrophic cells
Structure E.R. Siperstein and V.F. Allison, Endocrinol., 76 (1965)70 - K. Yamada and K. Yamashita, Z. Zellforsch., 80(1967)29
Cytochemistry (immunochemical ACTH identification) E.P. Bowie Anat. Rec., 172(1972)274 - G.C. Moriarty, Anat. Rec., 172(1972)370
Effects of adrenalectomy K. Kurosumi and Y. Kobayashi, Endocrinol., 78(1966)745 - B.L. Baker, Anat. Rec., 172 (1972)264
Effects of adrenal enucleation and regeneration I. Nakayama *et al.*, Lab. Invest., 21(2)(1969)169
Effects of gonadectomy and thyroidectomy K. Kurosumi and Y. Oota, Endocrinol., 79(1966)808

Thyrotrophic cells
M.G. Farquhar and J.F. Rinehart, Endocrinol., 55(1954)847 - P.C. Goldsmith, Anat. Rec., 175 (1973) 329.

Ciliated cells
Structure H.A. Dahl, Z. Zellforsch., 83(1967)169 - E.W. Millhouse, J. de Microscopie, 6(1967)671 - D.N. Wheatley, J. Anat., 101(3)(1967)479 - P. Dubois and C. Girod, Z. Zellforsch., 103(1970)502
Relationship to mitoses K.P. Dingemans, J. Cell Biol., 43 (1969)361

Follicular cells
M. Kagayama, Endocrinol., 77(1965)1053 - R.M. Bergland and R.M. Torack, Amer. J. Path., 57(2)(1969)273

Stellate cells
Structure and function R.R. Cardell, Amer. J. Anat., 126 (1969)429 - J. Schechter, Amer. J. Anat., 126(1969)477

Capillaries
J.F. Rinehart and M.G. Farquhar, Anat. Rec., 121(1955)207 - M.G. Farquhar, Angiology, 12(1961)270

Nerves
Vasomotor M. Mazzuca, J. de Microscopie, 5(1966)105
Secretomotor (in teleosts) L. Vollrath, Z. Zellforsch., 78 (1967)234

Posterior Pituitary

General
Structure D. Duncan, Anat. Rec., 125(1956)457 - W. Bargmann *et al.*, Z. Zellforsch., 47(1957)114 - S.L. Palay, The fine structure of the neurohypophysis. In: H. Waelsch, (Ed.), *Progress in Neurobiology, Vol. 2 (Ultrastructure and Cellular Chemistry of Neural Tissue)*, Hoeber, New York, 1957, p. 31 - B.G. Monroe, Anat. Rec., 142(1962) 260 - K. Lederis, Z. Zellforsch., 65(1965)847 - D.J. Campbell and R.L. Holmes, Z. Zellforsch., 75(1966)35 - T. Vanha-Perttula and A.U. Arstila, Z. Zellforsch., 108 (1970)437
Development E.K. Priyimak, Arkh. Anat. Gistol. Embriol., 56(1)(1969)34
Function (secretory process under various conditions, general) J.D. Green and V.L. Van Breemen, Amer. J. Anat., 97(1955)177 - M. Campanacci, Arch. Ital. Anat. Pat., 34 (1960)273 - R. Barer and K. Lederis, Z. Zellforsch., 75 (1966)201 - I. Dedov, 6th Intern. Congr. for Electron Microscopy, Kyoto, 2(1966)525
Effects of dehydration S.L. Palay, Anat. Rec., 121(1955)348 - J.L. Boudier *et al.*, Z. Zellforsch., 108(1970)357
Effects of adrenaline and pilocarpine H. Fujita and J.F. Hartmann, Z. Zellforsch., 54(1961)734
Effects of histamine J.F. Hartmann, Z. Zellforsch., 48(1958) 291
Effects of castration D. Zambrano and E. De Robertis, Z. Zellforsch., 86(1968)14
Effects of lactation B.G. Monroe and D.E. Scott, J. Ultrastruct. Res., 14(1966)497

Related neurosecretory neurons, pericarya
Structure D. Eichner and H. Themann, Z. Mikr.-Anat. Forsch., 74(1966)242 - J. Kawabata, Arch. Hist. Jap., 26 (1966)215 - W. Bargmann *et al.*, Z. Zellforsch., 77(1967) 282 - B.G. Monroe, Z. Zellforsch., 76(1967)405
Cytochemistry (immunochemical) C. Rufener and P.K. Nakane, Anat. Rec., 175(1973)432

Hering bodies
D. Bodian, Bull. Johns Hopkins Hosp., 118(1966)282 - H.D. Dellmann and E.M. Rodriguez, Z. Zellforsch., 111(1970)293

Neurosecretory axons and axon terminals
E. Bindler *et al.*, J. Cell Biol., 34(1967)185 - W. Wittkowski, Z. Zellforsch., 82(1967)434 - L. Vollrath, Z. Zellforsch., 107 (1970)311 - W. Wittkowski, Z. Zellforsch., 107(1970)499

Pituicytes
Structure J. Krsulovic and G. Brückner, Z. Zellforsch., 99 (1969)210 - S. Whitaker *et al.*, Z. Zellforsch., 111(1970) 493
Function (phagocytosis after stalk transection) G. Sterba and G. Brückner, Z. Zellforsch., 93(1969)74

Pars Intermedia

Structure D.S. Vincent and T.C. Anand Kumar, Z. Zellforsch., 99(1969)185
Possible function B. Ziegler, Z. Zellforsch., 59(1963)486 - Y. Kobyashi, Z. Zellforsch., 68(1965)155 - E.K. Perryman, Anat. Rec., 172(1972)382

Pineal

General
Structure E. Anderson, J. Ultrastruct. Res., Suppl., 8(1965)1 - J.C. Van De Kamer. In: J. Ariëns Kappers and J.P. Schadé (Eds.), *Structure and Function of the Epiphysis Cerebri* (Progress in Brain Research, Vol. 10), Elsevier, Amsterdam, 1965, pp. 30–48 - Y. Sano and T. Mashimo, Z. Zellforsch., 69(1966)129 - M.N. Sheridan and R.J. Reiter, Amer. J. Anat., 122(1968)357 - H. Wartenberg, Z. Zellforsch., 86(1968)74 - J.P. Collin, Arch. d'Anat. Micr., 58(1969)145 - J.C. Gregorek, Anat. Rec., 175(1973)333
Function (photoreception, secretion) R. Miline and R. Krstic, Z. Zellforsch., 69(1966)428 - M.B. Bishoff, J. Ultrastruct. Res., 28(1969)16 - R.J. Orts and B. Benson, Anat. Rec., 175(1973)403 - S. Sorrentino, Anat. Rec., 175(1973)448

Effects of continuous light W.B. Quay, Z. Zellforsch., 60 (1963)479
Effects of darkness R.J. Reiter, Anat. Rec., 172(1972)392

Pinealocytes (chief cells)
Structure D.E. Wolfe. In: J. Ariëns Kappers and J.P. Schadé (Eds.), *Structure and Function of the Epiphysis Cerebri* (Progress in Brain Research., Vol. 10), Elsevier, Amsterdam, 1965, pp. 332 - A.U. Arstila and V.K. Hopsu-Havu, Z. Zellforsch., 80(1967)22 - H.S. Lin, J. Cell Biol., 33 (1967)15 - A. Pellegrino de Iraldi, Z. Zellforsch., 101 (1969)408
Cytochemistry (5-hydroxytryptamine) G.J. Etcheverry and L.M. Zieher, Z. Zellforsch., 86(1968)393
Function (secretion) H. Leonhardt, Z. Zellforsch., 82(1967) 307

Axons and axon terminals
Structure A.E. Rodin and R.A. Turner, Lab. Invest., 14 (1965)1644 - J.P. Collin and A. Meiniel, Arch. d'Anat. Micr., 57(1968)275
Function (uptake of labeled 5-hydroxytryptophan) I.J. Bak *et al.*, Z. Zellforsch., 105(1970)167
Effects of reserpine A. Pellegrino de Iraldi and R. Gueudet, Z. Zellforsch., 91(1968)178

Thyroid

General and follicular epithelium
Structure B.G. Monroe, Anat. Rec., 116(1953)345 - B. Walthard, Bull. Schweiz. Akad. Med. Wiss., 11(1955)346 - R. Ekholm and F.S. Sjostrand, J. Ultrastruct. Res., 1 (1957)178 - M. Irie, Arch. Histol. Japon., 19(1960)39 - U. Waller, Acta Endocrinol., 35(1960)334 - S.L. Wissig, J. Biophys. Biochem. Cytol., 7(1960)419 - R. Stoll *et al.*, Ann. Endocrinol. Paris, 22(1961)282 - F. Yoshimura and M. Irie, Z. Zellforsch., 55(1961)204 - R. Ekholm and S. Smeds, J. Ultrastruct. Res., 16(1966)71 - B.A. Young, J. Anat., 100(1966)895 - V. Pantic, Z. Zellforsch., 81(1967) 487 - P. Neve *et al.*, Exp. Cell Res., 51(1968)68 - J. Youson and H. Van Heyningen, Amer. J. Anat., 122 (1968)377 - N.J. Nadler, Anatomy of the thyroid gland. In: S. Werner (Ed.), *The Thyroid,* 3rd edition, Harper and Row, New York, 1969 - L. Toujas and J. Guelfi, Z. Zellforsch., 94(1969)118
Cytochemistry (endogenous peroxidase) Y. Nakai and H. Fujita, Z. Zellforsch., 107(1970)104 - J.M. Strum and M.J. Karnofsky, J. Cell Biol., 44(1970)655
Cytochemistry (acid phosphatase) R. Seljelid, J. Ultrastruct. Res., 18(1967)237
Function (secretion (origin and fate of colloid droplets)) I. Noseda, Z. Mikr.-Anat. Forsch., 60(1954)192 - R. Stoll *et al.*, Ann. endocrinol. Paris., 19(1958)183 - K. Kurosumi, Int. Rev. Cytol., 11(1961)1 - W.C. Bauer and J.S. Meyer, Lab. Invest., 14(1965)1795 - R. Seljelid, Exp. Cell Res., 41 (1966)688 - R. Seljelid, J. Ultrastruct. Res., 18(1967)1 - R. Seljelid, J. Ultrastruct. Res., 17(1967)195 - R. Seljelid, J. Ultrastruct. Res., 17(1967)401 - A.A. Voitkevitsch and V.S. Zenzerov, Arkh. Anat. Gistol. Embriol., 55(10) (1968)21
Function (uptake and utilisation of labeled iodide) R. Ekholm, J. Ultrastruct. Res., 5(1961)575 - O. Stein and J. Gross, Endocrinol., 75(1964)787 - A. Tixier-Vidal *et al.*, J. Ultrastruct. Res., 28(1969)78
Function (uptake of labeled aminoacids and protein synthesis) R. Ekholm and U. Strandberg, J. Ultrastruct. Res., 16(1966)181 - R. Ekholm and U. Strandberg, J. Ultrastruct. Res., 22(1968)252
Function (uptake of labeled hexoses and incorporation into thyroglobulin) P. Whur *et al.*, J. Cell Biol., 43(1969)289
Development R. Stoll *et al.* In: *Proceedings of Conference on Electron Microscopy, Stockholm, 1956*, Academic Press, New York, 1957, pp. 173–176 - J.D. Feldman *et al.*, J. Biophys. Biochem. Cytol., 11(1961)365 - H. Fujita and M. Machino, Exp. Cell Res., 25(1961)204 - A. Porte and A. Petrovic, Compt. Rend. Soc. Biol., 155(1961)1701
Epithelial exfoliation F. Ehrenbrand, Z. Mikr.-Anat. Forsch., 78(1968)99
Effects of cold exposure E.W. Dempsey and R.R. Peterson, Endocrinol, 56(1955)46
Effects of hibernation E.A. Nunez, Amer. J. Anat., 131 (1971)227
Effects of irradiation H.A. McQuade *et al.*, Radiation Res., 4(1956)532 - H.A. McQuade and T.C. Evans, Radiation Res., 11(1959)520
Effects of transplantation M. Fabre and J. Marescaux, Z. Zellforsch., 84(1968)328
Effects of hormonal (TSH) stimulation L. Herman, J. Biophys. Biochem. Cytol., 7(1960)143 - B. Roos, Pathol. Microbiol. Scand., 23(1960)129 - S.L. Wissig, Anat. Rec., 139(1961)287 - H. Sheldon *et al.*, J. Cell Biol., 23(1964) 200 - B.K. Wetzel *et al.*, J. Cell Biol., 25(1965)593 - R. Seljelid, J. Ultrastruct. Res., 18(1967)479 - M. Kosanovic *et al.*, Exp. Cell Res., 52(1968)147 - P. Neve and J.E. Dumont, Z. Zellforsch., 103(1970)61

Parafollicular (calcitonin producing) cells
Structure R. Ekholm and L.E. Ericson, J. Ultrastruct. Res., 23(1968)378 - S.L. Teitelbaum *et al.*, Anat. Rec., 168 (1970)69
Cytochemistry A.G.E. Pearse, Proc. Roy. Soc. Biol., 164 (1966)478 - M.D. Gershon and E.A. Nunez, Anat. Rec., 172(1972)315
Function (production of calcitonin) G.V. Foster *et al.*, Nature, 203(1964)1029 - W.C. Bauer and S.L. Teitelbaum, Lab. Invest., 15(1966)323 - S. Taylor (Ed.), Calcitonin. In: *Proceedings of Symposium on Thyrocalcitonin and the C-Cells*, Heinemann, London, 1968 - S.C. Marks and D.G. Walker, Am. J. Anat., 126(1969)299 - B.A. Young *et al.*, J. Anat., 102(2)(1967)275
Development M.E. Stocckel and A. Porte, Z. Zellforsch., 106 (1970)251
Effects of cold exposure E.A. Nunez *et al.*, J. Cell Sci., 6 (1970)821
Effects of vitamin D C.C. Capen and D.M. Young, Amer. J. Path., 57(2)(1969)365
Effects of parathyroid hormone D.G. Walker, Z. Zellforsch., 72(1966)100 - A.S. Chan, Anat. Rec., 175(1973)288

"Third epithelial component"
K.A. Zufarov *et al.*, Arkh. Anat. Gistol. Embriol., 57 (9)(1969)76 - R. Calvert and H. Isler, Anat. Rec., 168 (1970)23

Capillaries
R. Ekholm, Z. Zellforsch., 46(1957)139

Ultimobranchial Body (in Birds, Amphibia, Fishes)

Structure D.R. Robertson, J. Anat., 105(1969)115 - M.E. Stoeckel and A. Porte, Z. Zellforsch., 94(1969)495 - M.E.

Stoeckel and A. Porte, Z. Zellforsch., 102(1969)376
Structure (nerves) D.R. Robertson, Z. Zellforsch., 78(1967) 328
Function (uptake of amines and production of calcitonin) D.H Copp *et al.*, Canad. J. Physiol. Pharmacol., 45(1967) 1095 - E. Malmgvist *et al.*, J. Ultrastruct. Res., 23 (1968)457
Effects of hypercalcemia D.R. Robertson, Z. Zellforsch., 85 (1968)441

Parathyroid

General and chief cells
Structure J.D. Lever, J. Anat., 91(1957)73 - J.D. Lever, J. Endocrinol., 17(1958)210 - J.S. Trier, J. Biophys. Biochem. Cytol., 4(1958)13 - B. Walthard, Arch. "De Becchi" Anat. Patol. Med. Clin., 31(1960)441 - R. Davis and A.C. Enders. In: R.O. Greep and R.V. Talmage (Eds.), *The Parathyroids,* Thomas, Springfield, Ill., 1961, pp. 76–92 - R. Lange, Z. Zellforsch., 53(1961)765 - A. Porte and A. Petrovic. Compt. Rend. Soc. Biol., 155(1961)2025 - H. Sheldon, J. Ultrastruct. Res., 10(1964)377 - J.D. Lever. In: P.J. Gaillard, R.V. Talmage and A.M. Budy (Eds.), *The Parathyroid Glands,* University of Chicago Press, Chicago, Ill., 1965, p. 11 - M.E. Stoeckel and A. Porte, Z. Zellforsch., 73(1966)488 - M.E. Stoeckel and A. Porte, Z. Zellforsch., 73(1966)503 - C.C. Capen and G.N. Rowland, Anat. Rec., 162(1968)327
Function (secretion) B.L. Munger and S.I. Roth, Anat. Rec., 142(1962)261 - S.I. Roth, Arch. Path., 73(1962)495 - B.L. Munger and S.I. Roth, J. Cell Biol., 16(1963)379 - C.C. Capen and G.N. Rowland, Z. Zellforsch., 90(1968) 495 - H. Rohr and B. Krassig, Z. Zellforsch., 85(1968)271 - W.J. Dougherty, Anat. Rec., 175(1973)309
Effects of calcium S.I. Roth and L.G. Raisz, Lab. Invest., 15(1966)1187
Effects of deficiency of calcium, phosphorus and vitamin D S.I. Roth *et al.*, Amer. J. Path. 53(1968)631
Effects of glycerophosphate G.L. Melson, Lab. Invest., 15 (1966)318
Effects of pregnancy C.C. Capen *et al.*, Lab. Invest., 14 (1965)1673
Effects of pinealectomy R. Krstic, Z. Zellforsch., 77(1967)8

Eosinophilic cells
S.I. Roth *et al.*, Lab. Invest., 11(1962)933

Adrenal Cortex

Endocrine cells
Structure (general) J.D. Lever, Amer. J. Anat., 97(1955)409 - T. Zelander, Z. Zellforsch., 46(1957)710 - E. Molbert and K. Arnesen, Beitr. Pathol. Anat. Allgem. Pathol., 122 (1960)31 - G. Cotte and N. Cotte, Z. Zellforsch., 54 (1961)182 - H. Fujita, Z. Zellforsch., 55(1961)80 - D.D. Sabatini and E.D.P. De Robertis, J. Biophys. Biochem. Cytol., 9(1961)105 - R.M. Brenner, Amer. J. Anat., 119 (1966)429 - A. Propst and O. Muller, Z. Zellforsch., 75 (1966)404 - J.A. Long and A.L. Jones, Amer. J. Anat., 120(1967)463 - J.A. Long and A.L. Jones, Lab. Invest., 17(1967)355 - J.M.B. Bloodworth and K.L. Powers, J. Anat., 102(3)(1968)457 - A. Kjaerheim, Z. Zellforsch., 91(1968)429 - T. Sato, Z. Zellforsch., 87(1968)315 - S. Malamed *et al.*, Z. Zellforsch., 107(1970)447 - S. Malamed *et al.*, Anat. Rec., 175(1973)381
Structure (mitochondria) W.D. Belt and D.C. Pease, J. Biophys. Biochem. Cytol., 2(1956)369 (Suppl.) - W.D. Belt, J. Biophys. Biochem. Cytol., 4(1958)337 - E. De Robertis and D. Sabatini, J. Biophys. Biochem. Cytol., 4(1958)667 - E. Lindner, Z. Zellforsch., 72(1966)212 - A. Kjaerheim, Exp. Cell Res., 45(1967)236 - M.M. Magalhaes and M.C. Magalhaes, J. de Microscopie, 7(1968)549 - J. Frühling *et al.*, J. de Microscopie, 7(1968)705 - D.N. Wheatley, J. Anat., 103(1)(1968)151 - S.E. Dietert, Anat. Rec., 165 (1969)41
Structure (lipids) G. Cotte, J. Ultrastruct. Res., 3(1959)186 - G. Cotte and D. Picard, Compt. Rend. Soc. Biol., 153 (1959)1221
Structure (microvilli, annulate lamellae and cilia) I.A. Carr, Nature, 182(1958)607 - G.A. Harrison, J. Ultrastruct. Res., 14(1966)158 - D.N. Wheatley, J. Anat., 101(2) (1967)223
Cytochemistry A. Kahri, Acta Endocrinol., 52(108)(1966)1 - K.A. Gruber and R. Gerstner, Anat. Rec., 175(1973)334
Function J.H. Luft and O. Hechter, J. Biophys. Biochem. Cytol., 3(1957)615 - C.T. Ashworth *et al.*, Amer. J. Path., 35(1959)425 - J.R. Hillman and W.G. Seliger, Anat. Rec., 175(1973)344
Development M.H. Ross *et al.*, J. Biophys. Biochem. Cytol., 4(1958)659 - M.H. Ross. In: A.R. Currie, T. Symington and J.K. Grant (Eds.), *The Human Adrenal Cortex*, Livingstone, Edinburgh, 1960, pp. 558–569 - M. Arnold and G. Hager, Z. Zellforsch., 83(1967)117 - G.G. Nussdorfer, Z. Zellforsch., 103(1970)382 - G.G. Nussdorfer, Z. Zellforsch., 103(1970)398
Ageing T. Samorajski and C. Rolsten, Anat. Rec., 163(1969) 473
Effects of sodium deprivation J.A. Long and A.L. Jones, Anat. Rec., 166(1970)1
Effects of inhibitors of cholesterol biosynthesis S.E. Dietert and T.J. Scallen, J. Cell Biol., 40(1969)44
Effects of corticotrophic and other stimulation T. Yamori *et al.*, Z. Zellforsch., 55(1961)179 - F. Giacomelli *et al.*, J. Cell Biol., 26(1965)499 - A.I. Kahri, J. Cell Biol., 36 (1968)181 - P.A. Nickerson, Anat. Rec., 166(1970)479
Effects of steroids T. Zelander, J. Ultrastruct. Res., 2(1959)1 (Suppl.) - A. Kjaerheim, Z. Zellforsch., 91(1968)456 - M.J. Finegold and L.E. Greene, J. Cell Biol., 45(1970)455 - P.A. Nickerson *et al.*, J. Cell Biol., 47(1970)277 - G.G. Nussdorfer and G. Mazzochi, Z. Zellforsch., 111(1970)90 - G.G. Nussdorfer, Z. Zellforsch., 106(1970)143
Effects of hypophysectomy T.L. Volk and D.G. Scarpelli, Lab. Invest., 15(1966)707
Effects of prostaglandins D.P. Penney *et al.*, Anat. Rec., 175 (1973)409

Nerves
K. Unsicker, Z. Zellforsch., 95(1969)608

Adrenal Medulla

Endocrine cells
Structure O. Eranko and L. Hanninen, Acta Pathol. Microbiol. Scand., 50(1960)126 - J.G. Wood and G. Callas, Z. Zellforsch., 71(1966)261 - F. Al-Lami, Anat. Rec., 168 (1970)161
Cytochemistry R.D. Yates, Anat. Rec., 149(1964)237 - J.G. Wood, Amer. J. Anat., 121(1967)671
Function (production of norepinephrine and epinephrine) J.Moppert, Z. Zellforsch., 74(1966)45 - F. Al-Lami, Anat. Rec., 164(1969)317
Function (release of catecholamines) J.D. Lever and J.A.

Findlay, Z. Zellforsch., 74(1966)317

Function (uptake of labeled Dopa) L.G. Elfvin *et al.*, J. Ultrastruct. Res., 14(1966)277 - K. Hempel and M. Kraft, Z. Zellforsch., 85(1968)322

Development L.G. Elfvin, J. Ultrastruct. Res., 17(1967)45

Effects of denervation J.D. Lever, Endocrinology, 57(1955) 621

Effects of insulin-induced hypoglycemia F.A. D'Anzi, Amer. J. Anat., 125(1969)381

Stromal cells

Function (phagocytosis) H. Eisold *et al.*, Z. Zellforsch., 99 (1969)336

Ganglion cells and axon terminals

Structure K. Unsicker, Z. Zellforsch., 76(1967)187 - K. Unsicker, Z. Zellforsch., 95(1969)86

Effects of splanchnic nerve stimulation E. De Robertis and A.V. Ferreira, J. Biophys. Biochem. Cytol., 3(1957)611

Extra-Adrenal Chromaffin Tissue and Paraganglia

G. Siegrist *et al.*, J. de Microscopie, 5(1966)791 - P. Bock, Z. Zellforsch., 105(1970)389

Islets of Langerhans

General

Structure P.E. Lacy, Diabetes, 6(1957)498 - P.E. Lacy, Anat. Rec., 128(1957)255 - S.A. Bencosme and D.C. Pease, Endocrinology, 63(1958)1 - W. Stoeckenius and J. Kracht, Endokrinologie, 36(1958)135 - P.E. Lacy and W.S. Hartroft, Ann. N.Y. Acad. Sci., 82(1959)287 - J.D. Lever and M. Jeacock, Anat. Rec., 136(1960)233 (Abstract) - J.P. Thiery and J.P. Bader, Ann. d'Endocrin. (Paris), 27(1966)625 - R. Lange, Z. Zellforsch., 82 (1967)156 - D.H. Lee, Z. Zellforsch., 77(1967)1 - K. Wolff, J. Cell Biol., 35(1967)468 - A.A. Like, Lab. Invest., 16(1967)937 - L. Boquist, Z. Zellforsch., 89(1968)519 - D. Grossner, Z. Zellforsch., 82(1967)82 - E. De Hoyos-Guevara, Z. Zellforsch., 101(1969)28 - A. Faller, Z. Zellforsch., 97(1969)226 - S.L. Howell *et al.*, J. Cell Biol., 41(1969)154 - L. Boquist, J. Cell Biol., 45(1970)532 - W.B. Rhoten, Anat. Rec., 167(1970)401

Development D. Ferreira, J. Ultrastruct. Res., 1(1957)14 - B.L. Munger, Amer. J. Anat., 103(1958)275 - K. Gaede *et al.*, Z. Zellforsch., 49(1959)690 - N. Björkman *et al.*, Z. Zellforsch., 72(1966)425

Effects of cobalt P.E. Lacy and A.F. Cardeza, Diabetes, 7 (1958)368

Effects of obesity-hyperglycemia N. Björkman *et al.*, Z. Zellforsch., 58(1963)803

Alpha cells

Structure J. Gomez-Acebo, J. Cell Biol., 36(1968)33

Function (secretion of glucagon) B.L. Munger, Lab. Invest., 11(1962)885 - C. Hellerstrom *et al.* In: *The Structure and Metabolism of the Pancreatic Islets,* Pergamon Press, New York, 1964, p. 117

Effects of sympathetic stimulation A.C. Esterhuizen and S.L. Howell, J. Cell Biol., 46(1970)593

Beta cells

General P.E. Lacy, New Engl. J. Med., 276(4)(1967)187 - P.E. Lacy, Amer. J. Med., 31(1961)851 - A. Martinez-Palomo and S.A. Bencosme, J. de Microscopie, 5(1966) 259 - L. Boquist, J. Cell Biol., 43(1969)377 - M.H. Greider *et al.*, J. Cell Biol., 41(1969)162 - S.L. Howell *et al.*, J. Cell Biol., 41(1969)167 - L. Boquist, Z. Zellforsch., 106(1970)69

Cytochemistry (fluorescent antibody studies) P.E. Lacy, Exp. Cell Res., 7(1959)296 (Suppl.)

Function (uptake of labeled aminoacids and formation of insulin) S.L. Howell *et al.*, J. Cell Biol., 42(1969)695

Function (release of secretion) S.S. Lazarus *et al.*, Lab. Invest., 16(1967)330

Regeneration after subtotal pancreatectomy M. Marx *et al.*, Z. Zellforsch., 110(1970)569

Effects of protracted glucose treatment J.R. Williamson and P.E. Lacy, Arch Path., 72(1961)637

Effects of sulfonylurea J.R. Williamson *et al.*, Diabetes, 10 (1961)460 - B.W. Volk and S. Lazarus, Arch. Path., 78 (1964)114

Effects of alloxan J.R. Williamson and P.E. Lacy, Arch. Path., 67(1959)102 - J.R. Williamson, Diabetes, 9(1960) 471 - B.W. Volk *et al.*, Lab. Invest., 14(1965)1375 - R.E. Hinkley and P.R. Burton, Anat. Rec., 166(1970)67

Effects of cortisone S.A. Bencosme and A. Martinez-Palomo, Lab. Invest., 18(6)(1968)746

Effects of glucagon P.E. Lacy *et al.*, Diabetes, 8(1959)36

Effects of glucagon P.E. Lacy *et al.*, Diabetes, 8(1959)36 - P.H. Smith, Anat. Rec., 175(1973)446

Effects of Cytochalasin B W.B. Rhoten, Anat. Rec., 175 (1973)423

Delta cells

S. Kobayashi and T. Fujita, Z. Zellforsch., 100(1969)340

Nerves

S.A. Bencosme, Lab. Invest., 8(1959)629 - P.G. Legg, Z. Zellforsch., 80(1967)307 - S.S. Shorr and F.E. Bloom, Z. Zellforsch., 103(1970)12

Gastrointestinal Endocrine Cells

General

W.G. Forssman *et al.*, J. Cell Biol., 40(1969)692 - G. Vassallo *et al.*, Z. Zellforsch., 98(1969)333

Enterochromaffine

Structure A.C. Schofield and D.G. Silva, J. Anat., 103(1) (1968)1 - A. Penttilä, Z. Zellforsch., 102(1969)193

Effects of reserpine I. Singh, Z. Zellforsch., 81(1967)501

14. SKIN

Skin

General

General structure and function W. Montagna, *The Structure and Function of Skin,* Academic Press, New York, 1956 - H. Gansler, Acta Neuroveget. Vienna, 18(1958)320 - E. Horstmann, Arch. Klin. Exp. Dermatol., 211(1960)18 - R. Olsson, Z. Zellforsch., 54(1961)90 - A.S. Zelickson, *Ultrastructure of Normal and Abnormal Skin,* Lea and Febiger, Philadelphia, 1967

Development L.T. Threadgold and R. Lasker, J. Ultrastruct. Res., 19(1967)238 - P.F. Parakkal and A.G. Matoltsy, J. Ultrastruct. Res., 23(1968)403 - P. Sengel and M. Rusaouen, Arch. d'Anat. Micr., 58(1969)77

Development (effects of prostaglandins) C.W. Kischer, Amer. J. Anat., 124(1969)491
Cyclic changes in sexual skin (guinea pigs) M.H. Burgos and G.B. Wislocki, Endocrinol., 63(1958)106

Epidermis

General, human
Structure A. Charles and F.G. Smiddy, J. Invest. Dermatol., 29(1957)327 - C.C. Selby, J. Invest. Dermat., 29(1957) 131 - G.F. Odland, J. Biophys. Biochem. Cytol., 4(1958) 529 - R.G. Hibbs and W.H. Clark, J. Biophys. Biochem. Cytol., 6(1959)71 - G.A. Edwards and L. Makk, Amer. J. Path., 37(1960)101 - G.F. Odland, J. Invest. Dermatol., 34(1960)11 - A.S. Zelickson and J.F. Hartmann, J. Invest. Dermatol., 36(1961)65 - I.N. Mikhailov and L.N. Mikhailova, Arkh. Anat. Gistol. Embriol., 50(5) (1966)73

General, rodent
E. Horstmann and A. Knoop, Z. Zellforsch., 47(1958)348 - G. Bargen, Z. Zellforsch., 50(1959)459 - K. Setala *et al.*, J. Natl. Cancer Inst., 24(1960)329 - A.S. Breathnach and D. Goodwin, J. Anat. 100(1)(1966)159 - R.J. Branson, Anat. Rec., 160(1968)109
Development M.G. Menefee, J. Ultrastruct. Res., 1(1957)49 - M.A. Bonneville, Amer. J. Anat., 123(1968)147

General, amphibian
Structure Y. Shinagawa *et al.*, Jap. J. Electr. Micr., 17(1) (1968)41
Histochemistry (ATP-ase) M.G. Farquhar and G.E. Palade, J. Cell Biol., 30(1966)359
Development C.R. Leeson and L.T. Threadgold, Acta Anat., 44(1961)159
Function (transport of Na^+ and K^+) J. Okamoto, Jap. J. Electr. Micr., 17(1)(1968)34 - C. Voute and H.H. Ussing, J. Cell Biol., 36(1968)625

Keratinocytes
Structure R. Snell, Z. Zellforsch., 79(1967)492 - M. Bell, J. Cell Biol., 41(1969)914

Melanocytes
Structure N.A. Barnicot and M.S.C. Birbeck, in: W. Montagna and R.A. Ellis (Eds.), *The Biology of Hair Growth*, Academic Press, New York, 1958, pp. 239–253 - W.H. Clark and R.G. Hibbs, J. Biophys. Biochem. Cytol., 4(1958) 679 - A. Charles and J.T. Ingram, J. Biophys. Biochem. Cytol., 6(1959)41 - P. Drochmans, J. Biophys. Biochem. Cytol., 8(1960)165 - M.S. Birbeck *et al.*, J. Invest. Derm., 37(1961)51
Cytochemistry (acid phosphatase) Y. Hori *et al.*, J. Ultrastruct. Res., 25(1968)109

Langerhans cells
Structure W.H. Clark *et al.*, Amer. J. Path., 39(1961)333 - Y. Mishima, J. Cell Biol., 30(1966)417 - R.W. Sagebiel and T.H. Reed, J. Cell Biol., 36(1968)595
Cytochemistry G. Niebauer *et al.*, J. Cell Biol., 43(1969)80
Function J. Kiistala and K.K. Mustakallio, Z. Zellforsch., 78(1967)427
Origin B. MacKay and J.L. Smith, Anat. Rec., 172(1972)362 - W.M. Reams, Anat. Rec., 175(1973)421

Membrane coating granules
Structure and function A.G. Matoltsy and P.F. Parakkal, J. Cell Biol., 24(1965)297 - A.G. Matoltsy, J. Ultrastruct. Res., 15(1966)510 - I.R. Martinez and A. Peters, Amer. J. Anat., 130(1971)93

Keratohyalin
Structure A.I. Farbman, Anat. Rec., 154(1966)275
Cytochemistry A.G. Matoltsy and M.N. Matoltsy, J. Cell Biol., 47(1970)593
Function (role in keratin formation) E.L. Laden *et al.*, J. Invest. Dermatol., 28(1957)325 - I. Brody, J. Ultrastruct. Res., 3(1959)84

Stratum corneum
Structure of keratin J.A.G. Rhodin and E.J. Reith, Ultrastructure of keratin in oral mucosa, skin, esophagus, claw, and hair. In: E.O. Butcher and R.F. Sognnaes (Eds.), *Fundamentals of Keratinization*, AAAS, Publication No. 70, Washington, D.C., 1962, pp. 61–94 - M.G. Dobb, J. Ultrastruct. Res., 14(1966)294
Function (the keratinization process) I. Brody, J. Ultrastruct. Res., 2(1959)482 - A. Charles, J. Invest. Dermatol., 33 (1959)65 - I. Brody, J. Ultrastruct. Res., 4(1960)264 - J.V. Frei and H. Sheldon, J. Biophys. Biochem. Cytol., 11(1961)719 - A.G. Matoltsy, Mechanism of keratinization. In: E.O. Butcher, and R.F. Sognnaes (Eds.), *Fundamentals of Keratinization*, AAAS, Publication No. 70, Washington, D.C., 1962, p. 1 - A.I. Farbman, Anat. Rec., 156(1966)269 - K. Fukuyama and W.L. Epstein, J. Cell Biol., 40(1969)830 - B.G. Stepanian, Arkh. Anat. Gistol. Embriol., 57(12)(1969)15

Basement membrane
Structure J.H. Cooper, Nature, 178(1956)643 - J.A. Swift and C.A. Saxton, J. Ultrastruct. Res., 17(1967)23
Development M.M. Salpeter and M. Singer, Anat. Rec., 136 (1960)27

Intraepithelial sensory nerves in the cat
Z. Halata, Z. Zellforsch., 106(1970)51

Dermis

Fibroblasts
Development K. Kajikawa, Jap. J. Electr. Micr., 10(3)(1961) 131
Effects of vitamin A overload M.R. Daniel *et al.*, J. Cell Biol., 30(1966)465

Matrix
C.W. Kischer, Anat. Rec., 175(1973)359

Anchor filaments
C.W. Kischer and J.S. Keeter, Amer. J. Anat., 130(1971)179

Elastic fibers
A. Charles, Brit. J. Dermatol., 73(1961)57

Histiocytes
K. Kajikawa and R. Hirono, Jap. J. Electr. Micr., 8(1960)50

Mast cells
G.E. Rogers, Exp. Cell Res., 11(1956)393 - D.E. Smith and Y.S. Lewis, J. Biophys. Biochem. Cytol., 3(1957)9 - R.G. Hibbs *et al.*, Amer. Heart J., 60(1960)121 - W. Gusek, Arch. Klin. Exp. Dermatol., 213(1961)573

Chromatophore (pigment) cells
Structure (general) A.S. Breathnach and S.V. Poyntz, J.

Anat., 100(3)(1966)549 - J.T. Bagnara *et al.*, J. Cell Biol., 38(1968)67

Structure of xanthophores, iridophores and melanophores (in reptiles) N.J. Alexander and W.H. Fahrenbach, Amer. J. Anat., 126(1969)41

Origin of premelanosomes (in Amphibia) G.E. Wise, Anat. Rec., 165(1969)185

Nerves

W. Reiter, Z. Zellforsch., 72(1966)446 - J.A. O'Daly and T. Imaeda, Exp. Molec. Path., 11(2)(1969)123

Hair Follicle

General

Structure of glassy layer G.E. Rogers, Exp. Cell Res., 13 (1957)521

Development A.S. Breathnach and J. Smith, J. Anat., 102(3) (1968)511 - E.J. Robbins and A.S. Breathnach, J. Anat., 104(1969)553

Changes in catagen phase of cycle P.F. Parakkal, J. Ultrastruct. Res., 29(1969)210 - P.F. Parakkal, Z. Zellforsch., 107(1970)174

Inner root sheath

Structure M.S.C. Birbeck and E.H. Mercer, J. Biophys. Biochem. Cytol., 3(1957)223 - G.E. Rogers, Exp. Cell Res., 14(1958)378

Function (keratinization) E.H. Mercer. In: W. Montagna and R.A. Ellis (Eds.), *The Biology of Hair Growth*, Academic Press, New York, 1958, pp. 91–111 - A. Charles, Exp. Cell Res., 18(1959)138 - B. Forslind and G. Swanbeck, Exp. Cell Res., 43(1966)191 - P.F. Parakkal, J. Cell Biol., 35(1967)473

Sensory nerve endings

T. Yamamoto, Jap. J. Electr. Micr., 15(3)(1966)158

Hair

Cuticle

M.S.C. Birbeck *et al.*, Exp. Cell Res., 10(1956)505 - M.S.C. Birbeck and E.H. Mercer, J. Biophys. Biochem. Cytol., 3 (1957)215

Cortex

M.S.C. Birbeck and E.H. Mercer, J. Biophys. Biochem. Cytol., 3(1957)203 - G. Patrizi and B.L. Munger, J. Ultrastruct. Res., 14(1966)329

Wool

G.E. Rogers, J. Ultrastruct. Res., 2(1959)309 - G.E. Rogers, Ann. N.Y. Acad. Sci., 83(1959)378

Arrector Pili Muscle

Structure (innervation) H.G. Wienker, Z. Mikr.-Anat. Forsch., 77(1967)197 - H.G. Wienker, Z. Mikr.-Anat. Forsch., 80 (1969)230

Feathers

B.K. Filshie and G.E. Rogers, J. Cell Biol., 13(1962)1

Scales

R.E. Waterman, Anat. Rec., 168(1970)361

Sebaceous Glands

Structure M. Bell, Anat. Rec., 166(1970)213

Function (lysosome role in holocrine secretion) D. Brandes *et al.*, Exp. Molec. Path., 4(1965)245

Sweat Glands

Small, "eccrine"

Structure T. Matsuzawa and K. Kurosumi, Jap. J. Electr. Micr., 12(3)(1963)175 - R.C. Henrikson, J. de Microscopie, 8(1969)767

Large, "apocrine"

B.G. Gross, J. Ultrastruct. Res., 14(1966)64

Antebrachial organ (Lemurs)

J.E. Kneeland, Z. Zellforsch., 73(1966)521

Steroidogenic Cells of Cutaneous Organ (Primates)

J. Sisson and W.H. Fahrenbach, Amer. J. Anat., 121(1967) 337

Mammary Gland

Secretory cells

Structure E. Knoop *et al.*, Milchwissenschaft, 13(1958)154 - R. Bässler and A. Schäfer, Z. Zellforsch., 101(1969)355

Function (milk secretion) W. Bargmann, Z. Zellforsch., 49 (1959)344 - K.H. Hollmann, J. Ultrastruct. Res., 2(1959) 423 - S.R. Wellings *et al.*, J. Natl. Cancer Inst., 25(1960) 393 - S.R. Wellings *et al.*, J. Natl. Cancer Inst., 25(1960) 423 - W. Bargmann *et al.*, Z. Zellforsch., 53(1961)545 - S.R. Wellings and K.B. Deome, J. Biophys. Biochem. Cytol., 9(1961)479 - L. Stockinger and J. Zarzicki, Z. Zellforsch., 57(1962)106

Regression (involution) H.J. Helminen and J.L.E. Ericsson, J. Ultrastruct. Res., 25(1968)193 - H.J. Helminen and J.L.E. Ericsson, J. Ultrastruct. Res., 25(1968)214 - H.J. Helminen and J.L.E. Ericsson, J. Ultrastruct. Res., 25(1968) 228 - H.J. Helminen *et al.*, J. Ultrastruct. Res., 25(1968) 240

Effects of prolactin M. Bousquet *et al.*, Z. Zellforsch., 96 (1969)418 - E.S. Mills and Y.J. Topper, J. Cell Biol., 44 (1970)310

Myoepithelial cells

E. Langer and S. Huhn, Z. Zellforsch., 47(1958)507 - F. Haguenau, Compt. Rend. Acad. Sci., 149(1959)182

Ductules

Effects of pregnancy T.M. Murad, Anat. Rec., 167(1970)17

15. SENSORY ORGANS

Sensory Organs - General

W.R. Loewenstein, Biological transducers, Sci. Amer., 203 (1960)98 - A.J.D. De Lorenzo, Studies on the ultrastructure and histophysiology of cell membranes, nerve fibers and synaptic junctions in chemoreceptors. In: Y. Zotterman (Ed.),

Olfaction and Taste (Wenner-Gren Center International Symposium Series) Vol. 1, MacMillan, New York, 1963, p. 5 - J. Babel *et al., Ultrastructure of the Peripheral Nervous System and Sense Organs. Atlas of Normal and Pathological Anatomy,* Thieme, Stuttgart, 1970

Eye

Lacrimal gland

Structure J.H. Abel Jr. and R.A. Ellis, Amer. J. Anat., 118 (1966)337 - A. Yamauchi and G. Burnstock, J. Cell Biol., 34(1967)917 - W. Kuhnel, Z. Zellforsch., 85(1968)408 - W. Kuhnel, Z. Zellforsch., 87(1968)504 - W. Kuhnel, Z. Zellforsch., 89(1968)550

Structure (nerves) G.L. Ruskell, Z. Zellforsch., 83(1967)321 - G.L. Ruskell, J. Anat., 103(1)(1968)65

Structure (sex difference) L. Luciano, Z. Zellforsch., 76 (1967)1

Effects of autonomic denervation G.L. Ruskell, Z. Zellforsch., 94(1969)261

Cornea, general

Structure D.M. Maurice, J. Physiol. London, 136(1957)263 - M.A. Jakus, The fine structure of the human cornea. In: G.K. Smelser (Ed.), *The Structure of the Eye*, Academic Press, New York, 1961, pp. 343–380 - M.A. Jakus, Invest. Ophthal., 1(1962)202 - W. Schwarz and D. Graf Keyserlingk, Z. Zellforsch., 73(1966)540 - S. Blümcke and K. Morgenroth, J. Ultrastruct. Res., 18(1967)502

Function (transport of ions and water) A. Donn, Invest. Ophthal., 1(1962)170

Function (transport of colloidal particles) G.I. Kaye, J. Cell Biol., 15(1962)241 - G.I. Kaye *et al.*, J. Cell Biol., 12 (1962)481

Cornea, Bowman's epithelium

Structure P. Stanka, Z. Mikr.-Anat. Forsch., 75(1966)461 - S. Blümcke *et al.*, Z. Zellforsch., 84(1968)176 - S. Blümcke *et al.*, Z. Zellforsch., 84(1968)189

Structure (innervation) M. Whitear, Experientia, 13(1957) 287

Regeneration S. Blümcke *et al.*, Z. Zellforsch., 93(1969)84

Cornea, substantia propria fibroblasts

Structure J.W. Smith *et al.*, J. Anat., 105(1969)382

Function (fibril formation) W. Schwartz, Anat. Rec., 136 (1960)275

Function (phagocytosis) S. Blümcke *et al.*, Beitr. Z. Path. Anat., 135(1967)213 - G.K. Klintworth, Amer. J. Path., 55(2)(1969)283

Cornea, Descemet's endothelium

Structure M.A. Jakus, J. Biophys. Biochem. Cytol., 2(1956) 243 (Suppl.) - M.L. Feeney and L.K. Garron, Anat. Rec., 136(1960)192 (Abstract)

Function (transport of colloidal particles) G.I. Kaye *et al.*, Anat. Rec., 139(1961)244 (Abstract)

Choroid

Structure L. Feeney and M.J. Hogan, Amer. J. Ophthal., 51 (1961)1057 - L. Feeney and M.J. Hogan, Amer. J. Ophthal., 51(1961)1084 - R. Sumita, Jap. J. Electr. Micr., 10(2)(1961)111

Structure (nerves) L. Feeney and M.J. Hogan, Amer. J. Ophthal., 51(1961)1072

Ciliary epithelium

Structure A. Holmberg, Arch. Ophthal., 62(1959)935 - A. Holmberg, Arch. Ophthal., 62(1959)952

Structure (nerves) Z. Lukas and K. Mazanec, Z. Mikr.-Anat. Forsch., 76(1967)530 - P.E. Pataky, Anat. Rec., 168 (1970)339

Function (aqueous humor production) G.D. Pappas and G.K. Smelser, Amer. J. Ophthal., 46(1958)299 - G.D. Pappas and G.K. Smelser, The fine structure of the ciliary epithelium in relation to aqueous humor secretion. In: G.K. Smelser (Ed.), *The Structure of the Eye*, Academic Press, New York, 1961, pp. 453–467 - A. Bairati and N. Orzalesi, Z. Zellforsch., 69(1966)635

Effects of hypothermia A. Holmberg and B. Becker, Amer. J. Ophthal., 49(1960)1134

Iris

Structure A.J. Tousimis and B.S. Fine, Amer. J. Ophthal., 48(1959)397 - T. Vegge and A. Ringvold, Z. Zellforsch., 94(1969)19 - A. Ringvold, Z. Zellforsch., 109(1970)306

Structure (nerves) J. Ochi *et al.*, Z. Zellforsch., 91(1968)90

Schlemm's canal

Structure L.K. Garron and M.L. Feeney, Arch. Ophthal., 62 (1959)966 - A. Holmberg, Arch. Ophthal., 62(1959)956 - T.S. Leeson and J.S. Speakman, Acta Anat., 46(1961)363 - T. Vegge, Z. Zellforsch., 77(1967)267

Retina, general

Structure F.S. Sjöstrand, Electron microscopy of the retina. In: G.K. Smelser (Ed.), *The Structure of the Eye*, Academic Press, New York, 1961, pp. 1–28 - F. Wald and E. De Robertis, Z. Zellforsch., 55(1961)649 - M. Yoshida, Jap. J. Electr. Micr., 14(4)(1965)285 - T. Samorajski *et al.*, J. Cell Biol., 28(1966)489 - V.I. Govardovsky and T.R. Kharkeievitch, Arkh. Anat. Gistol. Embriol., 52(3) (1967)53 - M.M. Magalhaes, Exp. Cell Res., 47(1967)628 - A.W. Clark and D. Branton, Z. Zellforsch., 91(1968)586 - A. Van Harreveld and F.I. Khattab, Anat. Rec., 161 (1968)125 - H.A. Hansson, Z. Zellforsch., 107(1970)23

Histochemistry (glycogen) D. Eichner and H. Themann, Z. Zellforsch., 56(1962)231

Function (the visual process) G. Wald, General discussion of retinal structure in relation to the visual process. In: G.K. Smelser (Ed.), *The Structure of the Eye*, New York, Academic Press, 1961, p. 101 - J.E. Dowling, Sci. Amer., 215(1966)78 - R. Hubbard and A. Kropf, Sci. Amer., 216(1967)64

Function (uptake of labeled glucose and glycogen synthesis) M.M. Magalhaes and A. Coimbra, J. Cell Biol., 47(1970) 263

Development J.R. Keefe *et al.*, Anat. Rec., 154(1966)759 - J.W. Sechrist, Amer. J. Anat., 124(1969)117 - N. Popoff and R.M. Ellsworth, J. Ultrastruct. Res., 29(1969)535

Effects of vitamin A deficiency J.E. Dowling and I.R. Gibbons. In: G.K. Smelser (Ed.), *The Structure of the Eye*, Academic Press, New York, 1961, pp. 85–99

Effects of sodium glutamate A.I. Cohen, Amer. J. Anat., 120 (1967)319

Retina, pigment epithelium

Structure E. Yamada, J. Biophys. Biochem. Cytol., 4(1958) 329 - E. Yamada *et al.*, Jap. J. Electr. Micr., 6(1958)42 - Y. Taniguchi, Amer. J. Ophthal., 48(1959)221 - K.R. Porter and E. Yamada, J. Biophys. Biochem. Cytol., 8

(1960)181 - A.J. Tousimis and B.S. Fine, Electron microscopy of the pigment epithelium of the iris. In: G.K. Smelser (Ed.), *The Structure of the Eye*, Academic Press, New York, 1961, pp. 441–452 - E. Yamada, The fine structure of the pigmented epithelium in the turtle eye. In: G.K. Smelser (Ed.), *The Structure of the Eye*, Academic Press, New York, 1961, pp. 73–84

Function (phagocytosis of degraded photoreceptor outer segments) R.W. Young and D. Bok, J. Cell Biol., 42(1969) 392 - T. Ishikawa and E. Yamada, Jap. J. Electr. Micr., 19(1)(1970)85

Function (transport of Vit. A to photoreceptors) R.G. Pourcho and M.H. Bernstein, Anat. Rec., 175(1973)415

Function (melanin synthesis) J. Zimmerman, Anat. Rec., 175 (1973)477

Development F. Moyer, Electron microscope observations on the origin, development, and genetic control of melanin granules in the mouse eye. In: G.K. Smelser (Ed.), *The Structure of the Eye*, Academic Press, New York, 1961, pp. 469–486 - A.S. Breathnach and L.M. Wyllie, J. Ultrastruct. Res., 16(1966)584 - W. Lerche and K.G. Wulle, Z. Zellforsch., 76(1967)452 - C.R. Braekevelt and M.J. Hollenberg, Exp. Eye Res., 9(1970)124

Regeneration J. Keefe, Anat. Rec., 172(1972)341

Retina, photoreceptors (general)

Structure A. Lasansky and E. De Robertis, J. Biophys. Biochem. Cytol., 7(1960)493 - M.F. Moody and J.D. Robertson, J. Biophys. Biochem. Cytol., 7(1960)87 - E. Yamada, Jap. J. Electr. Micr., 9(1)(1960)1 - E. De Robertis and A. Lasansky, Ultrastructure and chemical organization of photoreceptors. In: G.K. Smelser (Ed.), *The Structure of the Eye*, Academic Press, New York, 1961, pp. 29–52 - H. Fernandez-Moran, The fine structure of vertebrate and invertebrate photoreceptors as revealed by low-temperature electron microscopy. In: G.K. Smelser (Ed.), *The Structure of the Eye*, Academic Press, New York, 1961, pp. 521–556 - R.M. Eakin and J.A. Westfall, J. Ultrastruct. Res., 6(1962)531 - H. Klug and P. Lommatzsch, Z. Mikr.-Anat. Forsch., 77(1967)596 - S. Uga *et al.*, Jap. J. Electr. Micr., 19(1)(1970)71 - D.H. Dickson and M.J. Hollenberg, J. Morphol., 135(1971)389

Cytochemistry (OsO_4–ZnI_2 reactive sites) A. Pellegrino de Iraldi and R. Gueudet, Z. Zellforsch., 101(1969)203

Development S.E.G. Nilsson, J. Ultrastruct. Res., 11(1964) 581 - C.R. Braekevelt and M.J. Hollenberg, Amer. J. Ophthal., 69(1970)1032

Renewal of outer segments R.W. Young, J. Cell Biol., 33 (1967)61

Effects of iodoacetate A. Lasansky and E. De Robertis, J. Biophys. Biochem. Cytol., 5(1959)245

Retina, rods

Structure E. De Robertis, J. Biophys. Biochem. Cytol., 2 (1956)209 (Suppl.) - E. De Robertis, J. Biophys. Biochem. Cytol., 2(1956)319 - E. Yamada, J. Biophys. Biochem. Cytol., 6(1959)517 - A.I. Cohen, Amer. J. Anat., 107(1960)23

Cytochemistry (ATPase) T. Matsusaka, J. Cell Biol., 33 (1967)203

Function (uptake of labeled aminoacids, protein synthesis) R.W. Young, J. Ultrastruct. Res., 23(1968)462

Development K. Tokuyasu and E. Yamada, J. Biophys. Biochem. Cytol., 6(1959)225 - K. Tokuyasu and E. Yamada, J. Biophys. Biochem. Cytol., 7(1960)187

Retina, cones

Structure E. De Robertis and A. Lasansky, J. Biophys. Biochem. Cytol., 4(1958)743 - E.R. Berger, J. Ultrastruct. Res., 14(1966)143

Retina, photoreceptor-bipolar synapses

Structure E. De Robertis and C.M. Franchi, J. Biophys. Biochem. Cytol., 2(1956)307 - A.J. Ladman, J. Biophys. Biochem. Cytol., 4(1958)459 - F.S. Sjöstrand, J. Ultrastruct. Res., 2(1958)122 - E.M. Evans, Z. Zellforsch., 71(1966) 499 - A. Pellegrino De Iraldi and G.J. Etcheverry, Z. Zellforsch., 81(1967)283 - H.A. Hansson, Z. Zellforsch., 107 (1970)45 - S. Uga and H. Ikui, Jap. J. Electr. Micr., 19(3) (1970)278

Retina, synapses between rod and cone distal axons

E. Raviola and N.B. Gilula, Anat. Rec., 175(1973)421

Retina, outer nuclear layer

Structure G. Raviola *et al.*, Z. Zellforsch., 70(1966)532 - J.B. Sheffield, J. de Microscopie, 5(1966)173

Retina, inner plexiform layer

G. Raviola and E. Raviola, Amer. J. Anat., 120(1967)403

Retina, optic fiber layer and inner limiting membrane

A.I. Cohen, Amer. J. Anat., 108(1961)179

Retina, horizontal cells

C.E. Dieterich, Z. Zellforsch., 98(1969)277 - S. Uga and H. Ikui, Jap. J. Electr. Micr., 18(3)(1969)153

Retina, Müller's cells

Structure A.J. Ladman, Anat. Rec., 139(1961)247 (Abstract) - B.S. Fine and L.E. Zimmerman, Invest. Ophthal., 1 (1962)304

Function (possible "nursing" role) A. Lasansky, J. Biophys. Biochem. Cytol., 11(1961)237

Lens

Structure H. Hueck and O. Kleifeld, Graefe's Arch. Ophthal. 160(1958)20 - T. Wanko and M.A. Gavin, J. Biophys. Biochem. Cytol., 6(1959)97 - T. Wanko and M.A. Gavin, Cell surfaces in the crystalline lens. In: G.K. Smelser (Ed.), *The Structure of the Eye*, Academic Press, New York, 1961, pp.221–233 - H.A. Hansson, Z. Zellforsch., 107(1970)187 - N.S. Rafferty and E.A. Esson, Anat. Rec., 175(1973)418

Development A.I. Cohen, Amer. J. Anat., 103(1958)219 - N.R. Willis *et al.*, Canad. J. Ophthal., 4(1969)307 - E.E. Shubert *et al.*, Canad. J. Ophthal., 5(1970)353

Effects of irradiation T. Wanko *et al.*, Arch. Ophthal., 62 (1959)977

Zonula (suspensory lens ligament)

Structure H.A. Hansson, Z. Zellforsch., 107(1970)199

Function G.D. Pappas *et al.*, Arch. Ophthal., 62(1959)959

Vitreous body

Structure B.S. Fine and A.J. Tousimis, Arch. Ophthal., 65 (1961)95 - J.W. Smith and A. Serafini-Fracassini, J. Anat., 101(1)(1967)99 - H.A. Hansson, Z. Zellforsch., 101 (1969)323

Ear

Outer ear (tympanic membrane)

F.R. Johnson *et al.*, J. Anat., 103(2)(1968)297

Inner ear (general)
H. Engström and J. Wersall, Int. Rev. Cytol., 7(1958)535 - I. Friedmann, Brit. Med. Bull., 18(1962)209 - S. Iurato *et al.*, *Submicroscopic Structure of the Inner Ear,* Pergamon Press, Oxford, 1967

Vestibular ear (general)
H. Engström and J. Wersall, Exp. Cell Res., Suppl. 5(1958) 460

Vestibular ear (type I hair cells)
D.W. Hamilton, J. Ultrastruct. Res., 23(1968)98

Vestibular ear (cristae ampullares)
J. Wersall, Acta Oto-Laryngol., 126(1956)1 (Suppl.) - D.W. Hamilton, Anat. Rec., 164(1969)253

Vestibular ear (otolithic membrane)
M.D. Ross, Anat. Rec., 175 (1973) 429.

Vestibular ear (perilymphatic fibrocytes)
D.W. Hamilton, Anat. Rec., 157(1967)627

Cochlear ear (Corti's organ, general)
Structure and innervation C.A. Smith and E.W. Dempsey, Amer. J. Anat., 100(1957)337 - H. Engström, in: G.L. Rasmussen and W. Windle (Eds.), *Neural Mechanisms of the Auditory and Vestibular Systems,* Thomas, Springfield, Ill., 1961, pp. 48–64 - S. Iurato, Z. Zellforsch., 53(1961)259 - C.A. Smith and F.S. Sjöstrand, J. Ultrastruct. Res., 5(1961)184

Function (theoretical models)
M. Wharton Young, Anat. Rec., 175 (1973) 475.
Development L.K. Titova and F.G. Gribakin, Arkh. Anat. Gistol. Embriol., 53(8)(1967)40
Effects of sound K.A. Koitchev, Arkh. Anat. Gistol. Embriol., 56(1)(1969)43

Cochlear ear (Corti's organ, outer hair cells)
Structure and innervation C.A. Smith and F.S. Sjöstrand, J. Ultrastruct. Res., 5(1961)523 - R. Kimura and J. Wersall, Acta Oto-Laryngol., 55(1962)11 - E.L. Rodriguez-Echandia, Z. Zellforsch., 78(1967)30

Cochlear ear (Corti's organ, inner hair cells)
A.J. Duvall *et al.*, J. Cell Biol., 29(1966)497

Cochlear ear (Corti's organ, supporting cells and basilar membrane)
S. Iurato, Z. Zellforsch., 56(1962)40

Cochlear ear (Corti's organ, tectorial membrane)
S. Iurato, Z. Zellforsch., 52(1960)105

Cochlear ear (stria vascularis)
R. Hinojosa and E.L. Rodriguez-Echandia, Amer. J. Anat., 118(1966)631

Olfactory Epithelium

Structure A.J. De Lorenzo, J. Biophys. Biochem. Cytol., 3 (1957)839 - H. Brettschneider, Anat. Anz., 105(1958)194 - H.S. Gasser, Exp. Cell Res., Suppl. 5(1958)3 - T.S. Reese, J. Cell Biol., 25(1965)209 - K.H. Andres, Z. Zellforsch., 68(1966)140 - D. Frisch, Amer. J. Anat., 121 (1967)87 - M. Okano *et al.*, J. Ultrastruct. Res., 17(1967) 487 - K. Seifert and G. Ule, Z. Zellforsch., 76(1967)147 - R.A. Thornhill, J. Cell Science, 2(1967)591 - K.H. Andres, Z. Zellforsch., 96(1969)250 - G. Gemne and K.B. Doving, Amer. J. Anat., 126(1969)457
Function (reception of chemical stimuli) W. Le Gros Clark, Proc. Roy. Soc. London, Ser. B., 146(1957)299 - D. Ottoson. In: Y. Zotterman (Ed.), *Olfaction and Taste* (Wenner-Gren Center International Symposium Series, Vol. 1), MacMillan, New York, 1963, p. 35 - J.E. Amoore *et al.*, Sci. Amer., 210(1964)42
Regeneration B.D. Mulvaney and H.E. Heist, Amer. J. Anat., 131(1971)241 - P.P. Graziadei and R.S. Dehan, Anat. Rec., 175(1973)332

Taste Buds

Structure H. Engström and C. Rytzner, Ann. Otol. Rhinol. Laryngol., 65(1956)361 - O. Trujillo-Cenoz, Z. Zellforsch., 46(1957)272 - A.J. De Lorenzo, J. Biophys. Biochem. Cytol., 4(1958)143 - R.G. Murray and A. Murray, Anat. Rec., 138(1960)211 - R.G. Murray and A. Murray, J. Ultrastruct. Res., 19(1967)327 - H.A. Scalzi, Z. Zellforsch., 80(1967)413 - R.G. Murray *et al.*, J. Ultrastruct. Res., 27(1969)444 - A.I. Farbman and J.D. Yonkers, Amer. J. Anat., 131(1971)353
Structure (synapses between receptor cells and axons) S. Uga and K. Hama, Jap. J. Electr. Micr., 16(3)(1967)269
Development A.I. Farbman, J. Ultrastruct. Res., 19(1967) 514 - S. Fujimoto and R.G. Murray, Anat. Rec., 168 (1970)393 - C. Olivieri-Sangliacomo, Z. Zellforsch., 108 (1970)397

Touch Receptors and Meissner Corpuscles

Structure D.C. Pease and W. Pallie, J. Ultrastruct. Res., 2 (1959)352 - N. Cauna and L.L. Ross, J. Biophys. Biochem. Cytol., 8(1960)467 - G. Patrizi and B.L. Munger, J. Ultrastruct. Res., 13(1965)500

Pacinian and Herbst Corpuscles

D.C. Pease and T.A. Quilliam, J. Biophys. Biochem. Cytol., 3(1957)331 - P. Polacek and K. Mazanec, Z. Mikr.-Anat. Forsch., 75(1966)343 - R. Saxod, Arch. d'Anat. Micr., 57 (1968)379 - - P.H.J. Nafstad and A.E. Andersen, Z. Zellforsch., 103(1970)109

Muscle Spindles

Structure (general and intrafusal muscle fibers) S.G. Page, J. de Microscopie, 5(1966)101 - E. Andersson-Cedergren and U. Karlsson, J. Ultrastruct. Res., 19(1967)409 - H.J. Rumpelt and H. Schmalbruch, Z. Zellforsch., 102(1969) 601
Structure (intrafusal nerve endings) G. Hennig, Z. Zellforsch., 96(1969)275 - R. Mayr, Z. Zellforsch., 110(1970)97

Electroreceptors of Fish

A.W. Wachtel and R.B. Szamier, J. Ultrastruct. Res., 27 (1969)361

Subject Index